Register for Online Access

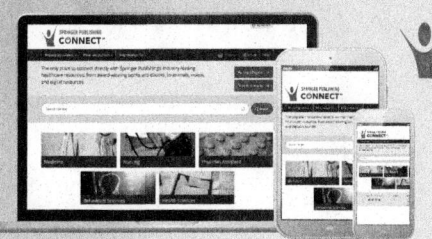

Your print purchase of *Physical Medicine and Rehabilitation Pocketpedia, Fourth Edition*, **includes online access to the contents of your book**—increasing accessibility, portability, and searchability!

Access today at:
http://connect.springerpub.com/content/book/978-0-8261-5628-0
or scan the QR code at the right with your smartphone. Log in or register, then click "Redeem a voucher" and use the code below.

G7DY9SRR

Scan here for quick access.

Having trouble redeeming a voucher code?
Go to https://connect.springerpub.com/redeeming-voucher-code

If you are experiencing problems accessing the digital component of this product, please contact our customer service department at cs@springerpub.com

The online access with your print purchase is available at the publisher's discretion and may be removed at any time without notice.

Publisher's Note: New and used products purchased from third-party sellers are not guaranteed for quality, authenticity, or access to any included digital components.

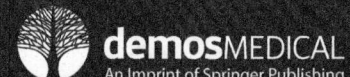

View all our products at springerpub.com/demosmedical

PHYSICAL MEDICINE AND REHABILITATION POCKETPEDIA

PHYSICAL MEDICINE AND REHABILITATION POCKETPEDIA

Fourth Edition

Leslie Rydberg, MD
Associate Professor of Physical Medicine and Rehabilitation
 and Medical Education
Associate Residency Program Director
Northwestern University Feinberg School of Medicine
Monika and Henry Betts Medical Student Education Chair
Shirley Ryan AbilityLab
Chicago, Illinois

Sarah Hwang, MD
Associate Professor of Physical Medicine and Rehabilitation
 and Obstetrics and Gynecology
Northwestern University Feinberg School of Medicine
Director of Women's Health Rehabilitation
Shirley Ryan AbilityLab
Chicago, Illinois

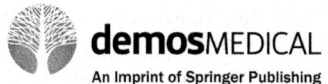

Copyright © 2023 Springer Publishing Company, LLC
Demos Medical Publishing is an imprint of Springer Publishing Company.
All rights reserved.
First Springer Publishing edition 2018.

No part of this publication may be reproduced, stored in a retrieval system, or transmitted in any form or by any means, electronic, mechanical, photocopying, recording, or otherwise, without the prior permission of Springer Publishing Company, LLC, or authorization through payment of the appropriate fees to the Copyright Clearance Center, Inc., 222 Rosewood Drive, Danvers, MA 01923, 978-750-8400, fax 978-646-8600, info@copyright.com or on the Web at www.copyright.com.

Springer Publishing Company, LLC
11 West 42nd Street, New York, NY 10036
www.springerpub.com
connect.springerpub.com/

Acquisitions Editor: Beth Barry
Compositor: Transforma

ISBN: 978-0-8261-5627-3
ebook ISBN: 978-0-8261-5628-0
DOI: 10.1891/9780826156280

22 23 24 25/ 5 4 3 2 1

Medicine is an ever-changing science. Research and clinical experience are continually expanding our knowledge, in particular our understanding of proper treatment and drug therapy. The authors, editors, and publisher have made every effort to ensure that all information in this book is in accordance with the state of knowledge at the time of production of the book. Nevertheless, the authors, editors, and publisher are not responsible for any errors or omissions or for any consequence from application of the information in this book and make no warranty, expressed or implied, with respect to the content of this publication. Every reader should examine carefully the package inserts accompanying each drug and should carefully check whether the dosage schedules therein or the contraindications stated by the manufacturer differ from the statements made in this book. Such examination is particularly important with drugs that are either rarely used or have been newly released on the market.

Library of Congress Cataloging-in-Publication Data

Names: Rydberg, Leslie, editor. | Hwang, Sarah, MD, editor.
Title: Physical medicine and rehabilitation pocketpedia / [edited by] Leslie Rydberg, Sarah Hwang.
Description: Fourth edition. | New York, NY : Springer Publishing Company, [2023] | Includes bibliographical references and index.
Identifiers: LCCN 2022035152 | ISBN 9780826156273 (paperback) | ISBN 9780826156280 (ebook)
Subjects: MESH: Physical Therapy Modalities | Rehabilitation–methods | Handbook
Classification: LCC RM700 | NLM WB 39 | DDC 615.8/2–dc23/eng/20221104
LC record available at https://lccn.loc.gov/2022035152

Publisher's Note: New and used products purchased from third-party sellers are not guaranteed for quality, authenticity, or access to any included digital components.

Printed in the United States of America by Gasch Printing.

Dedicated to the people who have supported us along the way:

Team Rydberg (Joe, James, and Ben) and the Harms family

Sarah's Squad (Peter, Oliver, and Amelia) and the Linn family

CONTENTS

Contributors xi

Preface xix

PART I. PRINCIPLES OF PM&R 1

1. Physical Medicine and Rehabilitation Fundamentals and Overview 3
   Michael V. Nguyen and Daniel A. Goodman

2. Neurologic Examination 8
   Ravi E. Kasi

3. Musculoskeletal Examination 18
   Daniel M. Cushman, Sarah F. Eby, and Meredith Ehn

4. The Care of People With Disability 26
   Nethra S. Ankam

5. Mobility: Gait, Assistive Devices, and Wheelchairs 34
   Martha M. Smith

6. Orthoses and Adaptive Equipment 50
   Kristi Turner, Kelly Breen, and Molly Henry

7. Therapy and Exercise Prescription 58
   Shane N. Stone, Kian Nassiri, and Patrick J. Barrett

PART II. MEDICAL REHABILITATION 67

8. Amputations 69
   Joan T. Le and Phoebe Scott-Wyard

9. Cardiac Rehabilitation 83
   Matthew C. Oswald, Christopher W. Lewis, and Eric W. Villanueva

10. Pulmonary Rehabilitation 90
    Vivian Roy, Julia Fram, and Leslie Rydberg

11. Burn Rehabilitation 97
    Mark E. Huang and Christopher W. Lewis

12. Cancer Rehabilitation 104
    Samman Shahpar, Ishan Roy, Eric W. Villanueva, and Madeline Flores

13. Transplant Rehabilitation 113
    Laura Malmut

14. Effects of Debility and Immobility 119
    Carley N. Sauter, Sarah Wineman, and Nethra S. Ankam

15. Medical Complications During Rehabilitation 122
    Kim Barker and Martin Laguerre

16. Rheumatologic Disorders and Osteoporosis 131
    Theresa J. Lie-Nemeth, Kimberly J. Mercurio, and Artelio L. Watson

17. COVID-19 Rehabilitation 140
    Jacqueline Neal, Rachna Soriano, and Jessica Dangelmaier

18. Surgical Orthopedics 148
    Mani Singh, Tracey Isidro, and Jennifer Soo Hoo

19. ICU Rehabilitation 156
    Julie Lanphere

20. Pediatric Rehabilitation 160
    Sarah Macabales, Mary Keen, and Larissa Pavone

PART III. NEUROLOGIC REHABILITATION 175

21. Spinal Cord Injury 177
    Allison Kessler and Natasha Bhatia

22. Traumatic Brain Injury 190
    Sangeeta Driver and Jamie Ott

23. Concussion 198
    Deena Hassaballa

24. Stroke 204
    Joseph Burris

25. Multiple Sclerosis 211
    Sarah M. Eickmeyer, Aimee Lambeth, and Khulan Sarmiento

26. Movement Disorders 217
    Priya V. Mhatre

27. Other Neurologic Disorders 223
    Haibi (Daniel) Cai and Nassim Rad

Contents | ix

28. Cognition 230
Sony Issac, Natalia Del Mar Miranda-Cantellops,
and Lauren T. Shapiro

29. Spasticity 236
Gary Vargas and Amy Mathews

30. Neurogenic Bladder and Bowel 243
Stephanie Hendrick and Ishaan Hublikar

31. Language, Speech, and Swallowing 251
Kathryn DeMarco and Kathleen Webler

PART IV. MUSCULOSKELETAL REHABILITATION 263

32. Electrodiagnostic Testing 265
Danielle Powell and Aleks Borresen

33. Ultrasound 280
Dayna M. Yorks, Matthew C. Sherrier, and Samuel K. Chu

34. Pain Medicine 287
Ai Mukai and Edward Kim

35. Spine 299
Jennifer G. Leet, Allen S. Chen, and David S. Cheng

36. Musculoskeletal—Upper Limb 306
Michael Catapano and Ashwin Babu

37. Musculoskeletal—Lower Limb 312
Theodora Lananh Swenson, James E. Gardner,
and Aaron Yang

38. Musculoskeletal—Sports and Performing
Arts Medicine 323
Daniel H. Blatz, G. Ross Malik, and Kevin Ozment

39. Peripheral Nerve Conditions 336
Kevin Huang, Benjamin Washburn, and Marco Masci

40. Pelvic Health Rehabilitation 349
Sarah Hwang

Index 352

CONTRIBUTORS

Nethra S. Ankam, MD, Associate Professor, Department of Rehabilitation Medicine, Sidney Kimmel Medical College, Thomas Jefferson University, Philadelphia, Pennsylvania

Ashwin Babu, MD, Sports Medicine Physiatrist, Massachusetts General Hospital, Associate Program Director, Spaulding/Harvard Physical Medicine and Rehabilitation Residency Training Program, Boston, Massachusetts

Kim Barker, MD, Associate Professor, Department of Physical Medicine and Rehabilitation, UT Southwestern Medical Center, Dallas, Texas

Patrick J. Barrett, MD, Assistant Chief, Physical Medicine and Rehabilitation Service, Jesse Brown VA Medical Center, Assistant Professor, Physical Medicine and Rehabilitation Department, Northwestern University Feinberg School of Medicine, Chicago, Illinois

Natasha Bhatia, MD, Attending Physician, Shirley Ryan AbilityLab, Assistant Professor of Physical Medicine and Rehabilitation, Northwestern University Feinberg School of Medicine, Chicago, Illinois

Daniel H. Blatz, MD, MPH, CAQSM, Attending Physician, Hospital for Special Surgery, Assistant Professor, Weill Cornell Medical College, New York, New York

Aleks Borresen, MD, Resident Physician, University of Alabama at Birmingham, Birmingham, Alabama

Kelly Breen, MS, OTR/L, BCPR, Max Näder Center for Rehabilitation Technologies and Outcomes Research, Shirley Ryan AbilityLab, Chicago, Illinois

Joseph Burris, MD, Chair, Department of Physical Medicine and Rehabilitation, University of Missouri, Columbia, Missouri

Haibi (Daniel) Cai, MD, Assistant Professor, Physical Medicine and Rehabilitation and Neurology, University of Texas Southwestern Medical Center, Dallas, Texas

Michael Catapano, MD, FRCPC, Department of Physical Medicine and Rehabilitation, Harvard University, Boston, Massachusetts

Allen S. Chen, MD, MPH, Associate Professor, Department of Orthopaedic Surgery, UCLA, Los Angeles, California

David S. Cheng, MD, Clinical Associate Professor, Department of Neurological Surgery, USC Keck School of Medicine, Los Angeles, California

Samuel K. Chu, MD, Assistant Professor, Department of Physical Medicine and Rehabilitation, Shirley Ryan AbilityLab, Northwestern Feinberg School of Medicine, Chicago, Illinois

Daniel M. Cushman, MD, Associate Professor, Physical Medicine and Rehabilitation, University of Utah, Salt Lake City, Utah

Jessica Dangelmaier, PA-C, Physician Assistant, Department of Physical Medicine and Rehabilitation, Shirley Ryan AbilityLab, Chicago, Illinois

Kathryn DeMarco, MS, CCC-SLP, Clinical Manager of Pediatrics, Shirley Ryan AbilityLab, Chicago, Illinois

Sangeeta Driver, MD, MPH, Section Chief, Brain Injury Medicine, Shirley Ryan AbilityLab, Assistant Professor of Physical Medicine and Rehabilitation, Northwestern Feinberg School of Medicine, Chicago, Illinois

Sarah F. Eby, MD, PhD, Associate Professor, Department of Physical Medicine and Rehabilitation, Harvard University, Boston, Massachusetts

Meredith Ehn, DO, DPT, Assistant Professor, Department of Physical Medicine and Rehabilitation, Shirley Ryan AbilityLab, Northwestern University Feinberg School of Medicine, Chicago, Illinois

Sarah M. Eickmeyer, MD, Associate Professor, Rehabilitation Medicine, Medical Director of Inpatient Rehabilitation, The University of Kansas, Kansas City, Kansas

Madeline Flores, MD, Resident Physician, Department of Physical Medicine and Rehabilitation, McGaw Medical Center, Northwestern University Feinberg School of Medicine, Chicago, Illinois

Julia Fram, MD, Resident Physician, Department of Physical Medicine and Rehabilitation, McGaw Medical Center, Northwestern University Feinberg School of Medicine, Chicago, Illinois

James E. Gardner, MD, Resident Physician, Department of Physical Medicine and Rehabilitation, Vanderbilt University Medical Center, Nashville, Tennessee

Daniel A. Goodman, MD, MS, Attending Physician, Department of Physical Medicine and Rehabilitation, Shirley Ryan AbilityLab, Chicago, Illinois

Deena Hassaballa, DO, FAAPMR, Clinical Assistant Professor, Department of Rehabilitation Medicine, UW Medicine, Seattle, Washington

Stephanie Hendrick, MD, Assistant Professor, Department of Physical Medicine and Rehabilitation, Shirley Ryan AbilityLab, Northwestern University Feinberg School of Medicine, Chicago, Illinois

Molly Henry, PT, DPT, NCS, Senior Physical Therapist, Spinal Cord Injury Innovation Center, Arms and Hands Lab Wheelchair Skills and Management, Shirley Ryan AbilityLab, Chicago, Illinois

Kevin Huang, DO, Attending Physician, Physical Medicine and Rehabilitation, Kaiser Permanente Woodland Hills Medical Center, Woodland Hills, California

Mark E. Huang, MD, Professor, Department of Physical Medicine and Rehabilitation, Northwestern University Feinberg School of Medicine, Shirley Ryan AbilityLab, Chicago, Illinois

Ishaan Hublikar, DO, Resident Physician, Marianjoy Rehabilitation Hospital, Wheaton, Illinois

Sarah Hwang, MD, Associate Professor of Physical Medicine and Rehabilitation and Obstetrics and Gynecology, Northwestern University Feinberg School of Medicine, Director of Women's Health Rehabilitation, Shirley Ryan AbilityLab, Chicago, Illinois

Tracey Isidro, MD, Department of Rehabilitation Medicine, NewYork-Presbyterian Hospital, New York, New York

Sony Issac, MD, Brain Injury Medicine Fellow, Department of Physical Medicine and Rehabilitation, University of Miami/Jackson Health System, Miami, Florida

Ravi E. Kasi, MD, Associate Professor and Residency Program Director, Department of Physical Medicine and Rehabilitation, Rush University Medical Center, Chicago, Illinois

Mary Keen, MD, Attending Physician, Marianjoy Rehabilitation Hospital, Wheaton, Illinois

Allison Kessler, MD, Section Chief, Division of Spinal Cord Injury, Shirley Ryan AbilityLab, Assistant Professor of Physical Medicine and Rehabilitation, Northwestern Feinberg School of Medicine, Chicago, Illinois

Edward Kim, MD, Fellow, UPMC Pain Medicine Program, University of Pittsburgh, Pittsburgh, Pennsylvania

Martin Laguerre, MD, Resident Physician, Department of Physical Medicine and Rehabilitation, UT Southwestern Medical Center, Dallas, Texas

Aimee Lambeth, DO, Resident Physician, Rehabilitation Medicine, The University of Kansas, Kansas City, Kansas

Julie Lanphere, DO, Associate Medical Director for Rehabilitation Services, Intermountain Health, PM&R Chairman for Intermountain Medical Center, Murray, Utah

Joan T. Le, MD, Department of Orthopedic Surgery, Division of Pediatric Rehabilitation Medicine, University of California, San Diego, Rady Children's Hospital San Diego, California

Jennifer G. Leet, MD, Pain Medicine Fellow, Department of Internal Medicine, David Geffen School of Medicine at UCLA, WLA VA Hospital, Los Angeles, California

Christopher W. Lewis, MD, Resident, Physical Medicine and Rehabilitation, McGaw Medical Center, Northwestern University Feinberg School of Medicine, Chicago, Illinois

Theresa J. Lie-Nemeth, MD, Attending Physiatrist, Schwab Rehabilitation Hospital, Clinical Assistant Professor, Department of Neurology and Rehabilitation, University of Illinois at Chicago, Chicago, Illinois

Sarah Macabales, DO, Resident Physician, Marianjoy Rehabilitation Hospital, Wheaton, Illinois

G. Ross Malik, MD, Sports Medicine Physiatrist, Mass General Brigham, Instructor, Spaulding/Harvard Department of Physical Medicine & Rehabilitation, Boston, Massachusetts

Laura Malmut, MD, Medical Director of Transplant Rehabilitation, Assistant Professor of Physical Medicine and Rehabilitation, MedStar National Rehabilitation Hospital, Georgetown University School of Medicine, Washington, DC

Contributors | xv

Marco Masci, MD, Attending Physician, Physical Medicine and Rehabilitation, Kaiser Permanente Panorama City Medical Center, Panorama City, California

Amy Mathews, MD, Assistant Professor, Department of Physical Medicine and Rehabilitation, University of Texas Southwestern Medical Center, Dallas, Texas

Kimberly J. Mercurio, MD, Attending Physiatrist, Fracture Liaison Service, Duly Health and Care, Westmont, Illinois, Attending Physiatrist, Schwab Rehabilitation Hospital, Chicago, Illinois

Priya V. Mhatre, MD, MS, Assistant Professor, Department of Physical Medicine and Rehabilitation, Northwestern University Feinberg School of Medicine, Attending Physician, Shirley Ryan AbilityLab, Chicago, Illinois

Natalia Del Mar Miranda-Cantellops, MD, Resident Physician, Department of Physical Medicine and Rehabilitation, University of Miami/Jackson Health System, Miami, Florida

Ai Mukai, MD, UT Dell-Austin Medical School, Texas Orthopedics Sports and Rehabilitation Associates, Austin, Texas

Kian Nassiri, DO, Resident Physician, Department of Physical Medicine and Rehabilitation, Northwestern University Feinberg School of Medicine, Chicago, Illinois

Jacqueline Neal, MD, MSE, Assistant Professor, Department of Physical Medicine and Rehabilitation, Northwestern Feinberg School of Medicine, Attending Physician, Department of Physical Medicine and Rehabilitation, Jesse Brown VA Medical Center, Chicago, Illinois

Michael V. Nguyen, MD, MPH, Assistant Professor, Department of Physical Medicine and Rehabilitation, McGovern Medical School, The University of Texas Health Science Center at Houston, Attending Physician, The Institute for Rehabilitation and Research–Memorial Hermann, Houston, Texas

Matthew C. Oswald, MD, Medical Director, Medically Complex Inpatient Rehabilitation, Shirley Ryan AbilityLab, Assistant Professor, Department of Physical Medicine and Rehabilitation, Northwestern University Feinberg School of Medicine, Chicago, Illinois

Jamie Ott, DO, Acting Assistant Professor and Attending Physician, Department of Rehabilitation Medicine, Harborview Medical Center, University of Washington, Seattle, Washington

Kevin Ozment, MD, Sports Medicine and Interventional Spine Fellow Physician, Department of Rehabilitation & Human Performance, Icahn School of Medicine at Mount Sinai, New York, New York

Larissa Pavone, MD, Program Director, Physical Medicine and Rehabilitation, Attending Physician, Marianjoy Rehabilitation Hospital, Wheaton, Illinois

Danielle Powell, MD, MSPH, Associate Professor, Department of Physical Medicine and Rehabilitation, University of Alabama at Birmingham, Birmingham, Alabama

Nassim Rad, MD, Assistant Professor, Physical Medicine and Rehabilitation, University of Washington Medical Center, Seattle, Washington

Ishan Roy, MD, PhD, Department of Physical Medicine and Rehabilitation, Shirley Ryan AbilityLab, Northwestern University Feinberg School of Medicine, Chicago, Illinois

Vivian Roy, MD, Assistant Professor, Department of Physical Medicine and Rehabilitation, Shirley Ryan AbilityLab, Northwestern University Feinberg School of Medicine, Chicago, Illinois

Leslie Rydberg, MD, Associate Professor of Physical Medicine and Rehabilitation and Medical Education, Associate Residency Program Director, Northwestern University Feinberg School of Medicine, Monika and Henry Betts Medical Student Education Chair, Shirley Ryan AbilityLab, Chicago, Illinois

Khulan Sarmiento, DO, Resident Physician, Rehabilitation Medicine, The University of Kansas, Kansas City, Kansas

Carley N. Sauter, MD, Department of Physical Medicine and Rehabilitation, Medical College of Wisconsin, Milwaukee, Wisconsin

Phoebe Scott-Wyard, DO, Department of Orthopedic Surgery, Division of Pediatric Rehabilitation Medicine, University of California, San Diego, Rady Children's Hospital San Diego, California

Samman Shahpar, MD, Assistant Professor, Department of Physical Medicine and Rehabilitation, Northwestern University Feinberg School of Medicine, Shirley Ryan AbilityLab, Chicago, Illinois

Lauren T. Shapiro, MD, MPH, Associate Professor and Vice Chair for Quality, Safety, and Compliance, Department of Physical Medicine and Rehabilitation, University of Miami Miller School of Medicine, Miami, Florida

Matthew C. Sherrier, MD, Assistant Professor, Department of Orthopaedics and Physical Medicine, Medical University of South Carolina, Charleston, South Carolina

Mani Singh, MD, Department of Rehabilitation Medicine, NewYork-Presbyterian Hospital, New York, New York

Martha M. Smith, PT, DPT, CLT, Clinical Manager, Nerve, Muscle & Bone Innovation Center, Shirley Ryan AbilityLab, Chicago, Illinois

Jennifer Soo Hoo, MD, Assistant Professor, Department of Rehabilitation Medicine, Weill Cornell Medicine and NewYork-Presbyterian Hospital, New York, New York

Rachna Soriano, DO, Assistant Professor, Department of Physical Medicine and Rehabilitation, Northwestern University Feinberg School of Medicine, Attending Physician, Department of Physical Medicine and Rehabilitation, Shirley Ryan AbilityLab, Chicago, Illinois

Shane N. Stone, MD, BS, Resident Physician, Department of Physical Medicine and Rehabilitation, Northwestern University Feinberg School of Medicine, Chicago, Illinois

Theodora Lananh Swenson, MD, Resident Physician, Department of Physical Medicine and Rehabilitation, Vanderbilt University Medical Center, Nashville, Tennessee

Kristi Turner, DHS, OTR/L, Regenstein Research Center for Bionic Medicine, Shirley Ryan AbilityLab, Chicago, Illinois

Gary Vargas, MD, Brain Injury Medicine Fellow, University of Texas Southwestern Medical Center, Dallas, Texas

Eric W. Villanueva, MD, Resident Physician, Department of Physical Medicine and Rehabilitation, McGaw Medical Center, Northwestern University Feinberg School of Medicine, Chicago, Illinois

Benjamin Washburn, MD, Attending Physician, Assistant Professor of Clinical PM&R and Orthopaedics, University of Missouri, Columbia, Missouri

Artelio L. Watson, MD, Attending Physiatrist, Pain Management, Schwab Rehabilitation Hospital, Chicago, Illinois

Kathleen Webler, MS, CCC-SLP, BCS-S, Senior Speech Language Pathologist, Shirley Ryan AbilityLab, Chicago, Illinois

Sarah Wineman, MD, Department of Physical Medicine and Rehabilitation, Medical College of Wisconsin, Milwaukee, Wisconsin

Aaron Yang, MD, Associate Professor, Department of Physical Medicine and Rehabilitation, Vanderbilt University Medical Center, Nashville, Tennessee

Dayna M. Yorks, DO, Department of Physical Medicine and Rehabilitation, Harvard Medical School, Spaulding Rehabilitation Network, Boston, Massachusetts

PREFACE

The fourth edition of the *Physical Medicine and Rehabilitation Pocketpedia* was a joy to work on. We especially enjoyed thinking about which important topics physical medicine and rehabilitation (PM&R) physicians face in their current clinical practice, collaborating with over 60 content expert chapter authors, and streamlining each submission to create a concise yet thoughtful chapter for each topic. Several new chapters have been included in this edition, including COVID-19 rehabilitation, transplant rehabilitation, caring for patients with disability, orthotics/adaptive equipment, and pelvic health, which help to showcase the breadth of expertise within the field of PM&R. We have also significantly expanded coverage of musculoskeletal rehabilitation and broken the book into topic-specific parts to make it easier to navigate.

We hope that you will enjoy using this updated *Pocketpedia* in the same way that we have enjoyed creating it, and that it will continue to be a convenient and succinct resource for ongoing education and clinical practice in our field.

Leslie Rydberg
Sarah Hwang

PART I

PRINCIPLES OF PM&R

CHAPTER 1

PHYSICAL MEDICINE AND REHABILITATION FUNDAMENTALS AND OVERVIEW

Michael V. Nguyen and Daniel A. Goodman

WHAT IS PHYSICAL MEDICINE AND REHABILITATION?

Physical medicine and rehabilitation (PM&R), also known as physiatry, is a medical specialty that promotes a patient-centered approach to improve function and quality of life. PM&R "focuses on the diagnosis, evaluation, and management of persons of all ages with congenital or acquired physical and/or cognitive impairments, disabilities, and functional limitations."[1] The specialty began in the late 1920s and was recognized by the American Medical Association in 1945. PM&R physicians, also known as physiatrists, have expertise and knowledge about the biomechanics of the human body and an extensive understanding and training on how mobility can impact quality of life. Physiatrists treat persons with a broad range of medical diagnoses related to illness, injury, or physical impairment using nonsurgical techniques. As experts in physical examination, physiatrists can design a unique treatment plan tailored to an individual's physical impairments, goals, and needs. Treatment goals can include restoration of function, but may also be supportive and accommodative, or through adaptive means. This chapter introduces the reader to the medical specialty of PM&R and includes information on a spectrum of patients cared for, care settings, care collaborators, and medical education training and certification.

EPIDEMIOLOGY

The number of individuals with disabilities in the United States is often underrecognized. According to the Centers for Disease Control and Prevention, greater than one in four individuals in the United States in 2020 identify as having a disability, accounting for 64 million people.[2] Over 11.1% of adults have a mobility-related disability, with nearly 11% reporting cognitive impairments. This makes this population one of the largest minority groups in the country.

LEVELS OF CARE

Physiatrists treat patients at all levels of care across the medical continuum. The appropriate medical setting for each patient is determined by their functional and medical needs. Patients often require a multidisciplinary team to optimize function and outcomes, and may be supervised by a physiatrist. The different levels of care are described in the following[3,4]:

- *Acute hospital:* Acute care hospitals treat patients who have developed an acute medical issue that may be life- or limb-threatening. These hospitals have access to the most advanced lifesaving equipment. Admission to acute care often occurs via the emergency department, but patients can also be directly admitted from the community if a physician deems their medical needs to be appropriate.
- *Inpatient Rehabilitation Facility (IRF):* This hospital-based rehabilitation setting provides at least 15 hours of therapy per week, 24-hour rehabilitation nursing care, and 24-hour access to a physician. This level of care is often referred to as acute inpatient rehabilitation. Specific criteria are required for admission to this level of care:
  o The patient requires frequent or daily physician evaluations.
  o The patient requires multiple therapy disciplines (physical therapist, occupational therapist, speech language pathologist, and orthotics and prosthetics) and is able to participate in 15 hours of weekly therapy.
  o The patient requires a coordinated team of providers.
  o The patient's function is expected to improve to support community discharge.
- *Long-term care hospital (LTCH):* LTCH is an acute care hospital for patients who require complicated recovery plan and prolonged hospitalization of 25 days or more. Patients are required to participate in therapies 5 days per week. Patients admitted to this level of care typically have two or more active medical issues that require three or more medical interventions, which *can* include:
  o Intravenous (IV) medications, continuous IV fluids, total parenteral nutrition (TPN) or tube feeds, or blood products
  o Ventilator weaning
  o Complex wounds or burns
- *Skilled nursing facility (SNF):* SNF provides postacute care to patients who are deemed appropriate for daily skilled nursing care or therapy. Care at this level is deemed appropriate by a physician and the care needs are related to a hospital-related medical condition *or* a condition that started while in this setting.
- *Day rehabilitation:* Day rehabilitation is an outpatient multidisciplinary therapy program for patients who require two or more therapy disciplines but do not require hospital admission.
- *Outpatient rehabilitation:* Outpatient rehabilitation is an individual therapy discipline focused on dysfunction of a focal anatomic region or a specific goal. Treatment is often in a series of visits.

- *Home health:* Home health is for patients deemed homebound by the medical provider, meaning it is extremely difficult for the patient to leave their home and/or needs help doing so. The patient needs skilled nursing services and skilled therapy care on an intermittent basis.

INTERDISCIPLINARY TEAM

Treating and managing complex medical and functional needs requires a team approach to optimize outcomes and function. The members of the multidisciplinary team are described in the following:.

- *Physiatrist:* A physiatrist is a physician who has completed residency in the field of PM&R. The physiatrist serves as the team leader responsible for coordinating patient services, setting realistic expectations for both the patients and their families, and developing a treatment plan to improve the functional status of individuals with acute or chronic impairments.
- *Neuropsychologist/rehabilitation psychologist:* This is a doctoral-level licensed provider who assesses how the brain and nervous system influence cognition and behavior. The provider can help provide guidance for optimal treatment of patients with acquired or congenital brain impairments.
- *Case manager:* Case managers coordinate referrals, discharge planning, and social or community services.
- *Rehabilitation nurse (RN):* An RN is a nursing professional who specializes in rehabilitation, with training on managing unique medical needs of patients with physical impairments or disabilities. Care can include medication management, wound management, bowel and bladder management, and education of patients and caregivers.
- *Occupational therapist (OT):* An OT helps develop, recover, improve, or restore function of patients experiencing impairments related to work or activities of daily living (ADLs). ADLs are activities needed for daily living and include feeding, bathing, dressing, grooming and hygiene, and toileting. An OT can help improve fine motor skills, handeye coordination, emotional control, and sequencing of complex tasks, as well as identify modifications to the task or the environment. Other roles include enhancing or improving patients' psychosocial, behavioral, cognitive, or sensory skills.
- *Physical therapist (PT):* A PT helps restore function in patients with mobility impairments, weakness, restricted range of motion, or pain. The role of the PT is to help develop gross motor skills, identify and provide training for mobility device needs, improve endurance, and increase joint range of motion or stability.
- *Speech-language pathologist (SLP):* An SLP works to assess and treat patients with cognitive, communication, speech, or swallowing deficits. An SLP performs instrumented studies to evaluate dyspha-

gia, which can include videofluoroscopic swallow studies (VFSS) or fiberoptic endoscopic evaluation of swallowing (FEES) studies.
- *Respiratory therapist (RT)*: An RT assists patients with impaired respiration and those who require devices to help with proper respiration. Devices can include tracheostomy, mechanical ventilator, or phrenic nerve stimulator. An RT has expertise in managing these tools as well as in administering medications or other treatments via the airways. The role of an RT includes education of patients and their families related to home care of their devices.
- *Vocational rehabilitation specialist (VR)*: A VR is a counselor or therapist who works with patients to develop work and educational plans, facilitates community reintegration, and provides guidance or strategies to achieve realistic work or educational goals.
- *Orthotist*: An orthotist is a professional who assists people with disabilities by customizing braces and splints used to stabilize joints or support impaired or injured body parts. They are trained to assess the unique needs of the individual, determine the technical specifications of prescribed devices, fabricate the devices, and evaluate device fit and outcome.
- *Prosthetist*: A prosthetist is a professional who fabricates and fits artificial limbs to improve the quality of life of individuals with amputations.
- *Patient care technician (PCT)*: Under the supervision of healthcare professionals, a PCT can provide basic medical care, including measuring vital signs and recording other important data. In a rehabilitation setting, a PCT may assist with ADLs.

TRAINING AND BOARD CERTIFICATION

- *Graduate medical training*: Training includes prerequisite completion of U.S. or Canadian medical school (MD or DO) or foreign medical school that meets certain requirements. A total of 48 months of clinical graduate training is required. Trainees must complete an initial 12 months of fundamental clinical skills residency program, followed by 36 months of PM&R medical training.[1]
- *Board certification*: The American Board of Physical Medicine and Rehabilitation (ABPMR) oversees diplomate training and certification. Board certification requires successful completion of a two-part examination.
- Subspecialty training: The ABPMR subspecialty training offers fellowship training on the following:
  - Brain injury medicine (12 months)
  - Neuromuscular medicine (12 months)
  - Pain medicine (12 months)
  - Pediatric rehabilitation medicine (24 months)

- Spinal cord injury medicine (12 months)
- Sports medicine (12 months)
* Additional fellowships without ABPMR certification include, but no limited to:
    - Musculoskeletal/spine fellowships
    - Stroke
    - Multiple sclerosis
    - Neurorehabilitation
    - Electrodiagnostic medicine
    - Cancer rehabilitation
    - Occupational and environmental medicine
    - Movement disorders

Physiatrists treat a variety of conditions, have the opportunity to treat patients throughout the spectrum of healthcare settings, and lead an interdisciplinary team of providers.

REFERENCES

The full complete reference list for this chapter appears in the digital version of the chapter, available at http://connect.springerpub.com/content/book/978-0-8261-5628-0/part/part01/chapter/ch01

CHAPTER 2

NEUROLOGIC EXAMINATION
Ravi E. Kasi

COGNITION

- *History:* Obtain premorbid cognitive functioning including any previous cognitive diagnosis (e.g., Alzheimer), education, and vocation.
- *Technical aspects:* Complete the examination with minimal distractions (ask family members to not answer questions for the patient), accommodate for hearing and language barriers, and perform the examination at the optimal time for the patient.
- *Orientation:* Ask the patient to provide their name, current location, and current date/time. Be mindful to avoid having the patient look at clues in the room (e.g., patient board) that may have this information.
- *Attention and concentration:* There is no specific bedside test for this, but it is a holistic observation of how the patient performs during your neurologic examination. At the conclusion of your examination, use descriptive words on what you observed: "easily distracted 5 seconds into a task needing redirection."
- *Short-term memory:* Have the patient recall three objects within 2 to 5 minutes. Provide a city the patient is not currently in, a color that is not present in the room, and an abstract word (e.g., truth). Ensure the patient can repeat the words to confirm registration (this can also assess their ability to repeat), then distract the patient with other aspects of the neurologic examination before asking them the three words 2 to 5 minutes later.
- *Long-term memory:* Ask the patient regarding information that can be confirmed on the chart or via conversation with the family, such as medical information (e.g., significant surgery from several years prior) and personal information (e.g., "where did you go to high school?").
- *Command following:* Advance the patient from a one-step (e.g., "raise your right hand") to a two-step (e.g., "grab a sheet of paper and fold it in half") command, to more complex commands. As you advance to two- or three-step commands (e.g., "grab this sheet of paper with your RIGHT hand, fold it in two, and place it on the floor"), you can also assess for right/left discrimination, concentration, short-term memory, apraxia, motor strength, and spatial orientation.
- *Apraxia:* Apraxia is the inability to complete a task due to deficits with motor planning. Ask the patient to complete a simple task (e.g., "grab the toothbrush and brush your teeth"). Be mindful of other factors that may mimic and/or impact their ability to complete a task (e.g., weakness, visual deficits, and hearing).

- *Writing:* Have the patient write a sentence and evaluate for sentence structure and meaning. Spelling errors should be evaluated within context. If history reveals the patient to be an English professor, spelling errors would be indicating a decline in function. The size of the lettering (e.g., micrographia in Parkinson) and legibility (e.g., tremors, weakness, fine motor deficits, and dysmetria) could be a sign of other neurologic conditions.
- *Abstract reasoning:* Ask the patient to explain a proverb (e.g., "it's raining cats and dogs").
- *Decision-making ability (competency vs. capacity)*[1,2]: Capacity is the ability of the patient to make a singular specific decision at a specific moment in time. This can be completed by anyone from the interdisciplinary team who assesses the patient's understanding of the risks, benefits, and alternatives of a singular decision. A patient's capacity can fluctuate based on their medical condition or the specific decision (e.g., simple vs. complex). Competence is a legal decision made by a judge following a legal proceeding, where information is presented regarding the patient's cognitive state. Competence is used to determine a patient's ability to stand trial, be a parent, make healthcare decisions, and so forth.

SPEECH

Speech and language can be analyzed by monitoring the rate, articulation, fluency, naming, word comprehension, repetition, writing, and reading during the examinations in Table 2.1. Dedicated testing is typically completed by speech language pathology and/or via neuropsychology testing.

CRANIAL NERVES[3]

Cranial Nerve I (Olfactory Nerve)

- *Function:* smell
- *Test:* Have the patient identify aromatic nonirritating products (e.g., soap, coffee) to each nostril while the other nostril is occluded.

TABLE 2.1 Language Deficits

Language Deficits	Explanation
Aphasia	Impairment of language
Alexia	Impaired reading comprehension
Agraphia	Impairment with writing
Acalculia	Impairment with calculations
Agnosia	Inability to recognize objects independent of issues related to vision, perception, comprehension, etc.
Neglect	Lack of acknowledgment

Using irritants (e.g., alcohol, ammonia) tests the nociceptors of the chemosensory system of cranial nerve (CN) V.

Cranial Nerve II (Optic Nerve)

- *Function:* vision acuity, visual field, pupillary light response, and color perception
- *Test:* Assess during vision testing (see the Funduscopic Examination section).

Cranial Nerve III (Oculomotor Nerve)

- *Function:* pupillary constriction, extraocular movements, and upper eyelid function (levator palpebrae superioris muscle)
- *Motor test:* Evaluate for upper eyelid strength or evidence of upper eyelid droop, as well as for extraocular movements (see the Funduscopic Examination section).

Cranial Nerve IV (Trochlear)

- *Function:* eye abduction, depression, and internal rotation via the superior oblique muscle
- *Test:* Evaluate for extraocular movements (see the Funduscopic Examination section).

Cranial Nerve V (Trigeminal Nerve)[4,5]

- *Function:*
  - Motor function of the temporalis and masseter muscles
  - Sensory innervation to the face: ophthalmic (V1), maxillary (V2), and mandibular (V3)
- *Sensory test:* Use pinprick or a wisp of cotton to test for sensation in all three quadrants (forehead, upper cheek, and jaw line). Sensory sparing of the angle of the jaw (C2 innervation) confirms CN V injury.
- *Motor test*[4,5]*:* Palpate the masseter muscle while the patient clenches their teeth and opens their mouth against resistance and observe the lateral movements of the jaw from side to side. Pterygoid muscle weakness will cause the jaw to deviate to the side of the CN palsy.[3]

Cranial Nerve VI (Abducens)

- *Function:* motor function to the lateral rectus muscle to assist with medial rotation of the eye
- *Test:* Evaluate for extraocular movements (see the Funduscopic Examination section).

Cranial Nerve VII (Facial Nerve)

- *Function:*
  - Motor to facial muscles for expression, closing the lower eyelid, and closing the mouth
  - Sensory innervation via taste of salty, sweet, sour, and bitter substances on the anterior two-thirds of the tongue

- *Motor test:* Ask the patient to smile, raise their eyebrows, frown, puff out their cheeks, and squeeze their eyelids together while looking for asymmetry. If there is facial weakness in the lower half of the face only, the etiology is likely central (e.g., stroke) rather than peripheral (i.e., the entire side of the face will be weak).
- *Sensory (taste) test:* Have the patient identify sweet, sour, salty, and bitter substances on one side of the tongue and compare with the other side.

Cranial Nerve VIII (Vestibulocochlear)

- *Function:* hearing (cochlear division) and balance (vestibular division)
- *Hearing test:* Rub your fingers in each ear and ask the patient to identify the side where they hear your fingers. Repeat this test several times (up to five times) to ensure accuracy. The Weber and Rinne tests can be done at bedside to distinguish between conductive and sensorineural hearing loss; however, the best test would be through a formal audiology referral.
- *Vestibular test*[6]*:* The most accurate test is a formal electronystagmography (ENG)/videonystagmography (VNG), rotary chair test, computerized dynamic posturography (CDP), and vestibular evoked myogenic potential (VEMP).

Cranial Nerve IX (Glossopharyngeal)

- *Function:*
  - Motor innervation to the pharynx
  - Sensory innervation including taste (salty, sweet, sour, and bitter) to the posterior portions of the eardrum and ear canal, the pharynx, and the posterior tongue
- *Motor test:* Have the patient say "ahh" while observing the posterior aspect of their mouth. If a patient has a stroke, the uvula will deviate away from the paretic side.

Cranial Nerve X (Vagus Nerve)

- *Function:*
  - Motor innervation to the soft palate (elevation), pharynx, and larynx
  - Sensory innervation to the pharynx and larynx
- *Motor test:* Test is the same as for CN IX.

Cranial Nerve XI (Spinal Accessory Nerve)

- *Function:* motor innervation to the sternocleidomastoid and the upper portion of the trapezius
- *Motor test (trapezius):* Shrug the shoulders against resistance. CN XI palsy can result in subacromial bursitis due to scapular dysfunction.

- *Motor test (sternocleidomastoid):* Turn the head against resistance while palpating the sternocleidomastoid muscle on the contralateral side to where the patient is turning toward.

Cranial Nerve XII (Hypoglossal Nerve)

- *Function:* motor innervation to the muscles of the tongue
- *Test:* Inspect the tongue for atrophy, fasciculations, or lesions. Ask the patient to move their tongue in all planes. Weakness due to a stroke will result in deviation toward the side of the lesion.

VISION

Funduscopic Examination

- *Visual acuity (CN II):* Test each eye (with the other eye covered) using the Snellen chart.
- *Color perception (CN II):* Color perception is tested using the HardyRandRittler plates.
- *Visual field (CN II)[4]:* Position yourself at a distance approximately the length of your hands away from the patient. Ensure they are looking directly into your eyes and not moving their eyes into the periphery. Move your hands to the outside quadrants of your visual fields and located halfway between you and the patient. Hold up any set of fingers that you can still see in your own peripheral vision and ask the patient to identify how many fingers they see. Be sure to ask them where they saw which fingers (e.g., two fingers on the right and three fingers on the left). Test all four quadrants of their visual field and double-check quadrants that have a field cut to ensure accuracy. Possible visual field deficits and their associated pathologies is noted in Table 2.2.
- *Pupillary light response (CN II/CN III):* Shine a light on the eye in a dimly lit room and observe both the eye being tested and the contralateral eye. CN II provides afferent (sensory) signals and CN III provides efferent (motor) response. CN II palsy will result in lack of pupillary constriction in both eyes when light is shined on the affected eye, but there will be pupillary constriction bilaterally when light is shined on the unaffected eye. CN III palsy will result in a dilated fixed pupil in the affected eye with no response to light regardless of the eye that has light shined on it. Shining a light on the affected eye will cause pupillary constriction in the contralateral eye.
- *Extraocular movements (CN III, CN IV, CN V):* Test eye movement by having the patient look up, down, right, and left (i.e., the eye should move in a horizontal H pattern). Evaluate for evidence of nystagmus or disconjugate gaze.
    - CN III deficit will result in the eye being *down* (superior oblique muscle action) and *out* (lateral rectus muscle action).
    - CN IV palsy results in the inability to look downward with the eye resting in upward gaze. This is also known as the "Pathetic

TABLE 2.2 Visual Field Deficits

Visual Field Deficit	Location of Injury	Visual Field Deficit Example
Bitemporal hemianopia	Optic chiasm injury most commonly due to pituitary adenoma. With pituitary expansion, CN III, IV, and VI could be impacted	
Homonymous hemianopia[7]	Injuries can involve the cerebral cortex (occipital lobe), optic radiations, and/or lateral geniculate nucleus. Specific types of HH can occur secondary to location of injury: optic tract (non-congruous, associated with motor deficits), temporal lobe (denser superiorly, associated with memory impairments), or parietal lobe (denser inferiorly, associated with language deficits)[8,9]	
Quadrantanopia	Usually is associated with occipital lobe injury. However, similar to subsets of HH, lesions can be associated with lesions to the temporal lobe (superior quadrantopia) or parietal lobe (inferior quadrantopia)[7]	

  Nerve" palsy due to the patient tucking their chin in (vertical diplopia) and side bends (torsional diplopia) to compensate and side bends (torsional diplopia) to compensate for blurred vision particularly when going downstairs (i.e., looking down).
  o CN VI palsy results in difficulty with laterally moving the eye, causing diplopia with lateral gaze.
- *Hemispatial neglect:* Neglect is being unaware of one side of one's visual field. This typically occurs following a brain injury. Testing is completed via observation during physical examination when the patient does not acknowledge or engage one side of the body. To confirm this diagnosis, ask the patient to identify the right and left sides of their body, point at objects on either side of their body in the room (e.g., window, door, and clock), have them draw a clock, and/or observe them eating a meal. Patients with hemispatial neglect will not be able to acknowledge anything on one side of their visual field, not draw one side of a clock, or only eat on one side of their plate.

MUSCLE TONE[10]

Flaccid tone can be (but not always) seen after an acute upper motor neuron (UMN) injury, such as acute spinal cord (e.g., during spinal shock) or stroke. It is also seen with lower motor neuron spinal cord injury (e.g., cauda equina), Guillain–Barré syndrome, polio, viral illness, and botulism. Spasticity is typically seen in lesions in the pyramidal tract (e.g., UMN lesions), such as stroke, spinal cord, and motor neuron disease. Clinically, there is a velocity-dependent increase in tone, with more resistance in one direction versus another (see Chapter 29 for a more detailed explanation). Rigidity is seen due to extrapyramidal lesionssuch as Parkinson (see Chapter 26) that result in sustained tone in all directions and not dependent on velocity.

MUSCLE STRENGTH GRADING[11]

Eliminating or including gravity: To include gravity when testing strength, ensure that the gravity vector is on the same plane and is opposing the vector of your muscle action (i.e., gravity is pulling against the motion of the extremity). Be mindful of the position of the patient (e.g., supine, head of bed partially up, sitting up, and standing) that will require you to adjust the position of the extremity to include or exclude gravity (see Table 2.3; Figure 2.1).

MUSCLE STRETCH REFLEXES[12]

Muscle stretch reflexes (MSRs) are completed by testing for muscle response by applying force on the muscle tendon using a reflex hammer. MSRs are graded from 0 to 4 (Table 2.4). Always complete MSRs in all four extremities and look for any asymmetry or isolated changes

TABLE 2.3 Motor Strength Scoring

Grade	Description
0	There is no muscular contraction.
1	Trace contraction is visible or palpable.
2	Full active ROM with gravity is eliminated (see Figure 2.1 for description).
3	There is full active ROM against gravity. With the extremity at 50% of the full ROM, the resistance you provide overcomes the patient's strength and you push the extremity to the start of the ROM.
4	There is full active ROM against gravity with minimal to moderate resistance. With the extremity at 50% of the full ROM, the patient is only able to maintain the extremity at that position.
5	There is full active ROM against gravity with maximal resistance. With the extremity starting at 50% of the full ROM, the patient can overcome the resistance that you provide and fully complete the action of the muscle.

ROM, range of motion.

Source: Stanford Medicine. Spasticity versus Rigidity (Stanford 25 Skills Symposium, 2015). 2015. https://stanfordmedicine25.stanford.edu/blog/archive/2016/Spasticity-versus-Rigidity-Stanford-25-Skills-Symposium-2015.html.

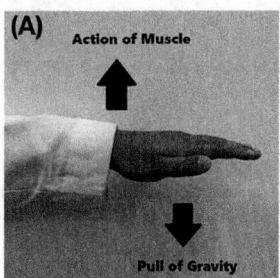 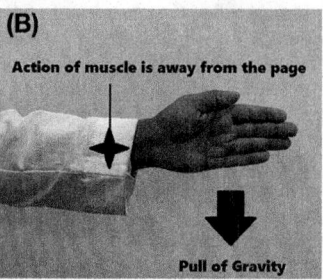

FIGURE 2.1 Eliminating or including gravity in motor strength testing. (A) Including gravity: During wrist extension, the action of the muscle is opposed by the gravity. (B) Excluding gravity: During wrist extension, the action of the muscle is away from the page and is on a different plane than the pull of gravity. Thus, gravity is eliminated.

TABLE 2.4 Muscle Stretch Reflexes

Grade	Description	Pathologic Condition
0	No response	Isolated finding typically due to LMN injury (e.g., radiculopathy) If discovered in the entire extremity could be due to plexus injury, polyneuropathy, or systemic LMN injury
1+	Diminished response: hypoactive	Possible pathologic response similar to grade 0 Could also be normal finding if it is symmetric throughout the body
2+	Normal response	
3+	Brisk response: hyperactive without clonus	Could be normal or due to UMN lesion
4+	Hyperactive with clonus	Occurs secondary to a UMN lesion with sudden rapid dorsiflexion of the foot at the ankle Comment regarding the number of beats of clonus and/or if it is sustained

LMN, lower motor neuron; UMN, upper motor neuron.

that indicate pathology. If reflexes cannot be elicited due to the patient tensing the muscle, distract the patient by having them look away or by performing the Jendrassik maneuver (i.e., hooking flexed fingers against one another).

Pathologic conditions can be superimposed on other pathologic conditions. A patient with an existing upper motor neuron (UMN) lesion (e.g, chronic spinal cord injury) can develop isolated diminished or absent reflex (i.e., 0 or 1 out of 4) due to an acute radiculopathy. A patient with severe peripheral neuropathy with chronically absent reflexes may not always develop hyperactive reflex (i.e., 3 or 4 out of 4) with an acute UN lesion due to chronic damage to the peripheral nerve.

Reflexes typically tested are the biceps (C5-6 but primarily C5), brachioradialis (C5-6 but primarily C6), triceps reflex (C6-C7 but primarily C7), patella or knee-jerk reflex (L2–L4 but primarily L4), medial hamstrings (L5–S1 but primarily L5),[13] and Achilles or ankle-jerk reflex (S1-2 but primarily S1).[14]

Other reflexes tested include the following:

- *Babinski:* Stroke the lateral sole of the foot from the heel to the ball with the end of a reflex hammer. A pathologic response indicating a UMN injury is extension of the big toe with fanning of the other toes ± knee and hip flexion.
- *Primitive reflexes:* These include snout, root, grasp, and palmomental reflexes.

SENSATION

- *Light touch:* This is completed with the cotton from the tip of a cotton swab pulled out. When testing, ensure that the tip of the cotton swab touches the skin and you do not apply pressure.
- *Pinprick versus dull:* This is completed with the sharp and dull aspects of a safety pin.
- *Temperature:* Use two different test tubes of hot and cold liquids.
- *Joint position or proprioception:* Move the patient's finger or toe holding the digit on the medial and lateral margins and test the ability to distinguish between the upward and downward movements. Ensure the patient is not looking at the joint.
- *Vibration:* Use a 128-Hz or 256-Hz tuning fork over a bony prominence and ask the patient when the stimulus ends.
- *Two-point discrimination:* Two-point discrimination tools are available online. Test by asking the patient to identify if they feel one or two pokes while rapidly randomly alternating between one and two points of the tool.
- *Stereognosis:* Place a common object in the patient's hand for identification.
- *Graphesthesia:* Draw a number or letter on the patient's palm for identification.

BALANCE AND COORDINATION

- *Finger-to-chin test:* This is a useful tool for assessment of not only cerebellar function but also other pathologic conditions. The best examination is with the patient sitting at the edge of the bed ± with truncal support (for a patient at high risk of fall, ensure there is someone present to catch the patient if they lean too far forward). Place your arm in a position distant to the patient that will require them to fully extend their hand ± body to touch the tip of your finger and return it back to their chin (avoid the nose as the patient may accidentally poke themselves in the eye). Repeat this examination several times in all four quadrants looking out for the following:

- Smooth pursuit but swings arm up quickly or inadequately- could be due to proximal shoulder pathology
- Dysmetria due to cerebellar injury
- Smooth pursuit but has difficulty hitting the target (e.g., your finger) due to visual spatial issues
- Body is falling to one side or another—impaired truncal control from unilateral weakness

- *Heel-to-shin test:* Ask the patient to place their heel on their knee and slide the heel down to their ankle. A pathologic finding would be inability to complete this task in a straight line, usually due to cerebellar deficits.
- *Pronator drift:* Ask the patient to keep their arm held up (i.e., supinated) with their eyes closed.
  - If the hand pronates ± and there is downward movement of the arm, there is an injury to the contralateral pyramidal tract (e.g., stroke). The arm simply moving downward could also be due to weakness.
  - If the arm moves upward, it is due to ipsilateral cerebellum injury.
- *Romberg test*[15,16]: Evaluate the patient's balance when they are standing with their feet together, eyes open, and arms held forward (i.e., horizontal to the floor) for 30 seconds. Repeat the same test but with the patient's eyes closed for 30 seconds to 1 minute. A positive test would be if the patient has a near fall (i.e., changes foot movement to prevent a fall) or if they fall (be sure to position yourself to avoid a fall from occurring). Swaying can be a normal physiologic proprioceptive correction[17] but the test can be positive if there is significant worsening of swaying with eyes closed. A positive test indicates either damage to proprioception (i.e., dorsal column of the spinal cord) or vestibular system.
- *Gait analysis:* See Chapter 5 for a more detailed explanation. Observe the individual walk down the hallway, do a tandem walk, walk on their heels/toes, hop on each foot, and perform shallow knee bend.

REFERENCES

The full complete reference list for this chapter appears in the digital version of the chapter, available at http://connect.springerpub.com/content/book/978-0-8261-5628-0/part/part01/chapter/ch02

CHAPTER 3

MUSCULOSKELETAL EXAMINATION

Daniel M. Cushman, Sarah F. Eby, and Meredith Ehn

CERVICAL SPINE

Inspection: head and shoulder posture, shoulder heights, lordosis/kyphosis, torticollis, scapular winging, and limb atrophy or ischemia

Palpation: spinous processes, facet joints, cervical paraspinals, occiput and suboccipital muscles, periscapular muscles, and lateral and anterior neck musculature

Range of motion (ROM): flexion (flex, 80°–90°), extension (ext, 70°), rotation (70°–90°), and lateral flex (20°–45°)

Special test (cervical spine): (see Table 3.1)

TABLE 3.1

Test	Explanation	Positive Finding
Spurling maneuver[1]	The patient extends and side-flexes the head; the examiner carefully applies axial compression.	Reproduction of radicular pain down the arm

SHOULDER

Inspection: head and shoulder posture, shoulder heights including the clavicles, scapula position, anterior glenohumeral fullness (anterior dislocation), and atrophy of rotator cuff and scapular girdle

Palpation: sternoclavicular (SC) joints, clavicles, acromioclavicular (AC) joints, ribs 1 and 2, scapula, greater and lesser tuberosities of the humerus, glenohumeral joint line, and long head biceps tendon in the bicipital groove

ROM: abduction (abd, 170°–180°), flex (160°–180°), external rotation (ER, 80°–90°), internal rotation (IR, 60°–100°); for the scapula, look for dyskinesis, winging, and asymmetry with active flex and abd

Special tests (shoulder): (see Table 3.2)

TABLE 3.2

Test	Explanation	Positive Finding
AC joint		
Cross-arm adduction (Apley scarf test, AC joint)	The patient flexes the arm to 90° and reaches to the opposite shoulder.[2]	Re-creation of localized pain at the AC joint
Rotator cuff		
Hawkins Kennedy (impingement)	The examiner forward-flexes the arm to 90° and then forcibly internally rotates the shoulder.[3]	Pain suggestive of supraspinatus tendon pathology or secondary impingement
Neer (impingement)	The arm is internally rotated and then passively elevated to end range in the scapular plane.[4]	Pain suggestive of supraspinatus tendon pathology or secondary impingement
Empty can test (supraspinatus)	The arm is abducted to 90°, horizontally adducted 30°, and internally rotated (thumb pointing toward the floor). The examiner then exerts an inferiorly directed eccentric force.[5]	Weakness and pain
Anterior dislocation		
Apprehension or crank (anterior dislocation)	The examiner abducts the arm to 90° and slowly and carefully externally rotates the patient's arm.[6]	Alarm or apprehension with further motion more so than pain (typically resembles what it felt like when it dislocated)
Biceps		
Speed test (biceps)	The arm is supinated and flexed to 90°. The examiner then applies an eccentrically directed force into extension.[7]	Increased tenderness in the bicipital groove suggestive of long head biceps tendinopathy

AC, acromioclavicular.

ELBOW

Inspection: bony alignment, carrying angle (11°–14° of valgus is normal for adult males and 13°–16° for adult females), effusion, soft tissue edema, muscular asymmetry/atrophy, and olecranon bursa

Palpation: cubital fossa, proximal shaft of the radius and ulna, radial head, medial and lateral epicondyles, ulnar collateral ligament, common flexor and extensor tendons, olecranon process and bursa, and triceps muscle and tendon

ROM: flex (140°–150°), ext (0°–10°), supination (90°), and pronation (80°–90°)

Special tests (elbow): (see Table 3.3)

TABLE 3.3

Test	Explanation	Positive Finding
Lateral epicondylitis		
Cozen test	The elbow is stabilized by the examiner's thumb over the lateral epicondyle. The patient makes a fist and pronates the forearm. The examiner resists wrist extension and radial deviation.[8]	Pain over the lateral epicondyle
Maudsley (middle finger) test	The examiner resists long finger extension distal to the PIP joint.[8]	Pain over the lateral epicondyle indicative of lateral epicondylitis while weakness with finger extension may be suggestive of posterior interosseous nerve entrapment
Medial epicondylitis		
Medial (tennis elbow shear) test	The patient flexes the elbow, pronates, and flexes the wrist. The examiner uses both hands to resist wrist flexion and pronation while the patient extends the elbow as if throwing.[9]	Pain at the medial epicondyle

PIP, proximal interphalangeal.

WRIST AND HAND

Inspection: deformity (e.g., mallet finger, boutonniere, swan neck, ulnar drift), bony alignment, soft tissue swelling or mass, joint effusion, muscular asymmetry/atrophy (intrinsic wasting, thenar/hypothenar atrophy), trophic changes, skin temperature, Heberden/Bouchard nodules, trigger finger, and Dupuytren contracture

Palpation: carpal, metacarpal, and interphalangeal joints, and carpals (including anatomic snuff box), metacarpals, phalanges, radial and ulnar styloids, distal radioulnar joint, and triangular fibrocartilaginous complex

ROM: radial deviation (15°), ulnar deviation (30°45°), wrist flex (80°–90°), wrist ext (70°–90°), finger flex (metacarpophalangeal [MCP] 85°–90°, proximal interphalangeal [PIP] 100°–115°, distal interphalangeal [DIP] 80°–90°), finger ext (MCP 30°–45°, PIP 0°, DIP 20°), finger abd (20°–30°), finger adduction (add, 0°), thumb flex (carpal-metacarpal [CMC] 45°–50°, MCP 50°–55°, interphalangeal [IP] 85°–90°), thumb ext (MCP 0°, IP 0°–5°), thumb abd (60°–70°), and thumb add (30°)

Special tests (wrist and hand): (see Table 3.4)

TABLE 3.4

Test	Explanation	Positive Finding
Stenosing tenosynovitis (de Quervain syndrome)		
Finkelstein (Eichhoff) test	The patient makes a fist with the thumb inside the fingers. The examiner ulnarly deviates the wrist.[10]	Pain over the abductor pollicis longus and extensor pollicis brevis tendons at the wrist
Carpal tunnel syndrome		
Phalen test	The patient's wrists are maximally flexed and pushed together over the dorsum of the hand for 1 minute.[11]	Tingling in the thumb, index finger, long, and lateral half of the ring finger
Tinel sign at the wrist	The examiner taps over the median nerve in the carpal tunnel.	Tingling in the thumb, index finger, long, and lateral half of the ring finger

LUMBOSACRAL SPINE AND PELVIS

Inspection: observe anteriorly, posteriorly, and laterally; normal gentle lumbar lordosis; posture (rigid, antalgic, and listing), head positioning, and shoulder asymmetry; iliac crest height asymmetry and lower limb asymmetry; observe gait

Palpation: spinous processes, paraspinal/gluteal musculature, posterior superior iliac spines, iliac crests, and greater trochanters

ROM: flex (50°–70°), ext (10°–20°), lateral flex (25°–35°), and axial rotation (25°–40°)

Special tests (lumbosacral spine and pelvis): (see Table 3.5)

TABLE 3.5

Test	Explanation	Positive Finding
Lumbar nerve roots		
Seated slump	The patient sits with the arms behind their back and legs together, slumped forward with full spinal and neck flexion; the examiner assists in extending the patient's knee.	Reproduction of radicular pain symptoms down the leg that is being extended
Straight leg raise	The patient lies supine and the examiner elevates the leg to 30°–70°.	Reproduction of radicular pain symptoms reproduced down the leg that is being extended
Lumbar facets		
Quadrant loading (extension quadrant/Kemp test)	The patient stands with their back to the examiner, who assists in extending the spine, with side flexion and rotation until symptoms are produced or the limit of motion is reached.	Narrowing of the neural foramen and increased stress on facet joint (on the side of flexion + rotation) yields painful symptoms[12]
Sacroiliac joints*		
Fortin finger	Ask the patient to point to the region of pain with one finger.	The patient localizing the pain with one finger and pointing immediately inferomedial to the posterior superior iliac spine

*Laslett's rule: sacroiliac pathology present if two to three sacroiliac provocation tests are positive (compression, distraction, sacral thrust, thigh thrust, Gaenslen, and posterior superior iliac spine pain).

HIP AND THIGH

Inspection: observe any soft tissue or bony asymmetries, lower extremity alignment, leg length discrepancy, or gait abnormalities; comparing with the contralateral side for all aspects of the examination is helpful

Palpation: anterior superior iliac spine, greater trochanter, iliac crest, posterior superior iliac spine, gluteal musculature, piriformis, and proximal hamstrings

ROM: flex (110°–120°), ext (10°–15°), abd (30°–50°), add (30°), IR (30°–40°), and ER (40°–60°)

Special tests (hip and thigh): (see Table 3.6)

TABLE 3.6

Test	Explanation	Positive Finding
Hip joint		
FABER/ Patrick test	The patient lies supine; the examiner bends the patient's knee on the side of interest, placing the patient's foot on top of the knee of the opposite leg, then slowly presses the knee toward the table.	Groin pain suggests intra-articular hip pathology; posterior pain suggests sacroiliac pathology.[13]
FADIR	The patient lies supine; the examiner flexes the patient's hip and knee on the side of interest to 90°, then maximally internally rotates and adducts the hip.	Groin pain due to impingement of the femoral neck against the acetabular rim is suggestive of hip impingement or labral lesion.
Stinchfield resisted hip flexion	The patient lies supine with legs straight and actively flexes at the hip to 20°–30°; the examiner applies resistance proximal to the knee.	Anterior groin pain suggests intra-articular hip pathology due to loading of the hip joint.[14]

KNEE

Inspection: observe lower extremity alignment (genu varum/genu valgum), leg length discrepancy, gait abnormalities, soft tissue or bony asymmetries, and joint effusion or erythema; comparing with the contralateral side for all aspects of the examination is helpful

Palpation: palpate for any effusion; patella, patellar tendon, quadriceps tendon, femoral condyles, medial joint line, medial collateral ligament, pes anserinus, lateral joint line, lateral collateral ligament, Gerdy tubercle/iliotibial band, posterior knee joint, gastrocnemii, and hamstrings

ROM: flex (135°–140°) and ext (0°–10°)

Special tests (knee): (see Table 3.7)

TABLE 3.7

Test	Explanation	Positive Finding
MCL		
Valgus stress test	The patient lies supine; the examiner holds the patient's relaxed, slightly bent leg, with the calf resting on their arm, the foot supported in their axilla, and their hand over the medial knee joint line, applying valgus stress (while not internally rotating the hip) and feeling for the medial articular surfaces snapping apart.	Medial tenderness is suggestive of MCL strain; medial articular surface gapping is suggestive of MCL tear.

(continued)

TABLE 3.7 (continued)

Test	Explanation	Positive Finding
ACL		
Lachman test	The patient lies supine; the examiner holds the patient's knee at 15° flexion, with one hand stabilizing the femur and the other firmly grasping the tibia. The examiner then translates the tibia anteriorly.	A soft endfeel with anterior translation of the tibia on the femur is suggestive of ACL tear.[15]
Anterior drawer test	The patient lies supine with hip on the affected side in 45° flexion, knee in 90° flexion, and foot resting on the table; the examiner grasps the patient's tibia with both hands, with thumbs on either side of the tibial tuberosity. The examiner then translates the tibia anteriorly.	Increased anterior tibial displacement is suggestive of ACL tear.[16]
PCL		
Posterior drawer test	The patient lies supine with hip on the affected side in 45° flexion, knee in 90° flexion, and foot resting on the table; the examiner grasps the patient's tibia with both hands, with thumbs on either side of the tibial tuberosity. The examiner then translates the tibia posteriorly.	Increased posterior tibial displacement is suggestive of PCL tear.[17]
Meniscus		
McMurray	The patient lies supine; the examiner holds the affected leg in 90° flexion at the hip and knee, with their thumb and index finger over the knee joint line and the patient's heel cupped in the other hand. To assess medial meniscus, the examiner externally rotates the tibia (at the heel) and extends the knee while applying a varus stress at the knee. To assess the lateral meniscus, the examiner internally rotates the tibia (at the heel) and extends the knee while applying a valgus stress at the knee.	The examiner feeling a snap or pop at the knee (via their thumb and index finger) is suggestive of meniscal tear.[18]

(continued)

TABLE 3.7 (continued)

Test	Explanation	Positive Finding
Patellofemoral		
Single-leg squat	The patient is in single-leg stance and the examiner asks them to do a partial squat (to 45°–60° knee flexion), then return to upright single-leg stance.	Dynamic knee valgus, seen when the knee shifts medially during squat, is suggestive of weak or poorly conditioned hip flexors, abductors, and external rotators and may contribute to painful knee symptoms, including patellofemoral pain syndrome.[19–21]

ACL, anterior cruciate ligament; MCL, medial collateral ligament; PCL, posterior cruciate ligament.

FOOT, ANKLE, AND LOWER LEG

Inspection: observe weight-bearing rearfoot and forefoot posture/alignment, both anteriorly and posteriorly (neutral, planovalgus, and cavovarus); observe any skin lesions, callouses, blisters, and nail abnormalities; observe overall bony alignment, any tissue swelling, or gait abnormalities; comparing with the contralateral side for all aspects of the examination is helpful

Palpation: medal malleolus, anterior talofibular ligament (ATFL), calcaneofibular ligament, posterior talofibular ligament, deltoid ligament, syndesmosis, Achilles tendon and insertion, and medial calcaneal tuberosity

ROM: plantarflexion (45°–50°), dorsiflexion (20°), inversion (35°–45°), and eversion (15°–25°); toe ext (hallux: 70°, others: 30°–40°)

Special tests (foot, ankle, and lower leg): (see Table 3.8)

TABLE 3.8

Test	Explanation	Positive Finding
Anterior drawer	The patient is seated with the knee flexed and the foot relaxed; the examiner grasps the tibia and fibula with one hand, while the other cups the heel to hold the foot in 20° plantarflexion, then translates it anteriorly.	Increased translation or the appearance of a dimple or suction sign over the area of the ATFL is suggestive of ATFL tear.[22]

ATFL, anterior talofibular ligament.

REFERENCES

The full complete reference list for this chapter appears in the digital version of the chapter, available at http://connect.springerpub.com/content/book/978-0-8261-5628-0/part/part01/chapter/ch03

CHAPTER 4

THE CARE OF PEOPLE WITH DISABILITY

Nethra S. Ankam

DEFINITIONS

About 26% of the U.S. population self-identifies as having a disability, making it the largest minority population in the country.[1] Physiatrists routinely care for people with disability; however, the sociopolitical and cultural implications of disability identity are not often taught, which can unknowingly compromise the care people with disability receive. Disability is a form of diversity and a social construct, rather than a biomedical designation. Medicine is fraught with systemic ableism, defined as structures of the healthcare systems prioritizing and valuing nondisabled bodies over disabled ones.[2] These biases are quite clear in the crisis standards of care developed during the COVID-19 pandemic, where people with disability were presumed to have lower quality of life and thus provided less medical care.[2] However, there are a multitude of less obvious examples in day-to-day practice as rehabilitation is inherently ableist when the goals of care are assumed—for example, assuming the goal for a particular patient is walking when they have used a wheelchair since a very young age. To combat this, physiatrists must practice person-centered, collaborative care, with shared decision-making and shared goal setting, elevating the person's voice in their own care. Physiatrists must also consider the concept of interdependence rather than independence being the goal of healthcare. Interdependence is the concept that every person needs varying supports to move through their life and thus people rely on each other as a community for care, which minimizes the role of care as a commodity.[2]

LANGUAGE CONSIDERATIONS

Generally, person first language is preferred. Person first language places the person before the disability and describes who the person is rather than their diagnosis. Examples of this language include "children with cerebral palsy" or "people with mental health conditions." Some people in the disabled community now feel that person first language erases their identity as a disabled person and thus prefer identity first language. Communities such as the Autistic community and the Deaf community have claimed identity first language. It is important to ask what language is preferred by the person. Not everyone who is thought to have a disability by the society identifies as having a disability. Of note, *nondisabled* is the preferred term for those without disability as it centers the disability identity.[3] For other examples

TABLE 4.1 Acceptable Versus Unacceptable Language

Words to Avoid	Acceptable Alternative Words
Mental retardation	Intellectual disability
Handicap	Disability, accessible
Insane, crazy	Mental health condition
Wheelchair-bound/confined to a wheelchair	Wheelchair user

of acceptable versus unacceptable language, see Table 4.1. For continuously updated information regarding acceptable language, visit the National Center on Disability and Journalism's Style Guide at https://ncdj.org/style-guide/.

MODELS OF DISABILITY

Biomedical Model of Disability

In this model, disability is caused by the health condition of the person and is mitigated only by the medical treatment of the health condition that results in cure.[4] This model is the conventional view of disability and creates harms for those with disability by not taking into account the resources of the person or the environment's interaction with the person. In this model, the impairments of the individual are solely responsible for the disability, and the model assumes treatment plans for individuals are driven by the diagnosis alone.[4] Adaptation in any individual situation is up to the individual without systems solutions and puts the solutions to disability within the medical realm, potentially removing a person's autonomy.[4] For instance, in this model, it is a given that a person with paralysis cannot go to the movie theater that has steps to enter, rather than considering the fact the movie theater should be accessible to wheelchair users.

Social Model of Disability

In this model, disability is a sociopolitical and cultural identity. Problems related to disability are caused by the way the society is organized, and in particular by the physical and attitudinal barriers in the environment. In this model, there is no need to intervene to fix the individual with disability, and the harms of disability are created by the exclusion of people with disability; thus, the solutions to the problem of disability are to change laws and policies to ensure the civil rights of people with disability.[4] In this model, the thought is if the society is organized using the universal design principles to include those with the most disability, all of the society benefits. For example, when the Americans With Disabilities Act (ADA) required automatic doors to stores, people who used wheelchairs clearly benefitted; however, those who had many packages or used strollers used the automatic doors more.[5] This model of disability draws its inspiration directly from the civil rights movement and is the basis of the philosophy of the Centers for Independent Living. For more information regarding the Centers for Independent Living, visit the Administration for Community Living at https://acl.gov/.

The World Health Organization's International Classification of Functioning, Disability, and Health

The International Classification of Functioning, Disability, and Health (ICF; Figure 4.1), created by the World Health Organization in 2001, is a biopsychosocial model.[6] In this model, disability exists in the interaction between the person and the environment, and disability is based on the functions that a person cannot do and would like to do.[6] Therefore, if there are adequate environmental supports, disability is not present. In this model, health conditions are defined as the disease or disorder. Body function and structure can be impaired and these impairments are additive. For instance, a person with thoracic spinal cord injury and emphysema will have the additive effects of these health conditions through impairments related to both conditions. Activity (defined as functions the person can do in an idealized environment, such as the gym) can be limited. Participation (defined as functions the person can do in the community) can be restricted. Activity limitations and participation restrictions together make up disability. Activity limitations and participation restrictions can be modified by environmental and personal factors, which can serve as barriers to or facilitators of function.[6]

The ICF is uniquely suited to the needs of physiatrists. Physiatrists should use their understanding of the person's health conditions and the environmental and personal factors in the context of the per-

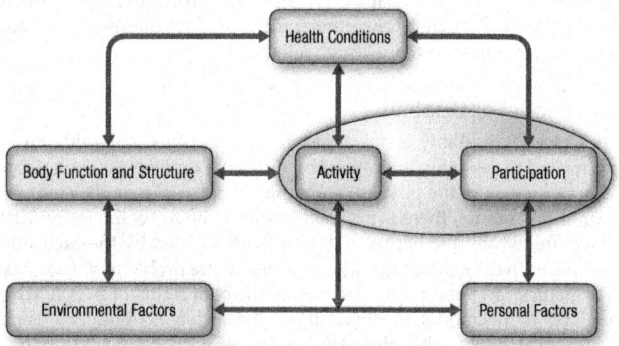

FIGURE 4.1 The World Health Organization's International Classification of Functioning, Disability, and Health.
Source: Reproduced with permission from World Health Organization, ed. *International Classification of Functioning, Disability and Health: ICF*. World Health Organization; 2001.

son's functional goals to develop interprofessional, collaborative treatment plans to help the person achieve their goals, the essence of the ICF. Physiatrists should understand that at different life stages, people with disability may need different engagement with the medical system versus environmental interventions to engage in life activities and achieve personal goals, and the ICF can serve as a reminder to consider all aspects of a person's care. For instance, someone with moderate knee osteoarthritis who has difficulty climbing stairs to do laundry might benefit from more biomedical interventions such as physical therapy and injections; however, they would also have improvement in life participation by altering their environment by obtaining help with laundry or moving the location of the machines.

LEGAL AND POLICY DEFINITIONS OF DISABILITY

Worker's Compensation

Worker's compensation typically uses an edition of the American Medical Association's Guides to the Evaluation of Permanent Impairment to define disability. Impairment is deviation or loss of use of any body function or structure in a person with a health condition.[7] Impairment is considered permanent when the person has reached maximum medical improvement.[7] Disability is functional loss in a person with a health condition.[7] However, many entities, when using these definitions to inform policies, equate the evaluation of permanent impairment to the definition of disability, anchoring their systems in the biomedical model of disability.

Social Security Administration

Impairment "results from anatomical, physiological, or psychological abnormalities which can be shown by medically acceptable clinical and laboratory diagnostic techniques."[8] Disability is "the inability to do any substantial, gainful activity by reason of any medically determinable physical or mental impairment, which can be expected to result in death or which has lasted or can be expected to last for a continuous period of not less than 12 months."[9] Again, this definition of disability anchors disability in the biomedical model.

Americans With Disabilities Act

Per the ADA, a disability is present if one of the following requirements has been fulfilled: A person can have a physical or mental impairment that limits at least one of their major life activities, which can include, but are not limited to, caring for oneself, performing manual tasks, seeing, hearing, eating, sleeping, walking, standing, lifting, bending, speaking, breathing, learning, reading, concentrating, thinking, communicating, and working. They can also have a record of such an impairment, or they can be regarded by others as possessing this sort of impairment.[10] For example, the deaf community does not see themselves as disabled, but others might regard them as having a disability, and as such they receive protections under the ADA. This definition of disability is anchored in the social model.

CONCEPTS ESSENTIAL TO CARE OF PEOPLE WITH DISABILITY

Person-Centered Care

Per the American Geriatrics Society Expert Panel on Person-Centered Care, person-centered care is care where the person's values and preferences guide all aspects of their healthcare.[11] Rehabilitation professionals see themselves as more person-centered than their patients note.[12] Elements essential to operationalizing person-centered care include creation of an individualized care plan based on the person's goals, with ongoing goal and care plan review, involvement of an interprofessional team including the person as a team member, and active coordination among all involved team members with a main point of

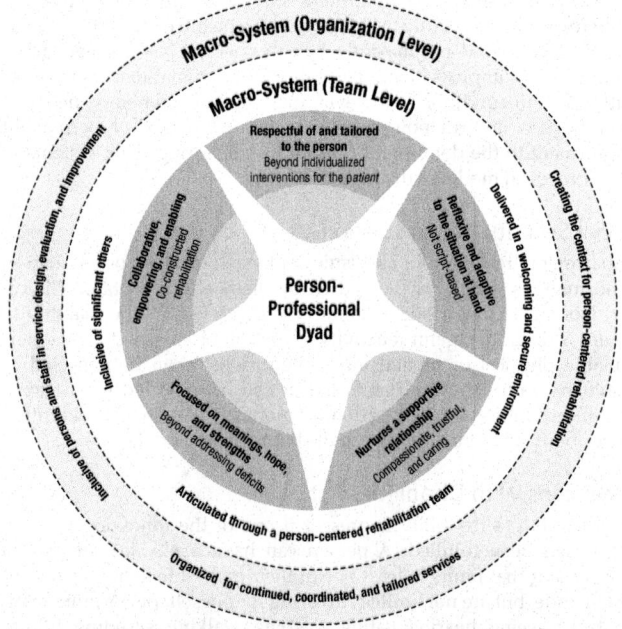

FIGURE 4.2 The Person-Centered Rehabilitation Model.
Source: Reproduced with permission from Jesus TS, Papadimitriou C, Bright FA, et al. Person-centered rehabilitation model: Framing the concept and practice of person-centered adult physical rehabilitation based on a scoping review and thematic analysis of the literature. *Arch Phys Med Rehabil.* 2022;103(1):106–120. doi:10.1016/j.apmr.2021.05.005.

contact for the person. To maintain the commitment to person-centered care and the person's autonomy, education and training of the care team and performance measurement and quality improvement using feedback from the person are required.[11] Person-centered rehabilitation builds upon the Person-Centered Care Model (Figure 4.2) and centers the rehabilitation on the care of the whole person, not just the impairments.[12] The model addresses the unique needs of the interprofessional rehabilitation team and the need for continual adaptation as the person progresses through rehabilitation.[12]

Shared Decision-Making

This model of decision-making is based on the idea that both healthcare professionals and patients bring expertise to the decision-making process.[13] A recent systematic review described the most common elements of shared decision-making models include describing treatment options and creating choice awareness, reviewing patient preferences and learning about the patient, tailoring information to the patient, reaching mutual agreement through deliberation, and then making the decision.[13]

Supported Decision-Making

Supported decision-making is a process where individuals with disabilities make their own choices with the support of a team of people of their choosing, operationalizing the concept of interdependence.[14] This is an alternative to guardianship, where the guardian makes the decisions for the person with disability.[14] This concept is grounded in the social model of disability. All people seek the counsel of trusted advisors to gather information to then make their own decisions. Supported decision-making is a formalized extension of this process for individuals with disabilities.[14] When treating a person with disability who utilizes supported decision-making, physicians should know the relationship of the support person to the patient and the role they will play.[15] The physician should adapt the discussion to the patient's needs, including providing sufficient time with adequate communication support in a comfortable environment.[15] During the conversation, the physician should assess the capacity of the patient to make the healthcare decision with support.[15] See http://supporteddecisionmaking.org/states for a list of states that have supported decision-making statutes.

PHYSICIAN OBLIGATIONS UNDER THE AMERICANS WITH DISABILITIES ACT

The ADA is a civil rights law grounded in the social model of disability. Disability civil rights protections prohibit discrimination and require physicians (and other entities) to take proactive steps to offer equal opportunities.[16] Clinical practices must provide equal access to care, accommodating all disability-related needs in collaboration with the patient, but ultimately based on the physician's judgment, and cannot refuse patients because of disability.[16] Practices must pay for accommodations, not patients.[16]

Accommodations and Disability Etiquette

Communication

Speak directly with the patient, not the support person. Speak to adults at an age-appropriate level. Avoid shouting when needing louder volumes as shouting changes facial expression. Provide extended time for answers and be prepared for apparent nonsequiturs as cognitive processing can take time. Provide access to American Sign Language interpreters and be sure to look at and speak to the patient when using the interpreter. Provide different forms of access to educational materials, such as Braille, large type, simplified language documents, descriptive picture captions on websites or electronic media, and so forth.

Physical Examination

Explain actions clearly and seek permission before you begin. Tell and show what you are going to do and why. Use concrete language that delineates the exact actions for the examination. You may need to use visual aids or use demonstrations of the examination maneuvers. Do not touch the assistive device without permission. Ensure patients are transferred to the examination table for a thorough examination. Collaborate with the patient to find out the best way to effect the transfer.

Accessible Office

An accessible office includes accessible parking, entryways, and bathrooms. There should be a patient lift device and staff trained to use it, along with a wheelchair-accessible scale. There should be at least one accessible examination room. For patients who are neuroatypical, they may need to be roomed right away to reduce stimulation. The ADA.gov website provides a guide to an accessible examination room (see Figure 4.3).

Accessible Office Policies

Schedule more time for people with disabilities, avoid fees for lateness, educate staff in disability etiquette, and have policies to alert staff to impairments and the type of accommodations required by the patient. Have review mechanisms to make sure the office remains accessible.

Further resources include the ADA.gov website, the Vanderbilt Kennedy Center Toolkit for Primary Care Providers (https://iddtoolkit.vkcsites.org/), and materials from the United Spinal Association on Disability Etiquette, located at https://unitedspinal.org/disability-etiquette/

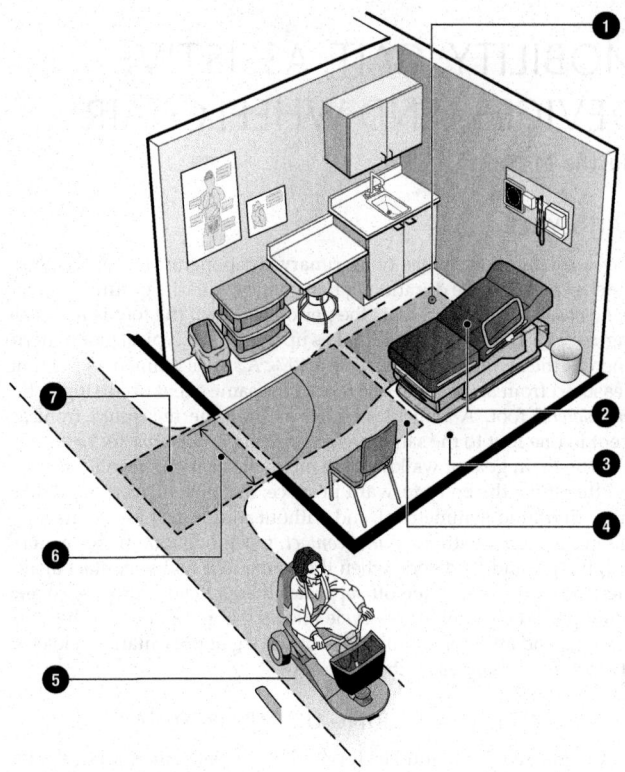

FIGURE 4.3 Guide to an accessible examination room. (1) A clear floor space, 30″ × 48″ minimum, adjacent to the examination table and adjoining accessible route, makes it possible to do a side transfer. (2) Adjustable height accessible examination table lowers for transfers. (3) Providing space between the table and the wall allows staff to assist with patient transfers and positioning. When additional space is provided, transfers may be made from both sides. (4) The amount of floor space needed beside and at the end of the examination table will vary depending on the method of patient transfer and lift equipment size. (5) Accessible route connects to other accessible public and common use spaces. (6) Accessible entry door has 32″ minimum clear opening width with a door that opens 90°. (7) Maneuvering clearances are needed at the door to the room.

Note: Additional clear floor space can be provided by moving or relocating chairs, trash cans, carts, and other items.
Source: From the U.S. Department of Justice Civil Rights Division. https://www.ada.gov/medcare_mobility_ta/medcare_ta.htm#accessibleexamrm.

REFERENCES

The full complete reference list for this chapter appears in the digital version of the chapter, available at http://connect.springerpub.com/content/book/978-0-8261-5628-0/part/part01/chapter/ch04

CHAPTER 5

MOBILITY: GAIT, ASSISTIVE DEVICES, AND WHEELCHAIRS

Martha M. Smith

GAIT CYCLE

The normal gait cycle has two primary components: the *stance phase*, which represents the duration of foot contact with the ground; and the *swing phase*, which represents the period in which the foot is in the air (Figure 5.1). The stance phase makes up 60% of the typical gait pattern, whereas the swing phase makes up 40%. A *step* is defined as the time measured from an event in one foot to the same event occurring in the *contralateral* foot. A *stride* is defined as the time measured from an event in one foot to the same event occurring in the *same* foot.[1]

The main goal of walking is to move the center of gravity (COG), and therefore, the body, forward in space; the most efficient pattern of gait is rhythmic, symmetrical, and without additional movements. The gait cycle begins with the *initial contact*, when one foot makes contact with the ground, and ends when that same foot makes contact again. The temporal event of toe-off separates the gait cycle into stance and swing periods. Defining this cycle allows the gait pattern to be standardized and allows the clinician to observe gait presentation and classify any abnormalities on the same scale.

MUSCLE ACTIVITY DURING UNIMPAIRED GAIT

Ankle dorsiflexors: These muscles (primarily the tibialis anterior, but also the extensor digitorum longus and the extensor hallucis longus) eccentrically contract to smoothly lower the foot from heel strike to foot flat. They also concentrically contract during the swing phase to dorsiflex the ankle and effectively shorten the swinging limb in order to clear the ground.

Ankle plantarflexors: The triceps surae act eccentrically during midstance to control ankle dorsiflexion caused by the body's forward momentum. At push-off, they act concentrically to lift the heel and toes off the ground (Figure 5.2).

Hip abductors: The gluteus medius and minimus contract eccentrically during the stance phase to limit pelvic tilt of the swing phase leg. Maximum contraction occurs after heel strike.

Hip flexors: The hip flexors (primarily the iliopsoas) contract eccentrically after the midstance phase to slow truncal extension caused by the ground reactive force (GRF) passing behind the hip. The tensor fasciae latae, pectineus, sartorius, and iliopsoas contract concentrically to flex the hip and shorten the limb for effective ground clearance during the swing phase.

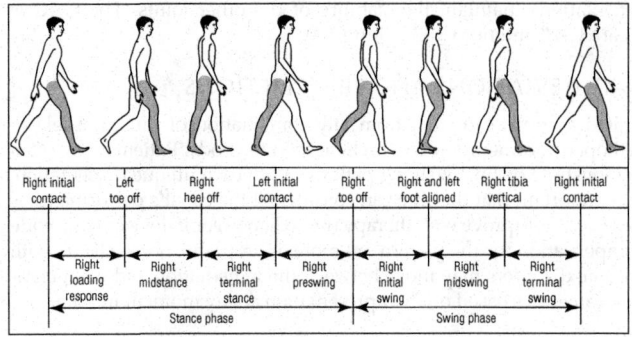

FIGURE 5.1 Components of the gait cycle.

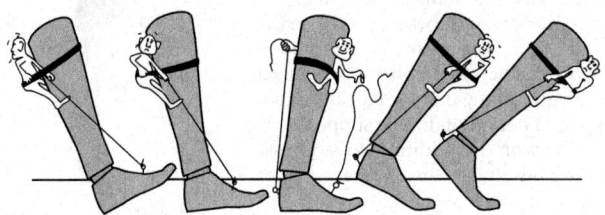

FIGURE 5.2 The actions of the ankle dorsiflexors/plantarflexors in normal gait.
Source: Inman V. *Human Walking*. Williams & Wilkins; 1981.

Hip extensors/hamstrings: The gluteus maximus and hamstrings start to eccentrically contract just before heel strike to maintain hip stability and slow down the forward momentum of the trunk since the GRF is anterior to the hip at this stage. The hamstrings have a double peak of activity. The first peak occurs during the swing phase, when there is an open kinetic chain (foot not in contact with the ground), decelerating the forward swing of the leg by eccentrically contracting during hip extension and flexing at the knee. At heel strike, the open kinetic chain is then converted to a closed kinetic chain (foot in contact with the ground), while the hamstrings act predominantly as hip extensors preventing both hip and knee buckling, while the gluteus maximus contracting propels the COG forward.

Knee extensors: The quadriceps act primarily to absorb shock as they eccentrically contract during heel strike to keep the knees stable. They are also active just before toe-off to help initiate the forward swing of the limb.

Standing: The gastroc-soleus complex (primarily the soleus) is the only muscle normally active during quiet standing. Ligaments and bony

GAIT DEVIATIONS AND PRESCRIPTIONS

Gait deviations can stem from any combination of musculoskeletal, orthopedic, or neuromuscular changes in the body. Patients may often demonstrate distinct walking patterns. With each unique presentation, it is important that the clinician considers if the client's performance is expected to improve with therapy (remediation) or if devices to provide compensation for the pattern are more appropriate. Some clients with chronic disorders may move between the remediation and compensation categories based on their presentation at any moment in time.

Muscle-Deficit Gait

Antalgic gait: To reduce pain, there is avoidance of weight-bearing (WB) on the affected limb. The examiner may note a decrease in the stance phase, a reduced step length on the unaffected side, and a prolonged period of double support.

Treatment: In addition to addressing the underlying cause of pain, use of assistive devices (e.g., walker, cane, or crutches) to reduce WB can help normalize the gait pattern and promote safety and balance.

Gastrocnemius gait: Weak plantarflexors during the terminal stance and toe-off prevent adequate heel lift. To limit drop in the COG that occurs without heel lift during the terminal stance, the step length of the contralateral leg is shortened.

Treatment: A solid or semisolid ankle–foot orthosis (AFO) with a full-length footplate can be considered to simulate plantarflexion during the terminal stance.

Gluteus medius–minimus (Trendelenburg) gait: In an uncompensated Trendelenburg gait (Figure 5.4A), there is contralateral pelvic drop secondary to the inability of the hip abductors to stabilize the pelvis during stance. In a compensated Trendelenburg gait (Figure 5.4B),

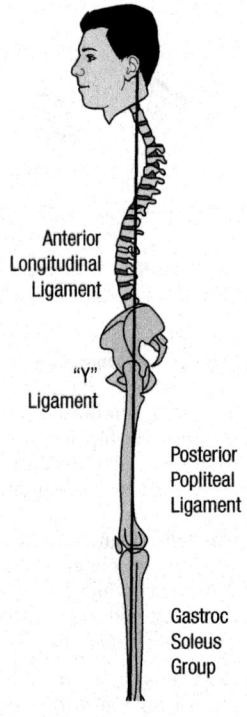

FIGURE 5.3 The center of gravity (COG) line.
Source: Cailliet R. *Low Back Pain Syndromes.* 5th ed. FA Davis; 1995.

5 Mobility: Gait, Assistive Devices, and Wheelchairs | 37

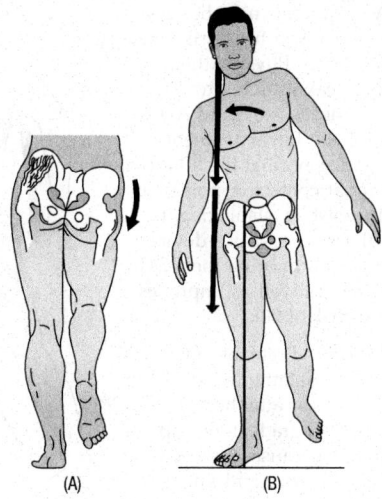

FIGURE 5.4 Uncompensated (A) and compensated (B) Trendelenburg gait.

weak abductors are compensated by a lateral lurch over the affected side to reduce the stress on the weak muscles.

Treatment: Referral to physical therapy for muscular strengthening in the pelvis, core, and hip girdle is beneficial. A cane used in the contralateral hand widens the base of support and decreases the hip abductor strength needed to keep the pelvis level. In bilateral abductor weakness, bilateral canes with a four-point gait may be used.

Gluteus maximus (extensor lurch) gait: This may be seen following injury to the inferior gluteal nerve or a subtrochanteric hip fracture. Weakened hip extensors are unable to decelerate the forward momentum of the body (hip flexion moment) at heel strike. To compensate, the subject adopts a prominent posterior lean and locks the hip joint in extension against the iliofemoral ligament, which keeps the body's COG behind the hip.

Treatment: Two crutches or canes are used for a three-point gait (Figure 5.5).

Quadriceps (back knee) gait: With weakness or inhibition of the quadriceps (e.g., distal femoral fracture, or following neurologic events such as a cerebrovascular accident [CVA]), buckling of the knee and general instability may be noted. The trunk may lurch forward at initial contact and the ankle plantarflexors strongly contract in order to bring the COG in front of the knee and force it into extension. These patients may compensate by using external rotation of the leg at initial contact and early stance to bring the medial collateral ligament anteriorly to prevent knee buckling.

Treatment: A knee brace may be used to provide knee stability at heel strike for truly orthopedic deficits. Physical therapy to strengthen the weak muscle groups is imperative, as well as trials of solid AFOs to further stabilize the lower segment of the leg. By reinstating normal tibial kinematics during initial contact, a posterior tibial force will assist in stabilizing the knee joint as well. Use of assistive devices promotes trunk flexion to bring the COG in front of the knee, as well as improves safety and reduces risk of fall.

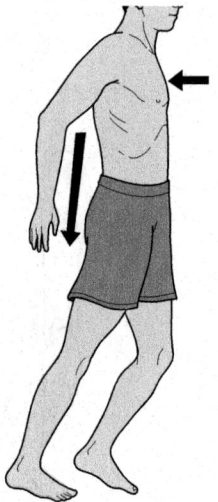

FIGURE 5.5 Gluteus maximus (extensor lurch) gait.

Tibialis anterior gait: Pretibial muscle weakness that is at least antigravity (≥3/5 grade) may cause *foot slap* after heel strike. If the muscles are <3/5 grade, foot slap is generally *not* heard because a steppage gait is more likely. The hip and knee are hyperflexed in a steppage gait to clear the foot during the swing phase, which may otherwise drag (Figure 5.6). The affected limb may alternatively be circumducted during the swing phase.

Treatment: A standard posterior leaf spring orthosis (PLSO) allows plantarflexion and assists in dorsiflexion. An AFO is often used both to prevent foot slap and to allow clearance of the foot during the swing phase. Note, however, that ankle plantarflexion stabilizes the knee. Thus, a standard hinged AFO (with plantarflexion posterior stop) may destabilize the knee.

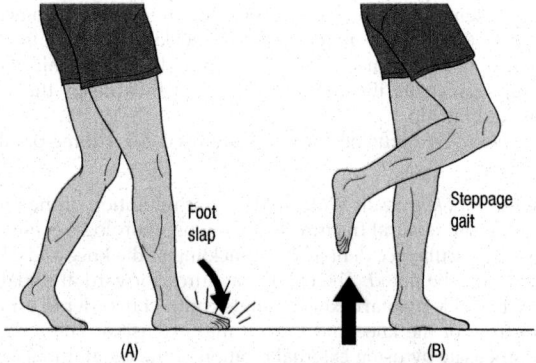

FIGURE 5.6 Tibialis anterior gait: (A) foot slap and (B) steppage gait.

Neuromuscular Impairments

Hemiplegic gait: Persons with extensor synergies may ambulate independently, but with impairments in balance and higher risk for falls. The typical extensor synergy pattern has a predilection for knee extension, ankle plantarflexion, and inversion. Therefore, extensor tone effectively makes the plegic limb longer than the nonplegic side. A circumduction gait compensates via exaggerated hip abduction to allow for toe clearance and ends with toe strike. Despite the circumduction, there is a decreased step length and swing phase on the plegic side. Gait speed will be reduced in order to maintain an acceptable rate of energy expenditure. Abnormal kinematics at the ankle with toe strike may lead to posterior forces at the knee, causing genu recurvatum.[4]

Treatment: A solid AFO or a hinged AFO with a posterior stop to decrease effective limb length may be helpful. Strengthening of the ankle muscles is imperative in therapy as the client is able.

Parkinsonian gait: The classic triad of Parkinson disease is tremor, bradykinesia, and instability, with at least the last two affecting gait. While standing, the knees, trunk, and neck are typically flexed and the body appears stiff. When there is ambulation, there is a characteristic shuffling gait with short quickening steps as if the patient is racing after the COG (festination). Turns are often made "en bloc" with reduced trunk rotation and decreased arm swing, which further compromises balance and safety and heightens risk of fall.

Treatment: Physical therapy intervention to address motor pattern impairments and postural issues at varying stages of the disease is helpful. Heel lifts and assistive devices may help improve safety. Specialty walkers with added weights or the U-Step walker may provide additional stability, as well as visual cues that can assist in reducing freezing.

Spastic paraplegia or diplegia/crouched gait: This gait pattern is often seen in persons with cerebral palsy, but also in some individuals with spinal cord involvement (spinal cord injury, multiple sclerosis, etc.). While standing, the hip and knees are flexed and internally rotated and the foot is held in equinovarus. With ambulation, the increased adductor tone at the thighs causes the knees to scissor in front of each other with each step. Hip adduction causes short step lengths, making the feet seem like they are sticking to the floor. Balance may be impaired as a result of a narrowing base of support. To compensate for this, there is a tendency to lean forward and toward the supporting side. The upper extremities tend to be semiflexed with elbows held out to the sides.

Treatment: AFOs can be used to address equinovarus. Botulinum toxin injection therapy may be helpful in addressing adductor scissoring and equinovarus. Use of an assistive device (e.g., a walker) may provide additional stability.

GAIT AIDS

Cane Basics

Cane length should be from the bottom of the shoe's heel to the upper border of the greater trochanter with the user standing. The shoulders should be level and the arm holding the cane should be flexed ~20° to 30° at the elbow to provide proper push-off. A cane can unload up to 20% of body weight off the affected lower limb, depending on cane design and the user's level of training. Canes may be single-point with a flat or curved handle, or they may have a quadruped base (either wide- or small-based) contacting the ground. It is essential that any cane has rubber stoppers in good repair on the bases in contact with the ground for safety and stability.

The basis for holding a cane on the opposite side of hip joint pathology is elegantly described in detail by Kottke and Lehmann.[5] The cane provides a rotatory moment (C in Figure 5.7) that counteracts the weight of the body (W) and reduces the force of the gluteus medius (F) necessary to maintain equilibrium at the hip fulcrum (H) when the affected lower limb is in single-support stance phase,[5] when advanced together with the affected limb in a three-point gait pattern. Stairs are usually ascended with the stronger lower limb first, then the cane and the affected limb. The affected lower limb and cane proceed down first during stair descent. (A frequently taught therapy mnemonic phrase for this is "Up with the good, down with the bad.") In practice, however, there are no hard and fast rules and the methods for use vary per individual patient needs.

Crutch Basics

Crutches have two points of contact with the body and are thus more stable than canes. The shoulder depressors (latissimus dorsi and pectoralis major) are the primary muscles used during ambulation with crutches. Other muscles include the triceps brachii, biceps brachii, quadriceps, hip extensors, and hip abductors. A patient *must* have sufficient abdominal and trunk musculature (core strength), as well as good balance, to safely ambulate with crutches, especially if reduced WB is to be safely maintained. These various

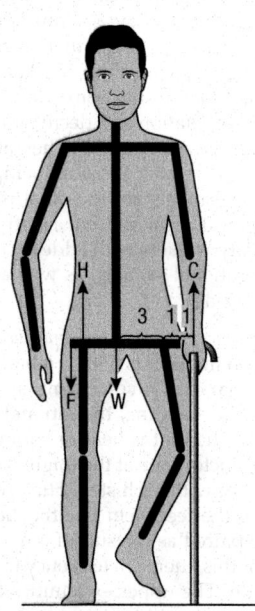

FIGURE 5.7 The basis for holding a cane on the opposite side of the affected hip.

C, cane; F, force of gluteus medius; H, hip fulcrum; W, weight.

5 Mobility: Gait, Assistive Devices, and Wheelchairs | 41

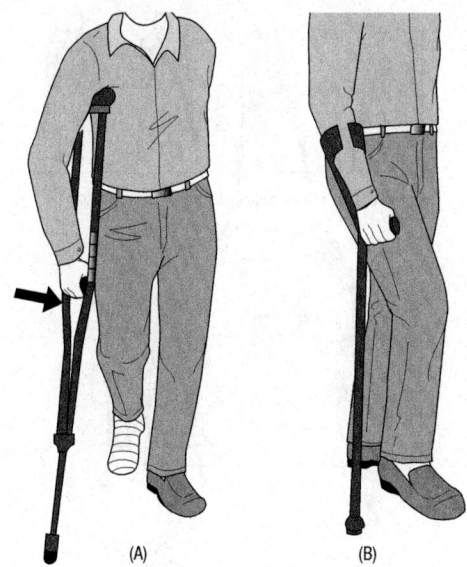

FIGURE 5.8 Crutches: (A) axillary crutch and (B) forearm crutch.

muscles may benefit from strengthening for optimal and better tolerated crutch use.

Axillary crutch (Figure 5.8A): Traditional axillary crutches are most often utilized and are fit to a patient's height and arm ratio. Use of heavy padding on the axillary area of the crutch, although a popular practice, should be discouraged. This encourages the habit of resting the body on the crutches, which increases the risk of *compressive radial neuropathies*. When used properly, bilateral crutches can provide total WB relief to a lower limb.

Forearm crutches (also known as Lofstrand or Canadian; Figure 5.8B): These provide less trunk support than axillary crutches but may be indicated if pressure in the axilla is contraindicated, for example, an open wound or compression neuropathy. A single forearm crutch can relieve up to 50% of body weight off a lower limb; bilateral forearm crutches, when used properly, can provide total WB relief to a lower limb.

Crutch gaits (Figure 5.9A): The crutches and the involved limb serve as point 1 while the uninvolved limb is point 2 in the *two-point* (or "hop-to") *gait*. In a *three-point gait* (i.e., the involved limb is partial WB), the crutches (point 1) and the two limbs (points 2 and 3) are advanced separately, with any two of the three points maintaining contact with

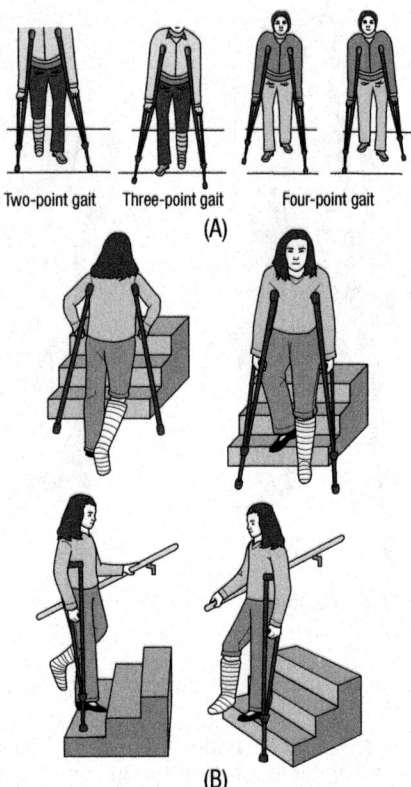

FIGURE 5.9 Crutch gaits: (A) two-, three-, and four-point gaits and (B) negotiating stairs using a banister for support.

the ground at all times. In a *four-point gait*, each individual crutch and lower limb is advanced separately. Efficiency is forsaken for increased stability or balance. When negotiating stairs without a banister, one method might be stronger limb → weaker limb → crutch → crutch for ascent and crutch → weaker limb → stronger limb for descent. A rail or banister, if present, replaces one of the crutches in this method (Figure 5.9B).

Walker Basics

Walkers (Figure 5.10A) provide a wider base of support and a generally safer gait than canes or crutches; there are many styles available, including options with wheels or platforms for upper extremities, as

5 Mobility: Gait, Assistive Devices, and Wheelchairs | 43

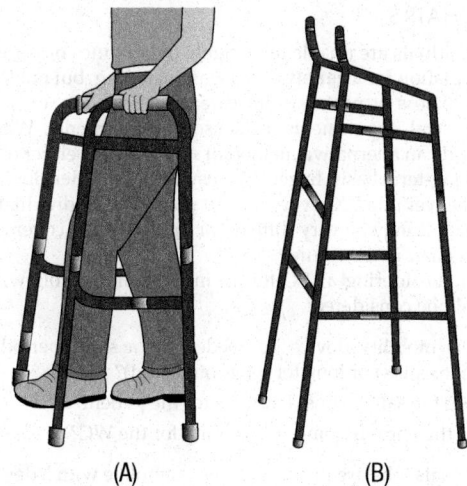

FIGURE 5.10 (A) Basic walker and (B) platform walker.

well as walkers with neurologic cues for individuals with movement disorders (U-Step). They allow up to 100% WB relief from an affected lower limb, depending on how they are used. A walker is fitted by placing it about 10" to 12" in front of the user. The proper height is set with the user standing straight, shoulders relaxed, and the elbows flexed about 20°. The main disadvantages of walkers include a slower gait cadence, risk of promoting bad posture, and overall bulk.

Rolling walkers are indicated for most persons who require significant support during ambulation due to impairments in strength or balance. This walker is pushed ahead, or along with, the individual as they ambulate, resulting in a smoother, more coordinated gait pattern and reducing the need for the individual to balance while lifting and advancing the walker in the forward plane. For individuals with good motor control and balance, a four-wheeled walker (rollator) with brakes and seat may be an option as well.

A *hemiwalker* can be used by an individual who requires more support than a cane, but is unable to use any bimanual support due to arm weakness or absence. It is wide-based, provides more lateral support than a quad cane, and is advanced on the individual's stronger side.

Platform walkers (Figure 5.10B) are used in a variety of situations, including distal upper extremity joint deformities, grip weakness, and flexion contractures of the elbow. They allow WB at the elbow, bypassing the hand, wrist, and part of the forearm, and may be useful to persons who have sustained injuries that preclude the use of a conventional walker.

WHEELCHAIRS

Many individuals are unable to navigate their homes or communities using ambulation for a variety of reasons, including, but not limited to, muscle weakness or paralysis, impaired balance, pain, orthopedic or musculoskeletal impairments, or sensory impairments. Wheelchairs (WC) provide an alternative method of safe mobility, either on a short-term or a long-term basis. In general, insurance providers in the United States will cover one WC every 5 to 10 years; if an individual has one type of chair, it may be very difficult or impossible to cover a secondary or new chair in the future.

When considering a WC for an individual, the following questions should be considered:

1. Will this mobility device be needed for a short period of time (e.g., <9 months) or long term (chronic need)?
2. What are the safety considerations for the patient?
3. What is the current home accessibility for the WC?

For individuals who are unable to safely ambulate with a device in the short term, consider a rental WC with a basic cushion to meet their needs during ongoing treatment or recovery. For individuals who will require a longer term mobility device, a referral to a WC seating clinic is recommended.

MANUAL WHEELCHAIRS

A comprehensive WC and seating evaluation includes assessment of medical history, cognition/communication, special sensory skills (vision and hearing), motor and sensory function, skin integrity, current seating/mobility device(s), WC skills, home environment/barriers, method(s) of available transportation, and level of community function (e.g., employment or school). A mat evaluation, which includes supine and sitting evaluations, helps determine postural deformities (e.g., joint contractures, pelvic obliquities, spinal kyphosis, or scoliosis), trunk/postural control, and pertinent range of motion findings. Important patient measurements include hip/trunk/shoulder width, knee-to-seat depth, knee-to-heel length, shoulder height, and axilla height (Figure 5.11). Following the evaluation, the seating therapist will work with insurance-approved vendors and adaptive therapy professionals (ATPs) to determine the best long-term WC solution for the individual and process the necessary paperwork to obtain this chair. It is important to note that it may take up to 6 months to finalize a custom WC order and delivery. A short-term solution and/or loaner WC may also need to be considered.

Prescription Considerations

Frame and weight: Folding frames are easier to transport, but may be heavier, less durable, and require more energy to propel. Rigid-frame

5 Mobility: Gait, Assistive Devices, and Wheelchairs | 45

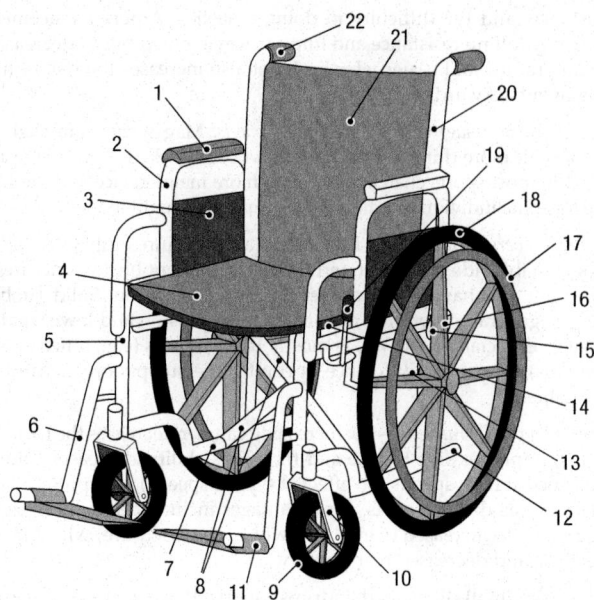

FIGURE 5.11 Components of a typical outdoor sling-seat wheelchair: (1) arm pad, (2) desk-style removable armrest, (3) clothes guard, (4) sling seat, (5) down tube, (6) footrest, (7) bottom rail, (8) cross brace, X bar, or X frame, (9) caster, (10) caster fork, (11) footplate, (12) tipping lever, (13) axle, (14) seat rail, (15) armrest bracket or hole for nonwraparound armrest, (16) armrest bracket or hole for wraparound arm rest, (17) handrim, (18) wheel, (19) wheel lock, (20) back post, (21) sling back, and (22) push handle.

chairs are more durable and energy-efficient during propulsion, but may be more difficult to transport. Rigid-frame WCs are not particularly useful for ambulatory persons because they do not typically come with swing-away footrests, making it difficult for them to perform sit-to-stand transfers. Decreasing the weight of a manual WC reduces rolling resistance, but does not necessarily reduce work of propulsion on level surfaces to a clinically significant degree. A difference, however, is appreciable on uphill grades. Lighter WCs are also easier for a user or caregiver to lift into vehicles for transport. Research has demonstrated statistically similar propulsion efficiencies for titanium, aluminum, and carbon fiber WC frames, although carbon fiber frames reduce vibration transmission in comparison with titanium and aluminum.[6]

Axle: Posterior placement is advantageous for users with poor trunk control, individuals with lower extremity limb loss/amputees, and reclining/posterior tilt WCs, but increases turning radius, rolling resistance, and the difficulty in doing wheelies. Anterior placement decreases rolling resistance and improves maneuverability (decreased turning radius and easier wheelies), but also increases the risk of tipping over backward.

Molded plastic (mag) versus wire-spoked wheels: Mag wheels are slightly heavier but more durable than spoked wheels. Spoked wheels are preferred in most sports chairs, but require more maintenance and are less safe for some individuals whose fingers may get caught in the spokes.

Pneumatic versus rubber tires: Pneumatic (air-filled inner tube) tires offer a comfortable ride on uneven terrain but are susceptible to punctures/going flat and have a higher resistance to propulsion. Solid rubber tires are generally preferred due to easier propulsion and lower maintenance, especially if the WC is mostly used indoors (e.g., office work, hospitals), where the difference in comfort versus pneumatic tires is negligible.

Camber (typically ranges 3°–5°): Increasing camber decreases the turning radius, improves side-to-side and forward stability, decreases rolling resistance at high speeds (no effect at typical speeds), and protects the user's hands during sports. Disadvantages include difficulty in tight spaces due to increased overall WC width, increased tire/wheel-bearing wear, and decreased rear stability.

Handrims: Small-diameter handrims (sports WCs) increase the distance covered with each stroke, but require greater force. Pegged handrims ("quad knobs") improve ease of use for tetraplegics and users with hand deformities, but increase risk of trauma during attempts to stop and may reduce accessibility. Many vendors also offer a variety of coatings or added rubberized grips for handrims to improve user efficiency and propulsion.

Casters: Small (≤5" diameter), narrow casters are appropriate for smooth, level surfaces and are less likely to shimmy. Smaller casters, however, are more likely to get caught in sidewalk cracks and elevator thresholds. Large (≥6" diameter), wide casters are advantageous in rougher, outdoor terrain, but have increased rolling resistance on smooth surfaces and are more likely to shimmy.

Cushions: Foam cushions are lightweight and inexpensive, but are not washable and dissipate heat poorly. These cushions do not offer adequate pressure relief. They are appropriate for ambulatory persons or users who are able to perform pressure relief independently with intact sensation.

Gel/foam combo cushions (e.g., Jay J2 and J3) consist of a firm gel emulsion on a contoured foam base, enclosed in a nonbreathable plastic. They provide good postural stability, are durable and easy to maintain and clean, and dissipate heat well. They are, however, expensive and heavy, and the contouring can interfere with transfers. *Air-filled villous cushions*, such as the ROHO, consist of multiple balloon-like air cells that assure maximum skin contact and provide the best pressure relief. The design is favorable for pressure ulcer prevention or healing. These cushions are lightweight, good at heat dissipation, and easy to clean and transport, but expensive and poor at providing postural stability. User vigilance is required to maintain optimal air pressure in each of the cells and to identify and repair punctures as needed.

Recline/tilt-in-space: Reclining and tilt-in-space WCs may be necessary in persons who lack the ability to otherwise achieve adequate pressure relief and in persons with orthostatic instability. Reclined positioning may also be beneficial for spasticity/spasm management and performing activities such as bladder catheterization or lower body dressing without having to transfer out of the WC. Users of reclining WCs may, however, be susceptible to increased spasms and shear forces during the actual reclining motion. Tilt-in-space WCs offer pressure relief without shear and also reduce the likelihood of triggering spasm during the tilt. Backflow of urine in the tilted position, however, may be an issue in users with indwelling catheters. Manual recline/tilt-in-space positioning requires caregiver assistance. These WCs are often prescribed as backups for persons who primarily use power WCs.

Special Wheelchairs or Wheelchair Modifications

"Hemichair": This may be an option for some users with hemiplegia due to stroke. The seat height is lowered ≈2" and a footrest is removed to allow the user to employ the neurologically intact foot for propulsion and steering.

Lower limb amputee: The rear axle is moved posteriorly ≈2" to compensate for the rearward displacement of the patient's COG. Turning radius is increased. A leg rest can be replaced by a residual limb support on the involved side.

One-arm drive: This is an option for persons with hemiplegia or unilateral arm amputation. Both handrims are on one side. Turning both rims propels the WC; one rim turns the WC. Overall WC width and weight are significantly increased. Good strength and coordination are required.

Power-assisted WC: This is a manual WC that operates by combining the force of the user and electrical power. It is indicated for users who are able to propel a manual WC, but have poor endurance, shoulder issues, or difficulty propelling on uneven surfaces. Power-assisted wheels increase the width of a WC and may reduce the precision of maneuvers in the WC.[7]

Standing WC: These WCs have frames that allow the user to assume a standing position with assistance from the framework of the WC. The standing position provides pressure relief and WB, may improve bowel/bladder function, and increases some accessibility (e.g., reaching cabinets). Standing WCs may also provide a psychological benefit to users, but are larger and heavier.

POWER MOBILITY DEVICES

Scooters

Indications: Scooters are for persons who can ambulate and transfer but have poor endurance or poor tolerance for prolonged manual WC use secondary to arthropathy or other conditions. Scooters are typically used for community mobility because their large turning radii often limit maneuverability within a household environment.

User requirements: Good sitting balance, intact cognitive and visuoperceptual skills, good hand–eye coordination, and adequate function of at least one upper limb to operate the controls are needed. Seating systems for scooters are very basic and offer little to no trunk support or stability, or specialized cushioning for pressure relief.

Caution: Some models tip over fairly easily, especially at high speeds. Scooters are not generally recommended for persons with progressive diseases, such as multiple sclerosis, as they do not have the ability to be significantly modified as function changes. Functional decline may soon preclude safe use of the scooter, but it may be pragmatically difficult to fund and procure a more suitable power mobility device in a timely fashion.

Power Wheelchairs

Indications: Power WCs are for users with physical limitations incompatible with manual WC propulsion (e.g., users with SCI at the C1–C4 level and many SCIs at the C5–C6 level) and for those with strength or endurance deficits (e.g., severe chronic obstructive pulmonary disease [COPD] and cardiac failure) who may not otherwise be candidates for a power scooter. Users may not have the postural stability/truncal control to use a power scooter and may require supportive features (e.g., custom seating and tilt-in-space functionality) not available in scooters. Power WCs have the ability for significant customization and adjustments to meet even the highest individual support needs, including management of ventilators or need for alternative drive controls, such as sip and puff, head controls, or microswitches.

User requirements: Users must have at least one reliably reproducible movement to access the control system, adequate cognitive and visuoperceptual function, proper safety awareness and insight, and motivation to use a power base. Candidates must undergo trials to determine if they can adequately and safely control a power WC.

Caution: An individual's home *must* be power WC-accessible in order for insurance to approve delivery; the individual must also require use of a power mobility device to function in their home in most cases. Power WCs must be charged regularly and require extra care and maintenance to ensure safe ongoing use. Methods of transportation must also be considered as power WCs are unable to fold for transport in standard vehicles. A power WC often weighs >350 pounds without the patient, so additional reinforcements may be needed for ramps and home surfaces as well.

REFERENCES

The full complete reference list for this chapter appears in the digital version of the chapter, available at http://connect.springerpub.com/content/book/978-0-8261-5628-0/part/part01/chapter/ch05

CHAPTER 6

ORTHOSES AND ADAPTIVE EQUIPMENT

Kristi Turner, Kelly Breen, and Molly Henry

INTRODUCTION

When there are limitations in range of motion, strength, or coordination, these will often coincide with difficulty in performing activities of daily living (ADLs) and with mobility. To combat these limitations, upper extremity orthoses, lower extremity orthoses, and adaptive equipment (AE) are commonly used in rehabilitation, especially in occupational therapy (OT) and physical therapy (PT).

UPPER EXTREMITY ORTHOSES

Upper extremity orthoses (commonly called splints) can be either static or dynamic, as well as custom-made or prefabricated. The purpose of orthoses can vary from immobilization of a particular joint(s) of the upper extremity, to providing slow stretch to a particular joint, to assisting in functional use of the upper extremity. In general, orthoses should maintain the integrity of the joints and arches of the hand and wrist, prevent muscle overstretching, prevent deformity, and promote as much function as possible.

Table 6.1 highlights few of the most common types of upper extremity orthoses utilized in patients with decreased functional use of their upper extremities, as well as the indications for use.[1,2]

LOWER EXTREMITY ORTHOSES

Lower extremity orthoses (commonly called braces) can be used to restrict excessive motion, assist with weak or absent motion, or transfer forces during the gait cycle.[3] Braces need to be evaluated based on the patient's impairments, including strength, sensation, presence or absence of spasticity, and gait deviations during the gait cycle. In general, lower extremity braces are used to increase function, manage pain, and reduce the risk of falling during ambulation. Therefore, the prescription and effectiveness of the brace must be assessed during ambulation to assess the loading forces occurring during the gait cycle for each individual. Orthoses are typically named by the joints that they are attempting to control.

Table 6.2 highlights few of the most common types of lower extremity orthoses utilized in patients who demonstrate pain or gait impairments.[4]

TABLE 6.1 Common Upper Extremity Orthoses

Orthosis	Indication	Diagnoses	Description
Hand			
Resting hand	Used when wrist and digit strength is absent or there is no volitional movement against gravity	High-level tetraplegia, tight finger flexors with pain, incomplete SCI, brain injury, and stroke	Used at night to maintain functional hand position
Wrist cock-up	Provide wrist stability, improve function, and reduce pain if present	Neurologic diagnosis (MS, stroke, SCI) and arthritis	Allows functional use of the hand while providing support[1]
Short opponens/ thumb spica	Patients with emerging or strong wrist extension, but no thumb extension	C6, weak C7 SCI –Thumb spica splint (similar look) often used to improve pain and reduce deformity in individuals with arthritis	Assists with functional tenodesis and protection of the thumb joint
Long opponens	Patients with 2–5 or below wrist extension fair and below Used infrequently; recent research suggests may impede bimanual grasp and U-cuff use when compared with standard wrist cock-up orthosis[2]	C5-weak, C6, weak C7 SCI, incomplete SCI, central cord	During the day when up in wheelchair and during functional tasks Utensil slot can be fabricated to accommodate eating or writing tasks
MP block/ lumbrical bar	Patients demonstrating reduced flexion at MP joints or hyperextension due to weakness in the intrinsic muscles of the hand	Incomplete SCI and peripheral nerve injury	Assists with preventing MP hyperextension and maintaining functional digit positioning at these joints

(*continued*)

TABLE 6.1 Common Upper Extremity Orthoses (continued)

Orthosis	Indication	Diagnoses	Description
Elbow			
Static progressive elbow orthosis	Used with decreased ROM at the elbow due to tissue shortening	SCI and posttraumatic elbow injuries	Provides low-load prolonged force to increase elbow flexion or extension
Pronation/supination strap	Used with limited ROM into pronation due to overactive bicep or other injuries	SCI, stroke, CP, brachial plexus, and arthritis	Strap applies a prolonged low-load force to mobilize the forearm into greater pronation or supination by wrapping it around the forearm
Shoulder			
GivMohr	Used when shoulder musculature is weak or flaccid to help reduce the risk of subluxation	Stroke, brain injury, SCI, ALS, brachial plexus injury, and neurologic conditions where shoulder muscle is weak or flaccid	Positioning device designed to support the UE into a functional position during activities such as standing or walking
McDavid shoulder support brace	Used when shoulder musculature is weak or flaccid to help reduce the risk of subluxation	Stroke, brain injury, SCI, ALS, brachial plexus injury, orthopedic conditions, and neurologic conditions where shoulder muscle is weak or flaccid	Positioning device designed to support the UE into a functional position during upright activities

ALS, amyotrophic lateral sclerosis; CP, cerebral palsy; MP, metacarpophalangeal; MS, multiple sclerosis; ROM, range of motion; SCI, spinal cord injury; UE, upper extremity.

TABLE 6.2 Common Lower Extremity Orthoses

Orthosis	Indication	Diagnoses	Description
Foot			
Heel wedge	Patients demonstrating excessive knee hyperextension during gait or have a plantarflexion contracture	TBI, SCI, stroke, CP, neurologic conditions with increased plantarflexion tone, and neurologic conditions with hypermobile knee joint ROM	Can be used to fill the space at the back of the heel for plantarflexion contractures Aids in faster transition of the center of gravity during the stance phase to prevent excessive knee hyperextension
Shoe lift	Patients with a leg length discrepancy of greater than .5 inches	History of a leg length discrepancy and history of lower extremity joint replacements or surgery	Can be inserted within the shoe up to 3/8 in or built up on the outside heel of the shoe for a more symmetrical weight shift
Ankle			
Solid AFO	Patients with significant limb weakness, absent ankle control, spasticity in weight-bearing, knee buckling, and foot drop	Stroke, TBI, incomplete SCI, Guillain–Barré, ALS, MS, and myopathy	Made of solid plastic and custom-molded to a person's leg Provides maximum stability while eliminating ankle ROM
Hinged solid AFO	Patients with significant lower leg weakness but have some tibial control in the sagittal plane to allow for faster and more efficient gait	Stroke, TBI, incomplete SCI, Guillain–Barré, CP, and MS	Solid AFO but hinged at the ankle allowing some sagittal plane movement (requires more strength to control) Provides maximum medial lateral stability from the brace but hinge contraindicated for spasticity
PLS	Patients with purely foot drop but have medial lateral control at the ankle and can control progression of the tibia	Lumbar stenosis with myelopathy, incomplete SCI, and stroke with only foot drop; foot drop affecting only sagittal plane	Thin, narrow plastic brace that allows for passive ankle dorsiflexion during ambulation while assisting with foot clearance during the swing phase

(continued)

TABLE 6.2 Common Lower Extremity Orthoses (continued)

Orthosis	Indication	Diagnoses	Description
Carbon fiber AFO	Patients with foot drop and decreased strength for limb advancement; patients need to have medial lateral stability and some tibial control to wear	Stroke, TBI, incomplete SCI, stenosis with myelopathy, MS, Guillain–Barré, and CP	Full-length, prefabricated off-the-shelf brace that can be trimmed to fit any patient Assists with foot clearance and limb advancement by providing energy return, with a design for a natural, efficient gait pattern Lightweight and durable
KAFO	Individuals with hip control but minimal control of the knee joint due to significant quadriceps and hamstring weakness	L1–L3 complete SCI, multitrauma with significant limb paralysis but intact hip movement	Full-length brace that locks the knee into extension throughout the gait cycle Mechanism present to unlock the knee for sitting Need some hip flexor strength to advance the limb as it is difficult with the limb in full extension High energy cost to ambulate long term with KAFO
Neoprene knee brace	Patients with significant knee joint pain due to osteoarthritis or instability during ambulation	History of knee pain during activity, unstable medial lateral knee due to ligamentous injury, and osteoarthritis	Provides a compression sleeve with medial lateral stability bars to provide increased support at the knee and manage knee pain during gait
Swedish knee cage	Patients with significant knee hyperextension during the stance phase of ambulation causing knee pain or potential damage to the posterior ligament structure	Stroke, incomplete SCI, Guillain–Barré, TBI, MS, peripheral nerve injury to the quadriceps, and previous ligament laxity/knee hyperextension	Limits the amount of extension at the knee joint to maintain ligament health and manage pain during period of significant quadriceps weakness

AFO, anklefoot orthosis; ALS, amyotrophic lateral sclerosis; CP, cerebral palsy; KAFO, kneefootankle orthosis; MS, multiple sclerosis; PLS, posterior leaf spring; ROM, range of motion; SCI, spinal cord injury; TBI, traumatic brain injury.

ADAPTIVE EQUIPMENT

AE is defined as any piece of equipment that is utilized to perform a specific functional task or ADL.[1] These devices are used to increase or improve functional abilities of individuals with disabilities and can be found commercially, can be custom-made, or a combination of both.[1] In addition, the device may be used to increase safety and prevent injury due to the patient's limitations or diagnosis. For example, individuals who have decreased balance may benefit from using a device like a reacher to pick up items that require them to reach out of midline in order to decrease the likelihood of falling. Individuals with arthritis may benefit from larger handled items to assist with joint protection, whereas individuals who have Parkinson disease may benefit from weighted utensils to assist with managing their tremors when eating.

Although specific AE may be commonly used for certain diagnoses or impairments, it is not appropriate for everyone and is only recommended after a thorough assessment of an OT. The evaluation allows the OT to identify the problem, determine what interventions are needed (e.g., environmental modification or other compensatory technique), and determine if an AE would be beneficial to address the functional impairment. Additionally, the OT provides education to the patient on the purpose and use of AE during functional tasks. Table 6.3 shows examples of some of the more common pieces of AE and their purpose. It should be noted that AE can often be utilized for a variety of tasks and contexts, but the table shows only the most common purpose.

TABLE 6.3 Common Adaptive Equipment

Adaptive Equipment	Purpose
Eating	
Universal cuff	To allow independence with holding utensils (e.g., fork, spoon, toothbrush, and pen/pencil) for individuals with weak or absent digit (grip) strength, may be placed over residual limb in individuals with upper limb loss.
Plate guard	To prevent food from sliding off the plate
Built-up silverware	To increase ability to grasp silverware and decrease the fine motor manipulation needed for regular silverware • Can come as a weighted option to reduce spillage from tremors • Option for utensil that can be bent to the left or right angle to decrease coordination needed for eating
Rocker knife	To cut food with gentle rocking motion versus forceful back and forth motion, which is required with a regular knife Useful for those with decreased hand strength and coordination or for joint protection

(continued)

TABLE 6.3 Common Adaptive Equipment *(continued)*

Adaptive Equipment	Purpose
Built-up foam tubing	Used to increase the circumference of a utensil to allow for a more gross grasp pattern for those with decreased strength or coordination of their hands, and can be useful for individuals with upper limb loss when learning to use their prosthesis for functional tasks • Also often used for building up toothbrush, razor, writing utensils, and stylus
Nonslip material	Used to stabilize items to prevent slipping Often used to hold plate in place for eating • Material can be cut in any size/shape allowing it to assist with stabilizing and increasing grip on any item with a slippery surface
Dressing	
Reacher	To be able to safely retrieve items outside the base of support for those with decreased range of motion or safety concerns
Dressing stick	To don/doff pants/undergarments and doff socks and shoes Useful for those with range of motion, strength, coordination, or safety concerns
Sock aid	To don sock or ted hose without having to bend down to the foot or bring the foot up to the lap
Long-handled shoe horn	To assist with donning shoe for those with decreased range of motion, coordination, or safety concerns
Elastic shoelaces	To eliminate having to tie shoelaces for individuals with limited fine motor coordination and strength Shoe able to be slipped on the foot once the elastic shoelaces are tied
Button hook	Fasten buttons by eliminating fine motor coordination involved Device hooks button and is pulled through the hole
Bathing and hygiene	
Long-handled sponge	To wash areas such as the feet and back for those with less reach outside the base of support due to safety concerns or decreased hand coordination
Wash mitt	To be able to wash the body without having to hold onto a washcloth or sponge Useful for those with decreased hand strength or coordination deficits, and may be used to go over residual limb for individuals with upper limb loss

(continued)

TABLE 6.3 Common Adaptive Equipment *(continued)*

Adaptive Equipment	Purpose
Toilet aid	To assist with wiping during perineal hygiene for those with decreased range of motion of the upper extremity and with safety concerns –Different models used for decreased hand strength and coordination and used for SCI and upper limb amputation
Long-handled comb/brush	To accommodate for decreased range of motion or strength of the upper extremity to reach the head
Flexible long-handled mirror	To allow independence for skin check on the back, peri area, or any area difficult to see Often used with individuals with SCI for self-cathing and skin checks and for individuals with lower extremity amputations to be able to fully inspect their residual limb
Miscellaneous	
Writing utensil holder	A writing device for individuals with weak finger or hand dexterity
Mouth stick	To allow individuals with limited strength and dexterity in their upper extremities to press buttons and turn pages using the stick in their mouth

SCI, spinal cord injury.

REFERENCES

The full complete reference list for this chapter appears in the digital version of the chapter, available at http://connect.springerpub.com/content/book/978-0-8261-5628-0/part/part01/chapter/ch06

CHAPTER 7

THERAPY AND EXERCISE PRESCRIPTION

Shane N. Stone, Kian Nassiri, and Patrick J. Barrett

THE THERAPY PRESCRIPTION

A useful therapy prescription should contain the patient's diagnosis, the type of therapy, the frequency and duration of therapy, the goals of therapy (including modalities if needed), and the safety precautions.[1]

1. Therapy Prescription Example 1
   - *Diagnosis:* left middle cerebral stroke on December 1, 2021, right hemiparesis, walking difficulty, cognitive impairment, and aphasia
   - *Physical therapy:* twice a week for 6 weeks
   - *Goals:* ambulation at the modified independent level with the least restrictive assistive device for >500 feet and teach fall prevention strategies and a home exercise program
   - *Safety precautions:* high risk of falling, poor safety awareness, and impulsive
2. Therapy Prescription Example 2
   - *Diagnosis:* mechanical low back pain and intervertebral disc injury
   - *Physical therapy:* twice a week for 6 weeks
   - *Goals:* McKenzie mechanical diagnosis and treatment, reduce pain, and teach proper body mechanics and a home exercise program
   - *Safety precautions:* activity as tolerated

Modalities

In some instances, it may be necessary to prescribe therapeutic modalities. If needed, the key components of a modality prescription include the diagnosis, impairments/disabilities, precautions, modality and settings (e.g., intensity and temperature range), area to be treated, frequency of treatment, duration of treatment, goals/objectives of treatment, and reevaluation date. For an overview of modalities, please see Table 7.1.

Heat (Thermotherapy): Heat can be applied to areas to reduce pain, relax muscles, and promote heating. Typically 40°C to 45°C is the therapeutic range. Heat can either be superficial, which means it penetrates up to 1 cm, or deep, which affects the tissue in the 3 to 5 cm range. Treatment duration should be from 5 to 30 minutes. Furthermore, there are three different ways to administer heat: conduction (direct contact),

TABLE 7.1 Summary of Modalities

Modality	Indication(s) for Use	Contraindication(s)
Heat	Pain relief, muscle relaxation, and promote healing	Acute hemorrhage, inflammation, malignancy, insensate skin, inability to respond to pain, atrophic skin, infection, and ischemia *Ultrasound:* over fluid-filled cavities, near pacemaker, laminectomy site, malignancy, and joint prosthesis with plastics *SWD and MWD:* children, metallic implants, contact lenses, and uteri that are either menstruating or pregnant
Cryotherapy	Pain relief	Ischemia, insensate skin, severe HTN, or cold sensitivity syndromes (e.g., Raynaud syndrome)
Traction	Nerve impingement	*General:* ligamentous instability, osteomyelitis, discitis, bone malignancy, spinal cord tumor, severe osteoporosis, and untreated HTN *Cervical:* never apply cervical in extension, vertebrobasilar artery insufficiency, rheumatoid arthritis, midline herniated disc, and acute torticollis *Lumbar:* restrictive lung disease, pregnancy, active peptic ulcers, aortic aneurysms, gross hemorrhoids, and cauda equina syndrome
TENS	Chronic low back pain (poor effectiveness evidence) and diabetic polyneuropathy (good effective evidence)	Not applied near pacemakers, carotid sinuses, or sympathetic ganglia Not used during pregnancy or on wounds
Massage	Pain relief	*Absolute:* malignancy, DVT, atherosclerotic plaques, and infected tissues *Relative:* incompletely healed scar tissue, anticoagulation, calcified soft tissues, and skin grafts
Phonophoresis	Osteoarthritis, bursitis, capsulitis, tendonitis, strains, contractures, scar tissue, and neuromas	Previous adverse reaction from the drug being applied *Ultrasound:* over fluid-filled cavities, near pacemaker, laminectomy site, malignancy, and joint prosthesis with plastics

(continued)

TABLE 7.1 Summary of Modalities (*continued*)

Modality	Indication(s) for Use	Contraindication(s)
Iontophoresis	Skin cancer, psoriasis, dermatitis, venous ulcers, keloid, and hypertrophic scars	Previous adverse reaction from the drug being applied Electrical contraindications such as pacemakers and embedded wires Orthopedic implants, skin lesions, impaired sensation, and pregnancy
Acupuncture	Pain relief, mental health conditions, and nausea primarily	Active skin infection, malignancy, and severe neutropenia

DVT, deep vein thrombosis; HTN, hypertension; MWD, microwave diathermy; SWD, shortwave diathermy; TENS, transcutaneous electrical stimulation.

convection (flow of heat), or conversion (apply nonthermal energy which causes the area to heat up). Examples of conduction include paraffin baths, hot packs, and electrical heat pads. Convection methods include fluidotherapy, whirlpool, and moist air. Examples of conversion are infrared, ultrasound (US), shortwave diathermy (SWD), and microwave diathermy (MWD). Contraindications to heat therapy include hemorrhage, inflammation, malignancy, insensate skin, inability to respond to pain, atrophic skin, infection, and ischemia. US should not be applied over fluid-filled cavities, near pacemakers, laminectomy sites, and joint prosthesis with plastics, or used in patients with malignancy. Furthermore, SWD and MWD should not be used in children, over any kind of metallic implants, contact lenses, or uteri that are either menstruating or pregnant.[1]

Cryotherapy: Ice packs and cold sprays can be applied to help reduce pain. Cold inhibits histamines and other vasodilators, causing vasoconstriction (occurs at about 10°C–15°C of skin temperature) and a decrease in nerve conduction velocity by prolonging Na^+ channel opening and thus a numbing/decreased pain sensation. Apply ice for 15 to 30 minutes maximum. After 30 minutes, the body will attempt to rewarm the area and this will negate the benefits of treatment. Cold is contraindicated in the setting of ischemia, insensate skin, severe hypertension (HTN), or cold sensitivity syndromes (e.g., Raynaud syndrome).[2]

Traction: Traction may help nerve impingement by increasing the intervertebral space up to 1 to 2 mm and widen the neural foramina temporarily. It can be performed both at the cervical spine and lumbar spine. Cervical traction is performed by applying 25 to 30 pounds of force. Greater amounts of force are needed (i.e., >50% of body weight) when applying lumbar traction due to the need to overcome the effects of friction when lying supine with the hips and knees flexed. Less force is needed when a split lumbar traction table is used because it virtually eliminates the frictional component. General contraindications to traction include ligamentous instability, osteomyelitis, discitis, bone malignancy, spinal cord tumor, severe osteoporosis, and untreated HTN.

Cervical traction should not be applied in extension due to risk of developing vertebrobasilar artery insufficiency. It should also be avoided if vertebrobasilar artery insufficiency is already present or if rheumatoid arthritis, midline herniated disc, and acute torticollis are present. Contraindications to lumbar traction include restrictive lung disease, pregnancy, active peptic ulcers, aortic aneurysms, gross hemorrhoids, and cauda equina syndrome.[3,4]

Transcutaneous electrical nerve stimulation (TENS): TENS is thought to provide pain relief based on the "gate theory," which proposes that stimulation of large myelinated fibers (A-beta and A-gamma) causes interneurons in the substantia gelatinosa to be excited, which then inhibits the lamina V, where the small unmyelinated A-beta and C pain fibers synapse with spinal neurons. There are two ways to administer TENS. The first is "Conventional" high-frequency (>50 Hz) TENS, which uses barely perceptible, low-amplitude, and short-duration signals that cause a tingling sensation. These TENS devices are often given to patients for home use. The second way to administer TENS is the "Acupuncture-like" type, which uses larger amplitude, low-frequency (1–10 Hz) signals, which may be uncomfortable, and are often applied in the office/clinic setting. Beta-endorphin release may play a role in the analgesic effects of "Acupuncture-like" TENS.

TENS is often used to treat chronic low back pain despite weak evidence that it is effective for this condition. It is also used to treat diabetic peripheral polyneuropathy, which conversely has good evidence that it works. TENS units should not be applied near pacemakers, carotid sinuses, or sympathetic ganglia, or used during pregnancy or directly on wounds.[5]

Massage: There are two major divisions of massage. There are Western techniques, which include effleurage (stroking), petrissage (kneading), tapotement (percussion), and Swedish massage (tapotement + petrissage + deep tissue massage), deep friction, and myofascial release, and there are also Eastern techniques, which include acupressure (Chinese), shiatsu (Japan), and Thai massage.

Absolute contraindications to massage include malignancy, deep vein thrombosis (DVT), atherosclerotic plaques, and infected tissues. Relative contraindications include incompletely healed scar tissue, anticoagulation, calcified soft tissues, and skin grafts.[6]

Phonophoresis: US is used to apply and cross transdermally topical medications such as steroids and other analgesic medications. It is used commonly to treat osteoarthritis, bursitis, capsulitis, tendonitis, strains, contractures, scar tissue, and neuromas.[1,7]

Iontophoresis: This is a method of administering medications by which electric currents are applied, causing the medication to go into the targeted area. The theoretical benefit of iontophoresis is that system side effects can be avoided since the medication is being applied locally. It is used to treat skin cancer, psoriasis, dermatitis, venous ulcers, keloid, and hypertrophic scars. Contraindications include previous adverse reaction to the drug being applied, electrical contraindications such as pacemakers and embedded wires, as well as orthopedic implants, skin lesions, impaired sensation, and pregnancy.[8]

Acupuncture

Technically acupuncture is not a modality, but rather part of the traditional Chinese medicine system that has been practiced for thousands of years. Acupuncture is included in the modality section since many conventional trained providers consider it to be one.[9] Acupuncture is the process of inserting and manipulating filiform needles into specified areas (acupuncture points) of the body for therapeutic purposes. Traditionally, it is understood that the points for treatment are selected based on a meridian system in which the internal organs, the vessels, and the spine are related to acupuncture points via meridians. It is thought that acupuncture cures disease by restoring the flow of vital energy (Qi) through this system.[1] Although the practice originated in China centuries ago, its poorly understood mechanism delayed its incorporation into Western medicine until the 21st century.[1] Investigations are ongoing, but the most prevalent theories are that pain is alleviated via the gate theory[10] (the stimulation of nonpain [A-beta] nerve fibers inhibits the pain [A-delta and C] fibers from relaying pain signals), as well as the increase in endogenous endorphins.[11]

The efficacy of this procedure for treatment of pain is an active area of research, but the strength of the studies is difficult to evaluate because of the inherent challenges of studying acupuncture. For example, researchers have struggled to blind participants, find a suitable sham option, or include large sample sizes of unique pathologies. Despite these limitations, there is enough evidence to support its use in some conditions. There is growing evidence that acupuncture can improve pain in patients with low back or neck pain, although the duration of benefit and the impact on function are still unclear.[12,13] There is also support for its use in migraine prevention,[12] as well as in myofascial pain.[13] Reviews have even found it can reduce pain as well as improve sleep in patients with fibromyalgia, although it does not improve fatigue.[12] Evidence has also demonstrated its benefit in shoulder pain, osteoarthritis, and rheumatoid arthritis.[13]

Although beyond the scope of this guide, it is important to briefly discuss the logistical considerations for the procedure. There are several needle sizes and lengths as well as techniques that are chosen based on the intention of the practice.[1] Overall, it is considered a safe procedure, with a worldwide incidence of .55 per 10,000 patients experiencing serious adverse events.[12] However, the risks and benefits should always be discussed with the patients.

As the body of evidence grows, it is important for providers to enhance their familiarity with acupuncture as more patients are seeking alternatives to opioids for pain relief. This is particularly true in the United States where the Congress has allocated funds to investigate alternatives, including acupuncture, to opioids for pain management due to the ongoing opioid epidemic.[14]

The Exercise Prescription

Exercise Recommendations

Per the U.S. Department of Health and Human Services, the general guidance for exercise of healthy adults is as follows:

1. 150 to 300 minutes of moderate-intensity *or* 75 to 150 minutes of vigorous-intensity aerobic physical activity (*or* an equivalent combination of the two) distributed throughout a week
2. Two or more days of muscle strengthening activities per week, involving all major muscle groups[15]

Additional recommendations to exercise include adjustments based on age and medical comorbidities.

Pre-Exercise Evaluation

The physician's evaluation should be comprehensive and include key elements of history, such as current and previous exercise patterns, motivations/barriers to exercise, discussion of risks/benefits of exercise, preferred types of activity, social support, and time and scheduling considerations. Special attention should be given to physical limitations, current and past medical conditions, current medications, history of exercise-induced symptoms (shortness of breath, asthma, hives, and chest pain), and a thorough review of cardiovascular, metabolic, and renal disease risk factors, including diabetes mellitus (DM), HTN, smoking, hyperlipidemia, sedentary lifestyle, obesity, and family history of heart disease before the age of 50 years.[1] Physical examination should include cardiovascular, pulmonary, and musculoskeletal assessments. In the setting of observable symptoms of cardiovascular, metabolic, or renal disease, individuals in need of medical clearance, exercise stress testing, and/or additional formal testing should be identified as per the American Heart Association (AHA) and American College of Sports Medicine (ACSM) guidelines. The most recent ACSM recommendations (2015) seek to reduce unnecessary barriers to adopting and maintaining a structured exercise program and/or regular physical activity.[16]

Components of an Exercise Prescription

The following five components apply to exercise prescriptions for persons of all ages and fitness levels. Careful consideration should be given to the health status, medications, risk factors, behavioral characteristics, personal goals, and exercise preferences.

Type is the particular form of exercise. Selection should be based on the desired outcomes and exercises or activities that are most likely to be enjoyed and sustained on a long-term basis. Ideally, every exercise program contains stretching, strengthening, and aerobic exercises.

Intensity is the relative physiologic difficulty of the exercise and should be tailored to the individual's goals. Intensity is calculated based on the heart rate (HR) and the rate of perceived exertion. The most commonly used scale is the Borg Scale of Perceived Exertion, which is scored from 6 (no exertion at all) to 20 (maximal exertion). A score of 9 is "very light" and consistent with a healthy person walking slowly. A score of 13 is "somewhat hard" and consistent with moderate-intensity exercise; it feels okay to continue. A score of 17 is "very hard" and consistent with a healthy person who can go on, but really has to push themselves. The Borg goal scores are based on the goals of the exercise program. A goal of 12 to 14, for instance, would be consistent with a moderate-intensity exercise program.

Duration (time) is the length of an exercise session. It may be continuous or intermittently accumulated during the day.

Frequency refers to the number of exercise sessions per day and per week.

Progression (overload) is the increase in activity during exercise training, which over time stimulates adaptation. This may be a change in frequency, intensity, and/or duration.[1]

Effectiveness of an Exercise Prescription

Regular exercise has been demonstrated to have a variety of health benefits, including promoting normal growth and development, improving overall quality of life, protecting against many chronic diseases, and reducing overall mortality, compared with sedentary individuals.[15] In determining an appropriate exercise program for an individual, it is important to consolidate multiple sources of information regarding the individual's health and preferences and collaborate on an effective plan to implement and maintain in order to reach their goals.

STRENGTH TRAINING

Isometric strengthening: Tension is generated without visible joint motion or appreciable change in muscle length (e.g., pushing against a wall). This exercise is most efficient when the exertion occurs at the resting length of the muscle and most useful when joint motion is contraindicated (e.g., status post tendon repair) or in the setting of pain or inflammation (e.g., rheumatoid arthritis). Injury risk is minimized. Isometric exercise should be avoided in older adults and in patients with HTN due to its tendency to elevate blood pressure (BP).

Isotonic strengthening: This is characterized by constant external resistance but variable speed of movement. Examples include free weights, weight machines (e.g., Nautilus), calisthenics (e.g., pull-ups, push-ups, and sit-ups), and TheraBand. The equipment is readily available, but there is potential for injury with this type of exercise.

Isokinetic strengthening: This is characterized by a relatively constant angular joint speed but variable external resistance. This exercise does not exist in nature; special equipment is required, for example, Cybex and Biodex. If the user pushes harder, the speed of the manipulated piece of equipment will *not* increase, but the resistance supplied by the machine will. This maximizes resistance throughout the length–tension curve of the exercised muscles and is beneficial in the early phases of rehabilitation. Injury risk is relatively low.

Concentric contractions versus eccentric contractions: Concentric contractions are characterized by active muscle shortening. The least amount of force is generated during fast concentric contractions. Eccentric contractions are characterized by active muscle lengthening, which generates high forces at low energy cost. The greatest amount of force is generated during fast eccentric, followed by isometric, slow concentric, and finally fast concentric contractions.

Plyometric exercise: A plyometric movement is a brief, explosive maneuver consists of an eccentric muscle contraction followed immediately by a concentric contraction (e.g., planting and jumping during sports). Plyometric training is aimed at increasing power.

Progressive resistive exercise: The *DeLorme axiom* posits that high-resistance, low-repetition (rep) exercise builds strength, while low-resistance, high-rep exercise improves endurance.[17] In the DeLorme method, a 10 repetition maximum (RM) is first determined. Ten reps of the exercise are performed in sets of 50%, 75%, and 100% of the 10 RM. The sessions are performed ~3 to 5 times per week and the 10 RM is redetermined approximately each week. In the *Oxford technique,* the order of the sets is reversed, so that 10 reps at 100% of the 10 RM are performed first, followed by sets of 75% and 50%. deLateur later demonstrated that for the most part, strength and endurance gains are equivalent for the two types of exercise as long as the muscles are exercised to fatigue.[18] High-resistance, low-rep exercise, however, achieves its results more efficiently (i.e., fewer reps, less time). Moritani and de Vries[19] demonstrated that gains in the first few weeks of strength training were mostly due to neural factors (e.g., improved coordination of muscle firing) and not muscle hypertrophy.

The *Daily Adjusted Progressive Resistance Exercise* (DAPRE) method involves four sets of exercise per muscle group, where the first set is 10 reps at 50% of 6 RM, the second set is six reps at 75% of 6 RM, and the third set is as many reps as possible at 6 RM. The weight for the fourth set is based on the reps completed during the third set. If five to seven reps of the 6 RM are completed, the weight remains the same. With fewer reps, the weight is decreased. With higher reps, the weight is increased. Adjustments to the working weight (6 RM) for the next training session are also made as needed.

AEROBIC AND ANAEROBIC EXERCISE

According to the ACSM, aerobic exercise refers to rhythmic activities that utilize large muscle groups and can be maintained continuously (relying on aerobic metabolism in order to extract energy in the form of adenosine triphosphate [ATP]).[20] Aerobic activities are diverse and can span a multitude of activities, including running, jogging, swimming, elliptical, dancing, and various sports (basketball, soccer, etc.). Aerobic capacity is the product of the capacity of the cardiovascular system to supply oxygen and the capacity of the skeletal muscle to utilize, and can be measured through obtaining peak oxygen consumption (VO_2).[20] The benefits of regular aerobic exercise have been well documented and there is significant correlation between reduction and prevention of cardiovascular disease and regular aerobic exercise.

Physiologically, aerobic exercise increases maximum oxygen consumption (VO_2max) and decreases resting BP. Other long-term cardiovascular adaptations/benefits of aerobic exercise include *increased* stroke volume (SV) with exercise, cardiac output (CO) during maximum exertion, work capacity, and high-density lipoprotein (HDL); and *decreased* resting HR, HR response to submaximal workloads, myocardial oxygen consumption at rest and submaximal activities, low-density lipoprotein (LDL), and triglyceride levels. The maximum HR does not change. Historically, aerobic exercise was felt to have a negligible effect on skeletal muscle mass, but more recently the mitigating effects of aerobic exercise on muscle mass loss and even hypertrophic/anabolic effects have been reported.[21] Diabetic patients benefit from reduced obesity and insulin requirements. Improvements in mood, sleep, immune function, and bone density may also be observed.

As a distinction to aerobic exercise, anaerobic exercise results when energy is obtained without the use of oxygen as the primary energy source and instead depends on glycolysis and fermentation, resulting in a buildup of lactic acid.[20] The *anaerobic threshold* signifies the onset of metabolic acidosis during exercise, traditionally determined by serial measurements of blood lactate. It can be noninvasively determined by assessment of expired gases during exercise testing, specifically pulmonary ventilation (VE) and carbon dioxide production (VCO_2). The anaerobic threshold signifies the peak work rate or oxygen consumption at which energy demands exceed circulatory ability to sustain aerobic metabolism.[1] Typically it is an intense physical activity of short duration and includes sprinting, high-intensity interval training, powerlifting, circuit training, and so forth, and has been demonstrated to have protective cardiovascular effects and favorable effects on the patient's lipid profiles.[22] Additional benefits have been demonstrated in building and maintaining both bone and muscle mass.[23]

REFERENCES

The full complete reference list for this chapter appears in the digital version of the chapter, available at http://connect.springerpub.com/content/book/978-0-8261-5628-0/part/part01/chapter/ch07

PART II

MEDICAL REHABILITATION

CHAPTER 8

AMPUTATIONS

Joan T. Le and Phoebe Scott-Wyard

EPIDEMIOLOGY, ETIOLOGY, AND LEVELS OF AMPUTATIONS

Physiatrists play an important role in the medical care of patients with amputations or congenital limb differences. In the United States, it is estimated that over 3.6 million people will be living with limb loss by year 2050.

Acquired Amputation

Each year, approximately 185,000 people undergo an amputation in the United States. The most common causes in adults include nonhealing wounds from peripheral vascular disease, diabetes mellitus, neuropathy, and trauma. Adult males outnumber females at 69% to 31%, and lower limb involvement exceeds upper limb amputation at 65% to 35%, respectively. Common causes of acquired amputations in pediatric patients arise from trauma or disease (e.g., neoplasm or infection).[1] The most common amputation in young children is finger amputation from getting their fingers caught doors. Power lawnmower accidents can cause lower limb amputations in young children. Other traumatic causes of amputations include motor vehicle accidents, firearms, fireworks, electrical or burn injuries, or farm equipment. Tumor types that may result in amputation include osteogenic sarcoma, Ewing sarcoma, and rhabdomyosarcoma.

Complications from infections may lead to amputations or complex limb deformities. Meningococcal septicemia and *Staphylococcus* or *Streptococcus* infections can result in infectious emboli or purpura fulminans. Amputation due to infarction, gangrene, or autoamputation may occur, skin grafts may be required for skin involvement, and growth plate involvement in pediatric patients may result in angular deformities of the limb during growth.[2]

The level of amputation depends on the extent of the tissue involved and vascular perfusion of the healthy intact soft tissue needed for coverage. The goal is to preserve limb length while ensuring residual limb healing with tissue viability and complete removal of all affected tissues. The levels of amputation in the upper limb, from proximal to distal, include forequarter amputation, shoulder disarticulation, *transhumeral* (TH) amputation (through the humerus, also known as above-elbow [AE] amputation), elbow disarticulation, *transradial* (TR) amputation (through the radius, also known as below-elbow [BE]), wrist disarticulation, and partial hand amputations. The levels of amputations in the lower body and limb, from proximal to distal, include hemicorporectomy, hemipelvectomy, hip disarticulation

(HD), *transfemoral* (TF) amputation (through the femur, also known as above-knee [AK] amputation), knee disarticulation, *transtibial* (TT) amputation (through the tibia; also known as below-knee [BK]), Syme, Boyd, and partial foot amputations (including Chopart, Lisfranc, and transmetatarsal).

Congenital Limb Deficiencies

It is estimated that 1 out of 1,900 babies are born with a congenital limb difference or deficiency, in a ratio of 2:1 upper to lower extremity.[3] Precise numbers are not known as limb length discrepancies or joint deformities (e.g., arthrogryposis) may not be included in these statistics. Limb differences are named as follows: *transverse* (normal limb development to a particular level, with no skeletal elements distally) or *longitudinal* (absence or reduction of an element within the long axis, with some distal skeletal elements present). Most causes of limb differences are unknown. Some medications linked to abnormal limb development include thalidomide, retinoic acid, and misoprostol. Other causes may include vascular malformations, vascular disruption sequence, genetic factors (point mutations), or disruptions in the uterine environment such as amniotic band syndrome (which can result in multilimb amputation, constriction rings, or acrosyndactyly). Maternal cigarette smoking, thrombophilia, or poorly controlled gestational diabetes can increase the risk of lower limb differences as well. There are limb deficiencies, usually in the upper limb, that are associated with syndromic patterns or congenital anomalies; therefore, further workup should be considered.

- *Associated with hematologic abnormalities:* thrombocytopenia-absent radius (TAR syndrome) and Fanconi anemia
- *Associated with cardiac defects:* Holt–Oram, Poland, and Roberts syndromes, to name a few
- *Associated with vertebral, gastrointestinal, and renal dysfunction:* VACTERL association (vertebral defects, anal atresia, cardiac defects, tracheoesophageal fistula, renal abnormalities, and upper limb difference)
- *Associated with craniofacial abnormalities:* Moebius syndrome (upper limb) or femoral-hypoplasia-unusual facies (lower limb)[4]

UPPER EXTREMITY AMPUTATIONS

Acquired upper extremity amputations are most commonly due to trauma, malignant tumors, and dysvascular disease. Congenital upper limb deficiencies make up two-thirds of all congenital limb differences. Those with unilateral upper limb amputations learn to become independent with most activities of daily living (ADLs). The most common transverse radial deficiency occurs in the upper third of the forearm, and the proximal radius at the elbow can be unstable, can hyperextend, and may subluxate anteriorly (see Figure 8.1).[2]

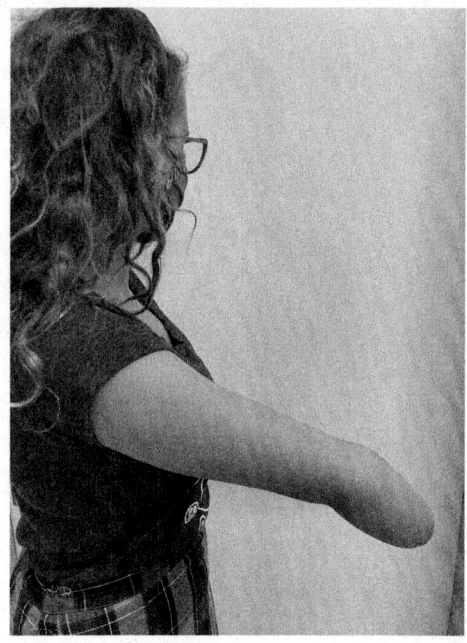

FIGURE 8.1 Hyperextension at the elbow seen in a patient with congenital right transradial deficiency.

For those with bilateral upper limb amputations, an occupational therapist can help them learn how to perform ADLs with their feet.

For children with congenital limb differences, age and developmental milestones should be considered when fitting a prosthesis. For example, when the baby pushes up in preparation for crawling around 6 to 8 months, a passive "banana arm" prosthesis can be fabricated to help the child get into a quadruped position.

For those with partial hand amputations, opposition posts/prostheses may be used to allow for grasp with intact fingers/palm.[5]

For those with a TR amputation, the longer the residual limb, the easier it is to flex the elbow and retain the ability to pronate/supinate the forearm, and this allows for optimal use of body-powered prostheses, which are more lightweight and durable compared with myoelectric prostheses. The prosthesis has a body harness that is attached to a cable, which is attached to the terminal device (TD) and allows body motions to operate the prosthetic components (Figure 8.2). The harness is either in a figure-of-8 or figure-of-9 configuration. The socket is connected to a wrist unit and a TD is attached at the end. The TD can be a hook, hand, or task-specific TD. The split-hook is the most common and practical TD. The two types of split-hooks are "voluntary

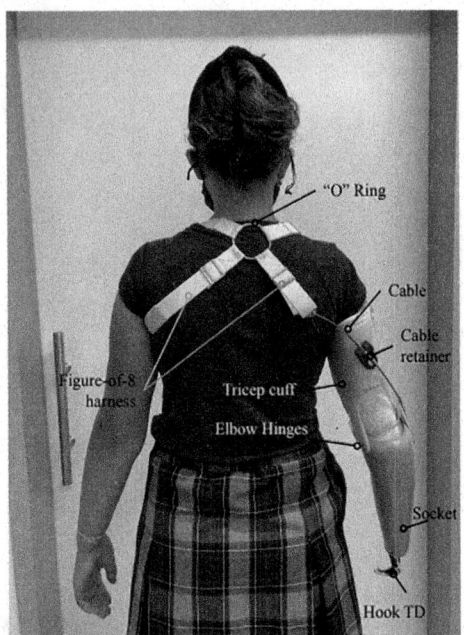

FIGURE 8.2 A below-elbow prosthesis worn by a patient with congenital right transradial deficiency.
TD, terminal device.

opening" (VO) and "voluntary closing" (VC) hooks. At rest, the VO hook is closed and the prehensile force is predetermined by the number of rubber bands placed on the hook. To open the VO hook, the wearer would provide tension on the cable by protracting the shoulders, performing glenohumeral flexion or biscapular abduction. For VC hooks, the hook is open at rest and the same movements close the TD. Some TDs have a locking mechanism for use with VC to avoid excessive force needed to keep the TD closed.

Externally powered myoelectric prostheses may be considered in those with upper limb amputations. The user's muscle contraction would be picked up by an electromyographic electrode, which sends the signal to the controller, resulting in the change in position or speed of the prosthesis. Increased weight, higher cost, and battery power are some factors to consider when prescribing this prosthesis. Myoelectric hands allow for palmar grasp with good grip force, but are not as durable as the hook TD.

For those with a TH amputation, the longer the residual limb, the better the lever arm. Their body-powered prosthesis would need a prosthetic elbow unit which can be locked in a flexed functional position.

In the elbow locked position, the motions that apply tension on the cable would operate the TD. The motions to unlock this elbow position are glenohumeral depression, residual arm extension, and abduction. While the elbow unit is unlocked, motions that apply tension on the cable would operate the elbow unit flexion/extension.

For those with TH amputations wanting to use an externally powered prosthesis, they may lack enough sites for which the electrodes can receive input when using the myoelectric prosthesis. Therefore, *targeted muscle reinnervation* (TMR) may be considered.[6] TMR is a surgical technique utilized for more intuitive control of a prosthesis, where multiple peripheral nerves are transferred to a target muscle to allow for electromyography signals to control a multifunctional myoelectric prosthesis. It is most suitable for upper extremity amputees with significantly impaired function, who have experience with a myoelectric prosthesis.[7] When compared with neurectomy, TMR has also been proven to both treat chronic limb and phantom pain as well as prevent its occurrence in amputees when done at the time of major limb amputation.[8,9]

If those with upper limb amputations choose to use a prosthesis, task-specific TDs can be switched in and used for unique activities, such as playing basketball, kayaking, weightlifting, biking, and so forth.

LOWER EXTREMITY AMPUTATIONS

Acquired lower limb amputations in adults are most commonly from peripheral vascular disease, diabetes, neuropathy, and trauma. In children, the most common cause of lower limb amputation is trauma or disease. One out of 1,900 babies born in the United States has a congenital limb deficiency and one-third of them have lower limb involvement.

Postamputation Rehabilitation

Residual limb care: Edema control is extremely important as this can have a negative impact on healing. Elevation and the use of rigid removable dressing with mild compression, followed by elastic prosthetic shrinker socks once the incisional wound is dry, worn 23 hours a day, can be beneficial until prosthetic fitting has taken place.

Contracture management/prevention: Contractures are easy to prevent, but hard to treat. For TT amputees, use of a knee extension board when in a wheelchair and avoidance of pillows under the knee when in bed are helpful in contracture prevention. In addition, use of rigid dressings with the knee in extension and prone positioning to prevent hip flexion contractures can be beneficial.[10]

Physical therapy: Preprosthetic or preoperative training to improve cardiopulmonary status, range of motion, contralateral leg strength, balance, and hip extensor and hip abductor strengthening can influence ambulation with a prosthesis. Physical therapy can also help with bed mobility, transfers, desensitization/scar management, contracture prevention, assistive devices, and gait training postoperatively.[11]

Prosthetic fitting: Once the incision site is healed and the edema is controlled, the prosthetist takes a cast of the residual limb to create a positive mold around which to shape the prosthetic socket. A clear "check" socket is fabricated from this mold and fitted onto the patient. A finalized socket is then fabricated and aligned with appropriate components and trialed on the patient, typically in parallel bars. Immediate postoperative prosthesis (IPOP) has previously been described to improve psychological and physical adaptation to a prosthesis; however, evidence to support its use is lacking and it is not ideal to evaluate adequate healing. Instead, it is recommended the team facilitate peer-based support and mentorship.

K-Level

K-Level is a rating system used to indicate a person's functional potential as an ambulator while using a lower limb prosthesis.

K0 = nonambulatory

K1 = ambulation on level surfaces with fixed speed

K2 = ambulation over low environmental barriers (stairs or uneven surfaces) with fixed speed

K3 = ambulation over environmental barriers with variable speed

K4 = ambulation with high impact, stress, or energy

PROSTHETIC SOCKET DESIGNS, SUSPENSION, AND COMPONENTS

The prosthetic socket is the most intimate interface with the patient's residual limb and acts as an extension of their body. The importance of good socket fit cannot be stressed enough as this prevents pain and skin breakdown, and encourages prosthetic proprioception and function. There are many different options for socket designs, including rigid outer socket with flexible inner socket, rigid frame with flexible inner socket, dynamic panel/windows with cable/ratchet system controlled by the patient, and flexible socket with embedded rigid frame. Prosthetic socks can be used to improve fit due to volume/weight changes.[12,13]

TT socket designs: These are typically fit with patellar tendon-bearing (PTB) socket, which uses the patellar tendon and soft tissues for weight-bearing (Figure 8.3), or total surface-bearing socket, which distributes pressure equally over the entire residual limb and used

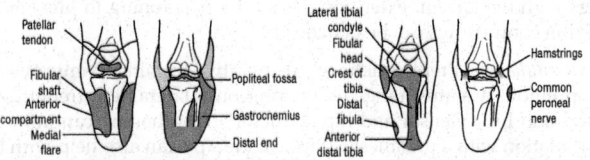

FIGURE 8.3 Pressure-tolerant/sensitive areas in the transtibial (TT) total contact socket.

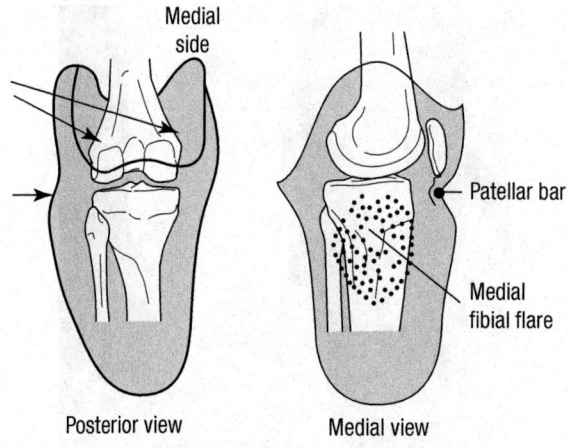

FIGURE 8.4 Total contact socket.

with a gel liner to apply constant pressure (Figure 8.4). Longer residual limbs with a widened distal end may benefit from a windowed design.

TT suspension: This can be achieved with anatomic lock (socket trimlines over the condyles), silicone locking liner (uses gel liner with mechanical connection: pin/shuttle lock, lanyard, or magnet; Figure 8.5), elastic sleeve (can be primary or secondary suspension), elevated vacuum suspension (Figure 8.6), or suprapatellar cuff.

TF socket designs: The socket is fit in 5° of flexion from maximum hip extension to provide mild hip extensor stretch and more efficient early stance phase. It is also typically set in adduction for improved femoral alignment and efficient single-limb support. Two common socket designs are the quadrilateral or ischial weight-bearing design (with narrow anteroposterior aspect, best for longer residual limbs) and the ischial containment design (with narrow mediolateral aspect, providing a "bony lock" of ischial tuberosity, pubic ramus, and greater trochanter; high proximal trimlines increase coronal stability for shorter limbs; Figure 8.7).[14]

TF suspension: As with TT suspension, elevated vacuum and silicone seal-in or locking liner can be used for suspension. Additionally, a pull-in socket with a pull sock or donning sleeve pulled through a hole at the bottom of the socket is an option. Belts can also be utilized (Figure 8.8) as auxiliary suspension, primary only if unable to use elevated vacuum suspension.

HD socket designs: HD prostheses have a much higher rejection rate due to increased energy cost. Prior to fitting, physicians should

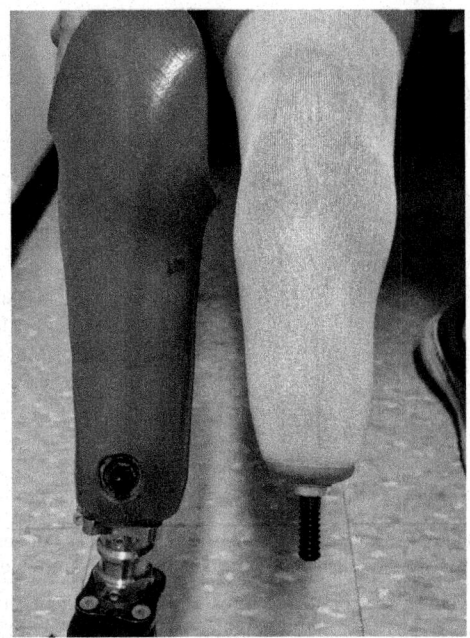

FIGURE 8.5 Example of silicone locking liner in a transtibial amputee.
Source: Used with permission from Jesus Mendoza, CPO.

evaluate motivation, single-leg balance, core strength, and weight-bearing tolerance within a socket. Design typically includes bucket-type socket with flexible inner socket, rigid laminated frame with belt, and suspended over iliac crests. Components include endoskeletal hip joint, with the knee and foot set posterior to the hip joint for increased stability. Length is also typically short due to decreased hip flexion and knee flexion in the swing phase.[15]

Partial foot socket designs: These are typically fit with a "prothosis," or anklefoot orthosis combined with a partial prosthetic foot insert, with carbon shank underneath to avoid midfoot breakage.

Bilateral TF amputations: The prosthesis should be short at first (or be fit with stubby-type prostheses without feet or knee units), and then height added as tolerated. Height can be estimated with arm span.

Osseointegration: Osseointegration is the surgical implantation of a direct skeletal attachment for prosthetic suspension, with improved osseoperception. Approximately 2,000 have been performed worldwide at the time of this writing. In the United States, *OPRA* (Osseointegration Prosthesis for the Rehabilitation of Amputees, a screw fixation

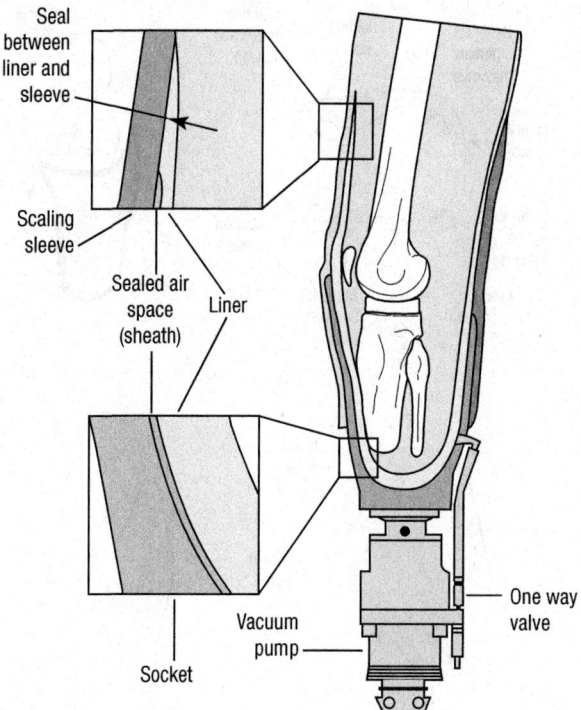

FIGURE 8.6 Elevated vacuum suspension.

implant) is the only Food and Drug Administration-approved device. Others, including press-fit and compression devices, are used under investigational device exemptions.

Most common use: bilateral amputees, extensive heterotopic ossification, short bony residuum, and need to eliminate socket issues associated with prosthetic failure

- *Benefits:* increased prosthetic use, increased walking speed, decreased energy cost, and improved quality of life
- *Risks :* soft tissue infections (however, most resolve by 1 year postoperatively); no high-impact activities; in TF amputees, subsequent prosthetic prescription to include microprocessor knee due to improved stance control and fewer falls
- *Exclusion criteria:* atypical bony anatomy, history of radiation or chemotherapy, peripheral vascular disease, diabetes with polyneuropathy, immune-compromised, systemic inflammatory disease, cognitive impairment, cardiorespiratory conditions that limit walking, and somatically unexplained pain[16]

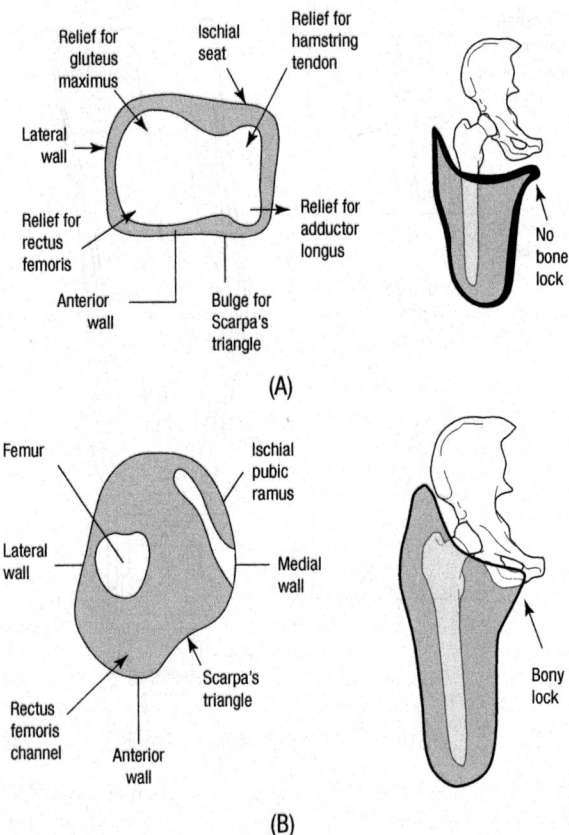

FIGURE 8.7 Transfemoral prosthetics sockets: (A) quadrilateral design and (B) ischial containment design.

Prosthetic Knees

Knee units range from very stable to very responsive, passive/body-powered to microprocessor-controlled (MPC). The prosthetic knee utilized will depend on the strength, stability, and activity level of the patient.[17,18]

Single-axis/constant-friction knee: This is used for single-speed walking and is very durable. It is also a good knee to use when you have a low build height (e.g., for children with limb deficiency who have close to the same leg lengths). It can also be used with a manually locking feature, which is

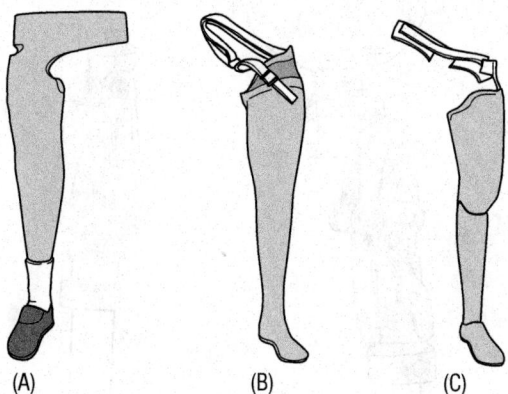

FIGURE 8.8 Three transfemoral belts: (A) total elastic suspension belt, (B) Silesian belt, and (C) hip joint with pelvic band.

helpful for bilateral TF amputees for increased stability (one knee unlocked at a time during gait training and allows for more comfortable sitting). In unilateral amputees, a locked knee does require circumduction in gait, or shortening the prosthesis by 1 cm for improved toe clearance during swing, which will also affect the stance phase cosmesis.

Weight-activated stance-control (WASC) knee: A WASC knee provides increased stability in weight-bearing, which locks the knee in extension, and is helpful in patients who have poor hip control. However, it must be unloaded to unlock the knee for sitting or flexion, causing a delayed swing phase.

Polycentric knee: Polycentric knee most commonly has four axis points (or four linkage bars; Figure 8.9). Due to the changing center of rotation, it is very stable during stance but does not disturb the swing phase. Some are also designed to be more cosmetically pleasing during sitting, which is useful for long TF or knee disarticulation amputees.

Fluid-controlled knee: Fluid-controlled knee utilizes oil or pneumatic cylinder with a piston. It is useful in patients with variable walking speed or cadence; hydraulic stance control also improves stability. It is heavier and more costly than other conventional knees and also requires more maintenance. It may be fabricated with microprocessor control component for more normal gait pattern.

MPC knee: This type of knee is controlled by an internal microprocessor, by creating either passive resistance or active propulsive movement. It allows for variation in both swing and stance phases on a moment-to-moment basis, based on data collected by sensors. In addition, it exhibits

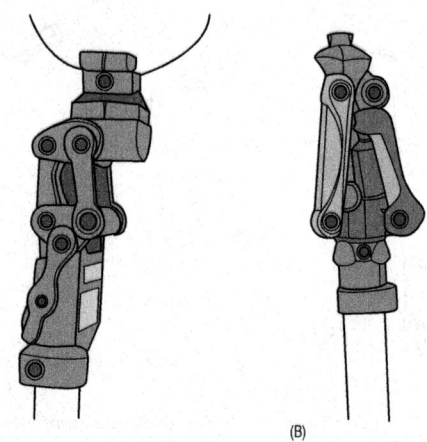

FIGURE 8.9 Two examples of polycentric knees: (A) is 7-bar linkage and (B) is a 4-bar linkage knee.

stumble control features that can prevent falls. Both active propulsive and myoelectric-controlled units are also being developed for the lower limb amputee population and a burgeoning area of research.

Prosthetic Feet

Prosthetic feet can vary from simple to very complex, and from passive to externally powered. The challenge is to balance stability with mimicking the dynamic footankle function in order to provide a smooth gait pattern and appropriate shock absorption. Hydraulic ankles (passive or MPC) are also available; however, these are not covered in the scope of this chapter.

Solid ankle cushioned heel (SACH) foot: A SACH foot typically includes a foam heel with solid wooden keel. It is inexpensive, durable, and simple. It is not energy-efficient but can be useful in less active amputees.

Single-axis foot: A single-axis foot allows movement in the sagittal plane with mechanical bumpers on either end to modulate flexion and extension. The rapid foot flat experienced can improve knee stability. This can also cause an abrupt knee hyperextension moment and is not advisable in TT amputees.

Multiaxial foot: A multiaxial foot allows movement in the sagittal plane, as well as some limited movement in the coronal and transverse plane, and can aid in walking on uneven surfaces. It can be costly and heavy.

Dynamic elastic response (DER) foot: This is also often called "energy-storing foot," which is a misnomer. It allows for more dynamic push-off and mechanical energy return. It is often made of carbon fiber, and can also be posterior-mounted to the socket for those with longer residual limb.

Complications

Skin issues: Skin issues are plentiful inside a prosthetic socket, such as fungal or bacterial infections, chronic choke syndrome or verrucous hyperplasia, and contact dermatitis. Treatment includes deferring prosthetic wear until completely healed, evaluating prosthetic fit, and reviewing hygiene of the prostheticskin interface.

Residual limb pain: This could be due to a multitude of causes, including neuroma or bursa formation, imbalance in myodesis, bony overgrowth, heterotopic ossification, or in the case of a cancer survivor a tumor recurrence. It is recommended that any stump pain be fully evaluated with appropriate imaging. If due to neuroma, consider TMR if available to avoid production of phantom pain with conventional neurectomy.

Phantom limb pain: This is defined as the sensation of pain in a limb that is no longer present and is very common in acquired amputees. Its exact cause is unknown; however, the prevalence is increased if there is preoperative uncontrolled pain. Treatment includes pharmacologic (opioids, antidepressants, nonsteroidal anti-inflammatory drugs, and anticonvulsants), surgical (neurectomy, deep brain stimulation, and TMR), psychological (biofeedback, relaxation, cognitive behavioral therapy, sensory discrimination training, hypnosis, virtual reality, and mirror therapy), continuous nerve blocks or epidural infusions, transcutaneous electric nerve stimulation (TENS), transcranial magnetic stimulation, spinal cord stimulation, use of a prosthesis, and acupuncture.

Overuse injuries: It is important to closely monitor for signs and symptoms of overuse or detrimental compensatory adaptations, such as carpal tunnel syndrome and back pain.

Prosthetic Gait

Generally, amputees with bilateral bilateral involvement or higher level amputations expend more energy in gait. A TF or HD amputee uses less energy to ambulate with crutches than with a prosthesis (Figure 8.10). The following are a few common prosthetic gait deviations and the likely causes.

Lateral bending: typically, toward the prosthetic side

- *Causes:* short prosthesis, abducted socket, hip abduction weakness, or contracture

Contralateral vault: excessive contralateral toe rise during the swing phase

- *Causes:* long prosthesis, excessive knee friction, and poor prosthetic suspension

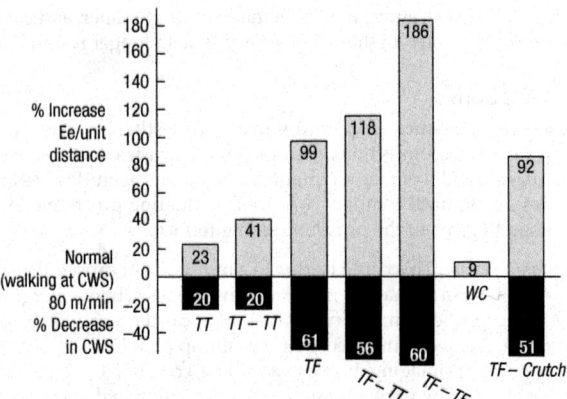

FIGURE 8.10 Graph showing the relationship of amputation level(s) with energy cost and speed. Comfortable walking speed (CWS) corresponds to the minimum energy cost per unit distance. Energy expenditure (EE)/unit distance and CWS for amputees using prostheses are compared with able-bodied subjects at a CWS of 80 m/min (≈3 mi/hr). The energy cost of ambulation at CWS for able-bodied subjects is 4.3 kcal/min.

TF, transfemoral; TT, transtibial; WC, wheelchair.

Heel whip: rapid medial or lateral rotational movement of the prosthetic heel at the initial swing phase

- *Cause:* malalignment of the knee or ankle joint

Abduction gait: prosthetic leg abducted during the stance phase;

- *Causes:* long prosthesis, hip abduction contracture, and high medial TF socket causing groin impingement

Circumduction gait: prosthetic leg swung outward in abducted arc and prosthetic knee flexion not engaged in swing phase

- *Causes:* long prosthesis, excessive knee friction inhibiting knee flexion in the swing phase, and hip abduction contracture

REFERENCES

The full complete reference list for this chapter appears in the digital version of the chapter, available at http://connect.springerpub.com/content/book/978-0-8261-5628-0/part/part02/chapter/ch08

CHAPTER 9

CARDIAC REHABILITATION

Matthew C. Oswald, Christopher W. Lewis, and Eric W. Villanueva

INTRODUCTION AND BENEFITS

Cardiac rehabilitation (CR) enhances the recovery and prevention of cardiac diseases through exercise programs, education, risk factor modification, and psychosocial counseling (Table 9.1).[1] CR is indicated following cardiac surgeries (e.g., coronary revascularization, valve replacements, cardiac transplantation, or left ventricular assist device [LVAD] implantation) and in patients with myocardial infarction (MI), systolic heart failure, chronic stable angina, or symptomatic peripheral artery disease.[2] Patients with diabetes, pulmonary artery hypertension, diastolic heart failure, or congenital heart disease may also be CR candidates.[3] Refer to Box 9.1 for contraindications to CR.

CR targets improvement in maximum oxygen consumption (VO_2 max), peripheral O_2 extraction, ST depression, and exercise tolerance. Physiologic goals also include lower blood pressure (BP), resting heart rate (HR), and myocardial O_2 demand. CR is also associated with improved glycemic control and favorable lipoprotein changes (e.g., reducing triglyceride [TG] and elevating high-density lipoprotein [HDL] levels). Studies show long-term CR increases the quantity of mitochondrial enzymes in "slow twitch" muscle fibers and increases the development of new capillaries in the muscles. CR may also improve left ventricular (LV) function and attenuate remodeling after MI.[4]

CR is associated with lower risk of cardiovascular death and hospital readmission in patients after acute MI.[5] Patients who complete CR are also found to have improved all-cause mortality after percutaneous coronary revascularization and coronary artery bypass grafting (CABG).[6,7] Formalized CR also correlates with long-term survival in patients after heart transplantation.[8] Patients with LVAD who undergo CR have improvement in exercise capacity and functional capacity.[9] Emerging data show CR is associated with lower hospital readmission rates and all-cause mortality among LVAD patients.[10] Additionally, CR can have a favorable effect on anxiety, depression, quality of life, and functional capacity.[11,12]

EPIDEMIOLOGY

The number of patients who can benefit from CR is increasing due to the prevalence of heart disease and its complications. Approximately .8 to 1.2 million MIs occur annually in the United States.[2,13,14] There are 6.3 million adults in the United States living with chronic heart failure.[15]

TABLE 9.1 Phases of Cardiac Rehabilitation[23]

Phases	Onset	Duration	Goals	Notes
Phase I (inpatient) Cardiac care unit Acute rehabilitation unit	Days 2–4 of hospitalization	1–2 wk	Prevent sequelae of immobilization Risk factor education Independent self-care and household ambulation	Telemetry monitoring until cleared by cardiology
Phase II (outpatient) Cardiac gym	After hospital discharge	8–12 wk	Return to normal activity (e.g., work, community activity, sexual activity)	Functional stress test for exercise prescription
Phase III (maintenance) Home or gym without supervision	After outpatient	Lifelong	Patient education (precautions, medications, disease) Risk modification	

Source: Data from Suler Y, Dinescu LI. Safety considerations during cardiac and pulmonary rehabilitation program. *Phys Med Rehabil Clin N Am.* 2012;23(2):433–440. doi:10.1016/j.pmr.2012.02.013.

EXERCISE PHYSIOLOGY AND PRESCRIPTION

The risk of cardiovascular complications from exercise training must be considered before beginning CR. The American Heart Association (AHA) stratifies patients into four classes (A–D) based on clinical characteristics and provides activity recommendations for each class.

- Class A individuals are healthy and have no evidence of cardiovascular risk with exercise.
- Class B individuals have established coronary artery disease (CAD) that is clinically stable. They have low risk of cardiovascular complications with vigorous exercise.
- Class C individuals are at moderate risk of complications during exercise due to history of multiple MIs or cardiac arrest, New York Heart Association (NYHA) Class III or IV congestive heart failure (CHF), <6 metabolic equivalent of task (METs) exercise capacity, or significant ischemia on exercise test (Table 9.2).
- Class D individuals have unstable cardiac disease and require restriction of activity; exercise is contraindicated.

Patients referred to CR are typically in Class B or C. There is minimal risk of adverse events with CR: The risk of any major cardiovascular complication (cardiac arrest, death, or MI) is one event in 60,000 to

> **BOX 9.1 Contraindications to Cardiac Rehabilitation**[25]
>
> - Unstable angina
> - Uncontrolled hypertension: resting SBP >180 mmHg and/or resting DBP >110 mmHg
> - Orthostatic BP drop of >20 mmHg, with symptoms
> - Severe or symptomatic aortic stenosis (aortic valve area <1.0 cm^2)
> - Uncontrolled atrial or ventricular arrhythmias
> - Uncontrolled sinus tachycardia (>120 beats per minute)
> - Uncompensated heart failure
> - Severe pulmonary hypertension
> - Third-degree atrioventricular (AV) block without pacemaker
> - Active pericarditis or myocarditis
> - Recent thromboembolism
> - Acute systemic illness or fever
> - Uncontrolled diabetes mellitus
> - Severe orthopedic conditions that would prohibit exercise
> - Other metabolic conditions, such as acute thyroiditis, hypokalemia, hyperkalemia, or hypovolemia (until adequately treated)
>
> BP, blood pressure; DBP, diastolic blood pressure; SBP, systolic blood pressure.
>
> *Source:* Adapted from Mampuya WM. Cardiac rehabilitation past, present and future: An overview. *Cardiovasc Diagn Ther.* 2012;2(1):38–49.

TABLE 9.2 NYHA Classification

NYHA Classification (for CHF and Angina)[24]
I. >7 METs tolerated asymptomatically, without functional limitation
II. <6 METs tolerated, but higher levels of activities cause symptoms
III. Asymptomatic at rest and with most ADLs; >4 METs not tolerated
IV. Symptomatic at rest and with minimal physical activities

ADLs, activities of daily living; CHF, congestive heart failure; METs, metabolic equivalent of task; NYHA, New York Heart Association.

Source: Data from Yancy CW, Jessup M, Bozkurt B, et al. 2013. ACCF/AHA guideline for the management of heart failure: A report of the American College of Cardiology Foundation/American Heart Association Task Force on Practice Guidelines. *J Am Coll Cardiol.* 2013;62(16):e147–e239. doi:10.1016/j.jacc.2013.05.019.

80,000 hours of supervised exercise.[16] Usual session duration/frequency is 40 to 60 minutes three to five times a week × 12 weeks or more when training at 70% of the maximum HR. For patients with severe deconditioning, shorter durations of daily training may be more practical.

The exercise prescription should address the type, intensity, content, duration, and frequency of exercise. Isotonic, aerobic, and rhythmic exercises involving large muscle groups should be emphasized. Isometrics and resistive exercises are relatively safe in patients with normal LV function, but are contraindicated in patients with CHF, severe valvular disease, uncontrolled arrhythmias, or peak exercise capacity <5 METs.

The MET (MET = 3.5 mL O_2 uptake/kg/min, or about 1 kcal/kg/hr) is the ratio of the energy expenditure of an activity relative to the resting metabolic rate (e.g., sitting quietly). Thus, a 5-MET activity uses five times the energy expended at rest. The METs for common activities include .9 for sleeping, ~1.5 for sedentary desk work, ~2.3 for slow walking on level ground, ~3.6 for fast walking, ~5.8 for sexual activity, and 7 for jogging. The maximum MET capacity is usually achieved between the ages of 15 and 30 years and progressively decreases with age. It can, however, increase with exercise and conditioning. A maximum capacity of 10 METs is typical of healthy but nonathletic middle-aged men. In young men, 12 METs is typical of maximal exercise. Distance runners can average 18 to 24 METs.

Exercise intensity can be determined by a variety of methods, but is commonly defined by calculating a *target HR*. The AHA method to calculate the *target HR* uses 70% to 85% of the maximum HR attained by cardiac stress testing. For young, healthy adults not undergoing formal exercise stress testing, the maximum HR is calculated using the patient's age (max HR = 220 bpm – patient age), which can then be multiplied by 70% to 85% to determine the *target HR*. This formula, however, does not apply if the patient has a history of MI. Note, the *target HR* is not precise and has an *SD* of 10 to 15 beats per minute (bpm). Additionally, this formula was derived from studies of men and may overestimate the HR in women. Therefore, in these cases it may be more accurate to measure the *peak exercise capacity*, which is the maximum ability of the cardiovascular system to deliver O_2 to exercising skeletal muscle and its ability to extract O_2 from the blood.

The *Karvonen formula* (target heart rate = (($HR_{max} - HR_{rest}$) × % desired intensity) + HR_{rest}) is beneficial in calculating a target HR zone to achieve during therapy. HR_{max} can be estimated by subtracting the patient's age from 220. Usually, the desired intensity for CR is between 40% and 85%. For more deconditioned patients, the exercise program should begin at the lower end of the spectrum (i.e., 40%–60%) and increase as fitness improves.

Peak exercise capacity can be calculated by clinically measuring O_2 uptake (VO_2), CO_2 production (VCO_2), and minute ventilation during exercise. The maximal O_2 uptake will eventually plateau despite increasing workload. Anaerobic threshold (AT) is another index used to estimate exercise capacity. AT is defined as the point at which minute ventilation increases disproportionately relative to VO_2 (often seen at 60%–70% of the VO_2 max). AT is an indicator of increase in lactic acid produced by working muscles and can be used to distinguish cardiac and noncardiac (e.g., pulmonary or musculoskeletal) causes of exercise limitation.

Borg's Rating of Perceived Exertion (RPE) Scale is particularly useful for patients taking medications that affect HR and for cardiac transplant patients because denervation of the orthotopic heart can make HR parameters unreliable. Resting HR is higher in heart transplant patients due to vagus nerve transection and subsequent denervation resulting in decreased parasympathetic tone. The traditional Borg's RPE scale is scored from 6 to 20, where 13 is rated as "somewhat hard" and corresponds with exercise intensity sufficient to provide training benefits but still allows conversation during exercise. A score of 12 to 13 corresponds to about 60% of the maximum HR, while a score of 15 corresponds to 85% of the maximum HR. Borg's scale may be confounded by psychological factors, but encourages independence in exercise (i.e., phase III CR) as external monitoring devices are weaned off.

For patients on beta-blockers, training at 85% of symptom-limited HR or 70% to 90% of the maximum workload determined by exercise testing is recommended.[17] Pacemakers do not necessarily preclude exercise training in a CR program.

ACTIVE MANAGEMENT AND PREVENTION OF COMPLICATIONS POST CARDIAC SURGERY

Patients who developed new significant functional deficits during their acute care hospitalization for a cardiac event often require inpatient rehabilitation. Patients with heart failure or recent cardiac surgery (CABG, valve replacement/repair, LVAD implantation) can successfully tolerate therapy early in the postoperative period and benefit from multidisciplinary inpatient rehabilitation due to loss of function in the context of a long hospital course and multiple comorbid chronic medical conditions. Furthermore, postsurgical patients benefit from training to accommodate sternal precautions while recovering strength and endurance for performance of activities of daily living (ADLs) and mobility. These patients also benefit from monitoring of acute complications including postoperative infections, pain, arrhythmia, heart failure, pericardial effusion, pleural effusion, and coronary artery graft failure. Establishing and maintaining collaborative relationships with local referring cardiology and surgical teams is important to optimize patient care and outcomes.

Heart Failure Exacerbation

Patients with a history of heart failure who present for CR require evaluation of specific clinical and laboratory markers to identify if they are having heart failure exacerbation (HFE). Patients with a history of heart failure should have a baseline weight measured on admission and subsequently tracked daily along with clinical volume assessments and measurements of intake and output. An increase of 2 to 3 pounds in a 24-hour period or 5 pounds in a week may indicate HFE. Patients may not develop symptoms until their weight increases by >10 pounds. Symptoms consistent with HFE include dependent edema, shortness of breath, cough, fatigue, and decreased therapy tolerance. If concerned about HFE, initial evaluation can include chest radiograph to evaluate for pulmonary edema. Laboratory assessments such as B-type natriuretic peptide may be helpful when compared with baseline. Patients with worsening function due to HFE may require hospitalization. Active clinical assessment and medication adjustments during inpatient rehabilitation can prevent rehospitalization during this critical recovery period.

Atrial Fibrillation With Rapid Ventricular Response

Patients at risk of developing atrial fibrillation with rapid ventricular response (RVR) include those with CAD, valvular heart disease (e.g., stenosis, regurgitation), rheumatic heart disease, heart failure, and hypertrophic cardiomyopathy. Symptoms include tachycardia, weakness, dizziness, reduced exercise capacity, dyspnea, angina, and presyncope. In the rehabilitation setting, the role of the clinician is to determine if the patient requires transfer for emergent medical evaluation. Patients are categorized by hemodynamic stability and symptoms: (a) hemodynamically unstable patients require emergent medical evaluation and consideration for emergency cardioversion, (b) symptomatic, hemodynamically stable patients require urgent physician evaluation and medical management, and (c) asymptomatic patients with a ventricular rate <120 bpm require physician assessment and management with oral medications.

Ventricular Assist Devices

LVADs provide continuous flow from the left ventricle to the aorta by means of a surgically implanted, extrinsically powered pump. LVADs are indicated in patients who have advanced refractory heart failure and either need a "bridge to transplant" or have contraindications to transplantation. The patient's exercise physiology significantly changes due to this device. Ventricular assistive devices have a fixed pump speed that does not change with exercise. Peak VO_2 following LVAD implantation averages 12 to 17 mL/kg/min.[18,19] Patients with an LVAD are at risk of postoperative bleeding, pump thrombosis, hemolysis, right heart failure, infection, aortic regurgitation, device failure, and neurologic complications including stroke.[20,21]

LVAD vital signs: Since an LVAD provides continuous flow, a palpable pulse is typically absent. As a result, BP often cannot be measured as a systolic and diastolic peripheral vascular resistance but rather a mean arterial pressure (MAP) through use of a Doppler. Long-term MAP goals for a patient with an LVAD may vary by surgical team and patient, but are typically 70 to 80 mmHg.[22]

LVAD parameters: In case of device malfunction due to thrombus formation within the pump, an interrogation would reveal an increase in pump power but no change in pump speed, volume status, or afterload reduction. The patient may concurrently display clinical and laboratory signs of hemolysis, including dark urine, anemia, and elevated lactate dehydrogenase (LDH) levels. In case of increasing edema or HFE, providers may observe increased flows in the context of increasing weights before onset of typical heart failure symptoms. Conversely, lower flow trends and declining weights may indicate overdiuresis and precede clinical signs of orthostasis or laboratory changes.

COMMON PRECAUTIONS

Sternal Precautions

Following a sternotomy, patients are typically instructed to follow sternal precautions for 6 to 8 weeks by avoiding reaching overhead or behind their back, pushing, pulling, or lifting objects. In the context of generalized weakness and deconditioning after surgery, these precautions can significantly limit functional independence and increase caregiver assist needs following surgery. During CR, precautions against prohibited movements and muscular activation are reinforced while safe movements are carefully practiced under the guidance of a therapist to optimize functional independence and safety.

Cardiac Precautions

Exercise should terminate in persons with CAD who experience new-onset cardiopulmonary symptoms, HR decreases >20% of baseline, HR increases >50% of baseline, BP increases above the target thresholds, or systolic blood pressure (SBP) decreases ≥30 mmHg from baseline or to <90 mmHg. O_2 saturation should be sustained above 92% at rest and with exertion.[23]

REFERENCES

The full complete reference list for this chapter appears in the digital version of the chapter, available at http://connect.springerpub.com/content/book/978-0-8261-5628-0/part/part02/chapter/ch09

CHAPTER 10

PULMONARY REHABILITATION

Vivian Roy, Julia Fram, and Leslie Rydberg

INTRODUCTION

Optimal function of the respiratory system is essential to successful rehabilitation. In this chapter, we discuss normal physiology, respiratory dysfunction in spinal cord injury (SCI), principles of pulmonary rehabilitation (PR), neuromuscular respiratory failure, and management of tracheostomies.

The skeletal muscles under voluntary control are involved in both the inspiratory and expiratory phases of respiration. The muscles involved in normal inspiration include the diaphragm (C3–C5; the primary muscle of inspiration), the external intercostals (T1–T12), and the accessory muscles (trapezii, sternocleidomastoid, scalenes, and serratus anterior). Expiration is typically a passive process. During active expiration, which may occur during coughing or exercise, the muscles involved include the internal intercostals (T1–T12) and the abdominal muscles (T7–L1; rectus abdominis, transversus abdominis, and internal and external obliques).[1,2] Therefore, with lesions causing SCI at or above the thoracic region, impaired cough reflex leads to retained secretions, mucous plugging, and pneumonia (which is the most common overall cause of death in SCI). Weakness of both muscles of inspiration and expiration also results in low vital capacity (VC), leading to atelectasis and decreased surfactant production.

The pulmonary system (specifically, the bronchial smooth muscle) is also controlled by the autonomic nervous system. Parasympathetic fibers to the bronchial smooth muscle are carried by cranial nerve X, also called the vagus nerve, and mediated by the neurotransmitter (NT) acetylcholine (ACh). Sympathetic fibers are carried by the spinal cord from T1 to L2 levels and mediated by ACh (preganglionic NT), as well as epinephrine and norepinephrine (postganglionic NT). Muscarinic ACh and adrenergic beta-2 receptors are present on the bronchial smooth muscle. During normal resting periods, the parasympathetic system activates the muscarinic ACh receptors, causing bronchoconstriction and mucous production. During periods of increased activity, the sympathetic system activates adrenergic beta-2 receptors, causing bronchodilation. In SCI above T1, the sympathetic nervous system is affected while CN X remains intact. This excess vagal tone causes the balance to shift toward bronchoconstriction (and subsequently bronchospasms) and excessive secretion production, both of which contribute to significant complications in SCI.

Management of the respiratory system in the rehabilitation setting, therefore, should center on expanding the lungs and clearing secretions. Bronchospasms can be reversed using beta-agonists such as albuterol or anticholinergics such as ipratropium. Noninvasive positive pressure ventilation can be used to expand the lungs and improve atelectasis. Invasive mechanical ventilation should be considered in patients with declining VC (approaching <10–15 mL/kg body weight), arterial blood gas measurement of $PaCO_2$ >50 mmHg or PaO_2 <50 mmHg on room air (signifying acute respiratory failure), significant atelectasis, or increased work of breathing. Secretion management should include mucolytics such as acetylcysteine, guaifenesin, or sodium bicarbonate to thin secretions in order to facilitate clearance. Secretion clearance can include suctioning (either using an oral suction tip or deep suction catheter through tracheostomy), assisted coughing (using manual quad cough technique or mechanical cough assist), or oscillating positive expiratory pressure devices (such as metanebulizing devices, which can simultaneously deliver aerosols).

PULMONARY REHABILITATION

Pulmonary disease leads to physical and psychological symptom burden that impairs physical function and quality of life. The goal of PR is to improve the symptoms associated with respiratory disease, optimize function, and facilitate healthy behaviors in patients with chronic respiratory illness. Documented benefits of PR include significant improvements in dyspnea, exercise capacity, anxiety and depression, health-related quality of life, and healthcare utilization.[3,4]

PR is typically an outpatient-based program. Interventions include exercise training, psychosocial support, and education. A PR plan must be comprehensive and individualized to the needs of each patient, including the psychological and social aspects of respiratory disease. PR requires a multidisciplinary team that may include physicians, exercise physiologists, nurses, physical therapists, occupational therapists, respiratory therapists, dieticians, and case managers.

Pulmonary diseases can be categorized as obstructive or restrictive disorders and pulmonary function testing (PFT) can help make this distinction (Figure 10.1). Additionally, exercise capacity testing prior to starting can be of benefit to planning a PR intervention. Testing options include the 6-minute walk test, shuttle walk test, and cardiopulmonary exercise testing.[5]

OBSTRUCTIVE DISORDERS

Obstructive pulmonary disease is characterized by the inability to exhale efficiently, resulting in decreased VC, forced expiratory volume (FEV), and increased residual volume (RV) on PFT (Table 10.1 and Figure 10.1). A postbronchodilator ratio of FEV in 1 second to forced vital capacity (FVC) <.7 is consistent with a diagnosis of chronic obstructive pulmonary disease (COPD), a condition that is defined by airflow obstruction and inflammation resulting in bronchitis and emphysema. Additional

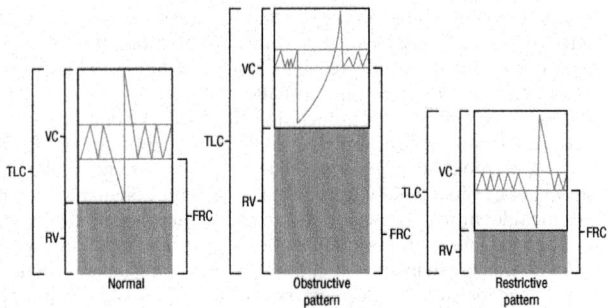

FIGURE 10.1 Lung volumes and capacities in ventilatory (restrictive) and obstructive disorders.

FRC, functional residual capacity; RV, residual volume; TLC, total lung capacity; VC, vital capacity.

TABLE 10.1 Characteristic Physiologic Changes Associated With Pulmonary Disorders

Measure	Obstructive Disorders	Restrictive Disorders	Mixed Disorders
FEV_1/FVC	Decreased	Normal or increased	Decreased
FEV_1	Decreased	Decreased, normal, or increased	Decreased
FVC	Decreased or normal	Decreased	Decreased or normal
TLC	Normal or increased	Decreased	Decreased, normal, or increased
RV	Normal or increased	Decreased	Decreased, normal, or increased

FEV_1, forced expiratory volume in 1 second; FVC, forced vital capacity; RV, residual volume; TLC, total lung capacity.

Source: Adapted from the Merck Manuals Online Medical Library. *The Merck Manual for Healthcare Professionals*. www.merckmanuals.com.

obstructive respiratory disorders include bronchiectasis, asthma, and cystic fibrosis.

The Global Initiative for Chronic Obstructive Disease (GOLD) utilizes the airway breathing circulation disability assessment tool to categorize the severity of COPD. PR may be appropriate at all stages of COPD. Evidence supporting the efficacy of PR is most prominent in patients with moderate to severe disease.[3]

Physical activity limitations in patients with obstructive lung disease are multifactorial. Hypoxemia and carbon dioxide retention lead to dyspnea and fatigue. Comorbid conditions such as coronary artery disease or arthritis further limit exercise tolerance and result in deconditioning. Additionally, medical treatments such as chronic steroid use or immunosuppressants can negatively impact peripheral muscle function.

PR consists of exercise training with the goal of improving cardiopulmonary fitness and peripheral efficiency. Of note, while symptomatic and functional improvement is frequently observed in PR, it does not directly improve the lung's ability to facilitate gas exchange. Exercise training includes aerobic and resistance training. Reaching the typical target range of 60% to 70% of maximal heart rate for aerobic exercise training can be difficult due to hypoxia, dyspnea, or even hypercapnia in severe disease. Oxygen saturation should be measured before and during exertion. Supplemental oxygen should be titrated to maintain saturation >88% to 90% during exertion and returned to baseline levels following exercise to prevent resting hypercarbia. Supplemental home oxygen may be indicated when PaO_2 is consistently <55 to 60 mmHg.

In obstructive respiratory disease, tachypnea and shallow breathing worsen shortness of breath by causing dead space ventilation. Breathing retraining is an important part of PR. Techniques including diaphragmatic and pursed lip breathing and therapies such as yoga and biofeedback promote slow, deep breathing. By decreasing the respiratory rate, a patient will have a longer time to exhale, reducing hyperinflation and dyspnea. COPD can also present with cough and sputum production; secretion management therapy and education (as discussed in the Introduction) should be incorporated into a PR program.

Tobacco cessation counseling is a key component of PR in patients with COPD who continue to smoke. Clinicians should assess behavioral readiness and consider pharmacologic tools, including nicotine replacement therapies and centrally acting medications such as bupropion and varenicline. Additional topics covered in PR include disease course and treatments, nutrition, immunizations, symptom management strategies, supplemental oxygen devices, and advanced care planning. PR can help prepare patients for lung volume reduction surgery or lung transplantation, providing education and optimizing functional outcomes prior to surgery.

RESTRICTIVE DISORDERS (INTRINSIC)

In restrictive lung disease, patients have difficulty expanding the chest wall, which leads to small lung volumes. This difficulty can be due to an extrinsic cause, such as a neuromuscular disorder, as discussed in the following section, or can be intrinsic to the lung tissue (e.g., interstitial lung disease [ILD]). ILD can be caused by infection, occupational and environmental exposures, connective tissue disorder, or idiopathic etiologies. Examples of ILD are idiopathic pulmonary fibrosis, sarcoidosis, and scleroderma. Decreased lung volumes, poor pulmonary compliance, and poor diffusion capacity are characteristic of

ILD. Typically, a total lung capacity below 80% of the predictive volume is observed. Common features of ILDs are dry cough and dyspnea on exertion. Patients with significantly reduced diffusion capacity are at risk of severe hypoxemia and hypercarbia. Patients with advanced disease can develop pulmonary hypertension and cor pulmonale. Although the PR model was developed for COPD, there is increasing evidence demonstrating that PR in ILD is safe, feasible, and efficacious. Documented benefits include improved dyspnea and fatigue, quality of life, and healthcare utilization.

NEUROMUSCULAR RESPIRATORY FAILURE

Multiple forms of neuromuscular disease can result in respiratory failure and require mechanical ventilation. This can occur with acute neuromuscular disease or with chronic progressive neuromuscular conditions. Some common diagnoses associated with neuromuscular respiratory failure include myasthenia gravis, Guillain–Barré syndrome (GBS), muscular dystrophy, and amyotrophic lateral sclerosis.

Patients present with symptoms of fatigue, excessive daytime sleepiness, or morning headaches; in the more acute phase, patients may have dyspnea, shallow breathing, restlessness, staccato speech, and dysphagia, and may not catch enough air and may struggle to breath. On examination, patients may have tachycardia, tachypnea, hypoxemia, and prominent use of accessory muscles.

Neuromuscular respiratory failure occurs when there is weakness in the respiratory muscles. Weakness or paralysis of the bilateral diaphragm forces the accessory muscles of inspiration to take over, increasing work of breathing. Expiration is affected as well. Although normal expiration predominantly occurs by passive recoil of the thoracic cage, the internal intercostals and abdominal wall muscles are involved with forced expiration and can be affected by neuromuscular weakness.[6]

Neuromuscular diseases produce a restrictive pattern of respiratory failure. First, patients develop atelectasis at the lung bases, causing blood shunting, leading to mild hypoxia. As patients become more fatigued, they develop alveolar hypoventilation, with increased respiratory rate and normal PCO_2 levels. In the later stages of respiratory failure with worsening weakness, the alveoli continue to collapse and the tidal volumes get progressively smaller, leading to a mixed hypoxemichypercapnic respiratory failure, with worsening ventilation–perfusion mismatch and increasing work of breathing, overloading the already fatigued muscles.[7]

Respiratory values include FVC, maximum inspiratory pressure (MIP)/negative inspiratory force, and maximum expiratory pressure (MEP). An FVC of <20 mL/kg or a 30% decline or more over 24 hours, an MIP of <30 cm H_2O, and an MEP of <40 cm H_2O are indicators of impending respiratory failure (also known as the 20/30/40 rule).

Treatment for neuromuscular respiratory failure includes secretion management and ventilatory support. In the acute setting, patient distress, inability to clear secretions, decline in VC, tachypnea, hemodynamic instability, and abnormal arterial blood gases may suggest the need for ventilatory support. Some patients may be safely treated with noninvasive ventilation (NIV), while many will require intubation. NIV should be avoided in patients with acute GBS with rapidly progressive weakness due to the severity of diaphragm weakness.

NIV can improve survival and quality of life in patients with chronic neuromuscular diseases. It is preferred by patients over tracheostomy for speech, sleep, swallowing, comfort, appearance, and security. Limitations of NIV include discomfort from the close-fitting mask, sleep disturbances, leaks, and gastric distention. Positive airway pressure can help overcome upper airway resistance and keep the alveoli open, thus improving gas exchange. Bilevel airway pressure (BIPAP) is more effective at providing rest for the fatigued respiratory muscles. Depending on their needs, patients may use BIPAP with a backup rate versus volume-assured pressure support. Patients with more severe chronic neuromuscular respiratory failure may progress to tracheostomy placement with mechanical ventilation, which requires increased healthcare support services as well as highly trained home professionals or caregivers.[8]

TRACHEOSTOMY MANAGEMENT IN REHABILITATION

Tracheostomy tubes are commonly encountered in the rehabilitation setting and are used for airway patency, mechanical ventilation, prevention of aspiration, and for ease of access to the lower respiratory tract to allow for secretion management. Tracheostomies are available in multiple shapes, lengths, and diameters. Choosing the right tracheostomy tube is essential to maintaining an unobstructed airway and preventing complications. A tube that is too small in diameter will cause increased resistance and difficulty with air movement, as well as increase the cuff pressure required for adequate seal; conversely, a tube that is too large will be difficult to pass through the stoma and decrease the ability for leak speech. Curved, angled, and extra-length (both horizontal and vertical) tracheostomy tubes are available to conform to patients with different body habitus. Tracheostomies can also be cuffed or uncuffed. Cuffed tubes allow for mechanical and positive pressure ventilation and prevent aspiration events, while cuffless tubes help facilitate airway clearance but do not protect against aspiration. Tight-to-shaft tracheostomy tubes, for which the cuff conforms to the shape of the tube, are particularly useful when progressing through tracheostomy weaning as these can simulate both cuffed and uncuffed states.[9]

Tracheostomy weaning begins with the cuff inflated so that air travels through the open stoma, often with the aid of humidified supplemental oxygen, delivered through a tracheostomy mask. After the patient tolerates activity off oxygen, an attachment called heat moisture exchanger can be placed to help thin secretions and facilitate clearance of secretions. During this process, the speech and language pathologist often begins working on phonation with the patient. In order to do this, the air must travel through the vocal cords using either a one-way speaking valve or a cap. It is imperative to use a cuffless tracheostomy tube (or, if using a cuffed or tight-to-shaft tube, the cuff should be deflated) with a one-way speaking valve or cap. Monitoring can include pulse oximetry, carbon dioxide monitoring, negative inspiratory force, and VC. An overnight pulse oximetry study can be obtained after a patient has been capped for >24 hours prior to considering decannulation. Once decannulated, the stoma can be covered with a gauze dressing to allow for healing. Otolaryngology consult should be obtained if there is difficulty tolerating one-way speaking valve or cap. Close communication with respiratory and speech language therapists is essential to a successful tracheostomy weaning.

REFERENCES

The full complete reference list for this chapter appears in the digital version of the chapter, available at http://connect.springerpub.com/content/book/978-0-8261-5628-0/part/part02/chapter/ch10

CHAPTER 11

BURN REHABILITATION

Mark E. Huang and Christopher W. Lewis

EPIDEMIOLOGY

In the United States, 486,000 burn injuries require medical attention each year, with approximately 40,000 requiring hospitalization and 30,000 requiring care at a burn center.[1,2] Causes of burns include heat (the most common agent), cold, chemicals, electricity, and radiation. In the United States, most patients admitted to acute burn centers are males (mean age 30 years old) with total body surface area (TBSA) burns of <10%. Almost all (>95%) of burned and hospitalized individuals survive.[1] Complications from severe burn injuries include contractures, scarring, hypermetabolic response, pruritus, heterotopic ossification, pain, and psychiatric morbidity. Predictors of mortality include older age (with increased risk most significant after 60–70 years old), higher TBSA burn involvement, and involvement of an inhalation injury. Notably, burns are among the leading causes of accidental death in younger children.

DESCRIBING BURNS

Individual burns are categorized by the thickness of the injury through the skin. Superficial burns involve only the epidermis and are characterized as being red, painful, and with little or no exudate. A common example of a superficial burn is a sunburn with redness only and no peeling. Partial-thickness burns involve the epidermis and the dermis, leading to the formation of a blister and can have mild to moderate exudate. Full-thickness burns involve the epidermis and the dermis and may include subcutaneous tissue (fat, muscle, and bone). Full-thickness burns may have significant exudate and often form eschars that must be debrided for adequate wound healing (Figure 11.1).

When describing burns on a patient, it is important to estimate the TBSA of the burn to convey severity and prognosis. A common method for estimating the TBSA is called the "rule of nines," where the front and back of the head (9%), each arm (9%), each leg (18%), anterior trunk (18%), and posterior trunk (18%) each accounts for 9% (or a multiple of nine) of the TBSA and the perineum for the remaining 1%.

In pediatric patients, the method for calculating the TBSA will vary depending on the age of the patient. The Lund and Browder chart[3,4] is an alternative method for estimating the TBSA that accounts for anatomic changes in proportions of the head, body, and extremities based on age. As children age, their head becomes a smaller proportion of their TBSA and their extremities become larger (Figure 11.2).

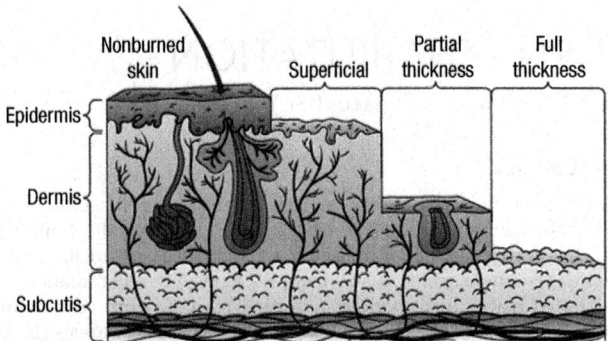

FIGURE 11.1 Anatomy of the skin, including the epidermis (superficial burn), dermis (partial-thickness burn), and subcutaneous tissue (full-thickness burn).

Source: From Murphy KP, McMahon MA, Houtrow AJ. *Pediatric Rehabilitation: Principles and Practice*, 6th ed. Springer Publishing Company; 2021; Figure 27.2.

Burn severity (minor, moderate, and major) is based on the TBSA and the type of burns present. Minor burns include patients with partial-thickness burns involving <10% of the TBSA (<5% TBSA in patients <10 years or >50 years of age) or full-thickness burns in <2% of the TBSA and typically can be managed as an outpatient. Moderate burns are partial-thickness burns that cover 10% to 20% of the TBSA in adults (5%–10% in patients <10 years or >50 years of age) or 2% to 5% of the TBSA full-thickness burn and typically require hospital admission. Major burns are partial-thickness burns that involve >20% of the TBSA in adults (>10% in patients <10 years or >50 years of age) or full-thickness burn in >5% of the TBSA and typically require referral to a burn center. Major burns also include any significant burn to the face, eyes, ears, genitalia, hands, feet, or major joints.[5]

WOUND CARE

There is no consensus regarding wound care other than the need to remove the necrotic tissue and ensure healthy granulation tissue base at the wound bed. The primary goal of wound care is to create an ideal environment for tissue growth. This is accomplished by multiple interventions including removal of the necrotic and devitalized tissue, managing moisture quantity, preventing infection with regular change of dressing, and protecting the wound from shear and trauma. Types of debridement include autolytic (e.g., alginates, honey-impregnated dressings, hydrocolloids, hydrogels, and hydrofibers), mechanical (e.g., irrigation, abrasion, and wet-to-dry dressings), sharp/surgical (e.g., removal of necrotic tissue via curette, scalpel, and scissors), and enzymatic (e.g., chemical liquefaction of necrotic tissue). Comparison between these methods has been limited in the literature.[6] Multiple

11 Burn Rehabilitation | 99

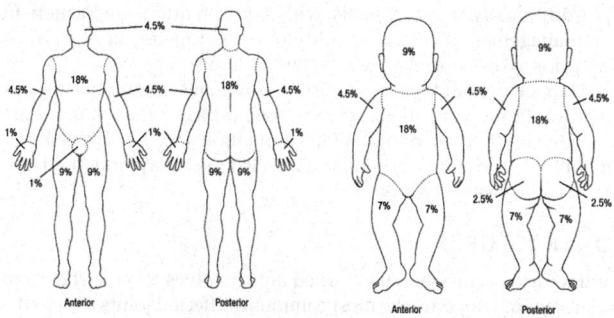

Area	Age 0	1	5	10	15	Adult
A = ½ of head	9 ½	8 ½	6 ½	5 ½	4 ½	3 ½
B = ½ of one thigh	2 ¾	3 ¼	4	4 ½	4 ½	4 ¾
C = ½ of one lower limb	2 ½	2 ½	2 ¾	3	3 ¼	3 ½

FIGURE 11.2 The top Panel Shows the Percentage of the total body surface area (TBSA) Among Adult (left) and Pediatric (right) patients. The Bottom Panel was Adapted from the Lund and Browder Chart Describing the Method for Estimating the Percent TBSA in Pediatric Patients with Burns as They Grow from Age 0 to Age 15 and Subsequently Adulthood.[3,4]

Source: From Veenema TG. *Disaster Nursing and Emergency Preparedness: For Chemical, Biological, and Radiological Terrorism and Other Hazards*, 4th ed. Springer Publishing Company; 2018; Figure 25.1.

methods are often used in combination. For patients with refractory second- and third-degree burns that will not close with primary or secondary intention healing, skin grafts performed by a surgeon should be considered. Common reasons for poor healing include wound size, infection, and poor vascularization.

To ensure a moist wound base for healing, Xeroform or wound veil is often combined with a moisturizing antimicrobial ointment such as bacitracin. Silver sulfadiazine has been classically used as it is inexpensive. For wound areas that have hypergranulation tissue, silver impregnated foam with silver sulfadiazine twice daily as well as focal treatment with silver nitrate can help reduce raised granulation tissue. As part of daily wound care process, a nonimmersion burn shower during dressing changes can help with wound cleansing before new dressings are applied. An antimicrobial wash such as chlorhexidine is often used as part of the shower.

Additionally, most patients with burns require medication for pain management. Scheduling additional pain medications immediately prior to dressing changes is often required.

Management of blisters in burn care remains controversial in the literature. From a functional perspective, a blister that is tense and associated with pain or functional limitation can be drained. The remaining epidermis overlying the affected area may often be left in place as a protective barrier.

CONTRACTURES

Contractures occur when the burned area involves a joint. The shoulder, elbow, and knee are the most commonly affected joints. The pathophysiology of contracture is potentially a result of scar formation with myofibroblasts and free actin. Prevention of contractures includes splinting, positioning, and range of motion (ROM) exercises. These interventions can be started early in the patient's recovery. A burned area can be splinted while a patient is either sedated or asleep to minimize edema and discomfort. Splints can be removed for dressing changes and ROM exercises. These splints are usually made from low-temperature thermo-moldable plastics that can be molded in hot water or with a hair dryer.

Positioning of a patient while being managed in an acute care or rehabilitation setting is important to prevent and minimize contracture formation. For burns involving the arms and hands, a wrist hand orthosis can be used to minimize the risk of development of the intrinsic minus position of the wrist and fingers. Axillary contractures are very common in post-burn recovery and evidence supports positioning the axilla in 90° of flexion with 10° or less of horizontal adduction to minimize stress on the brachial plexus.

SCARRING

The risk of scarring depends on multiple factors, including the depth and severity of the burn. Burns that are limited to the epidermis are at low risk of scarring. The skin may be noted to have pigmentation changes long term. However, full-thickness burns that involve the epithelial layer and the subdermal structures are at high risk of scarring. Treatment of full-thickness burns includes surgical debridement of the necrotic tissue and autologous transplantation of the dermal tissue depending on the extent of the wound.

Hypertrophic scarring is a condition where scar tissue proliferates and is characterized by raised, red, painful, pruritic, and often contracted skin overlying the area of injury. This is the most common complication after burn injuries, with a prevalence of 67%.[7] Patients at higher risk of hypertrophic scarring include younger age, darker skin pigmentation, prolonged wound healing phase, and open wounds >3 weeks.[7,8]

Prevention of hypertrophic scarring begins with appropriate wound care. If scars form, aggressive and early treatment with nonevaporative topical emollient cream (4–6 applications daily). Once the wounds have healed, primary avoidance of sun exposure through use of protective clothing is preferred. Pressure garment treatment prior to wound healing initially minimizes wound edema, and after wound healing the pressure garment (with or without silicone gel sheeting) can apply pressure to the scarring tissue and promote flatter scar formation. If initial preventive and treatment modalities are not satisfactory, corticosteroid injections (triamcinolone and 5-fluorouracil) and use of pulsed dye laser treatment can be considered.

HYPERMETABOLIC RESPONSE

The hypermetabolic response to burn injury is a syndrome characterized by increased metabolic rates, multiorgan dysfunction, muscle protein degradation, blunted growth, insulin resistance, and increased risk of infection. This response is most associated with patients who are suffering from severe burn injuries (TBSA >40%) and is mediated by surges in catecholamine and cortisol levels that can last up to 9 months after the burn injury.[9,10] Additionally, a patient's basal metabolic rate of energy expenditure can increase as much as 180% from the typical estimated rate from sex, age, height, and weight.[10,11]

Appropriate treatment for patients with large TBSA burns includes anticipatory medical management with anabolic agents and beta-blockers, in addition to exercise. Immediately post burn, patients can be started on oxandrolone (synthetic anabolic steroid, typical starting dose 10 mg twice daily or .1 mg/kg for pediatric patients), which has been shown to reduce mortality and hospital length of stay.[12] As burn patients are often persistently in a hypermetabolic state after their burns have healed, oxandrolone can be continued to maintain lean body mass and bone mineral density after discharge from acute care or inpatient rehabilitation. The body's stress response with increased catecholamines and cortisol is typically managed with beta-blockers (e.g., propranolol) with a goal to reduce the patient's heart rate by 20%. This can help with retention of lean body mass, wound healing, and reduction of risk of posttraumatic stress disorder (PTSD). Blood glucose levels should be monitored and insulin is often required in the acute post-burn phase to maintain euglycemia (blood glucose 80–130 mg/dL preprandial and <180 mg/dL postprandial).

PRURITUS

The complication of pruritus overlying burns typically presents 3 months after the burn injury. Patients' urge to scratch pruritic sites may be quite severe; education and treatment can help prevent infection and delayed wound healing. Initial treatments for localized symptoms include application of a topical moisturizer multiple times a day, titrated to the patient's pruritic symptoms. Other topical treatments include colloidal oatmeal as a protective barrier and for moisturizing and easing the inflammation. For larger treatment areas, oral medications may be more practical and efficacious. Medications include antihistamines (e.g., diphenhydramine, hydroxyzine, cetirizine) and other agents such as doxepin and gabapentin.[13] Hydroxyzine pamoate is useful both for its antipruritic and anxiolytic properties. Additional nonpharmacologic treatments include laser therapy, massage, and transcutaneous nerve stimulation. The best evidence exists for pulsed dye laser therapy,[13] but there is limited evidence to delineate between the efficacy of these nonpharmacologic treatments when treating pruritus.

HETEROTOPIC OSSIFICATION

Heterotopic ossification (HO) is the formation of ectopic bone in the soft tissue. Risk factors for HO include >30% of the TBSA burn injury. Presenting symptoms of HO include palpable firmness of the skin, pain, and erythema. Patients most commonly develop HO in the posterior elbow of the affected limb. Pharmacologic management remains controversial. While bisphosphonates have been traditionally a recommended treatment, the evidence for their use remains mixed. There is some suggestion that nonsteroidal anti-inflammatories show promise for treatment and prevention, more specifically cyclooxygenase-2 variants, due to less gastrointestinal toxicity.[14] The efficacy of surgical interventions depends on the timing and volume of soft tissue involvement. Surgical resection of the involved tissue has been shown to improve the ROM of the elbow and a small number of recurrences the year following the operation.[15] Aggressive ROM has been discouraged as this may potentially exacerbate the risk of HO development and progression.[14]

PSYCHIATRIC COMPLICATIONS

There is an increased incidence of psychological disorders in burn survivors. Depression and anxiety prevalence can be as high as 65%.[16] Patients often develop acute stress disorder during their acute care hospitalization and continue to have symptoms through rehabilitation. Patients are also at high risk of developing PTSD, with an incidence between 25% and 45%.[17] PTSD can emerge during the rehabilitation phase. Early intervention by psychology and psychiatry is essential to assist in the management of psychological symptoms. Treatment regimens include cognitive processing therapy and prolonged exposure therapy. Many patients also suffer from an altered body image. Body image satisfaction is typically associated with gender as well as percent of TBSA involvement. Referral for peer-to-peer counseling and support groups such as the Phoenix Society for Burn Survivors are important resources for these patients.[18]

COMMUNITY REINTEGRATION

Community reintegration is an important aspect of burn rehabilitation. In pediatric patients, male gender, length of hospitalization, and age were found to be associated with longer time until return to school.[19] Negative predictors of return to work at 12 months include prolonged hospital stay, need for inpatient rehabilitation, electrical burns, and burns at work.[20] For patients who are burned in the work environment, PTSD often remains a significant barrier for return to their original work environment. Other barriers include pain, neurologic problems, and impaired mobility. Early psychiatric intervention can be integral to a successful transition to work in these patients by employing treatments such as cognitive processing therapy and prolonged exposure therapy.

REFERENCES

The full complete reference list for this chapter appears in the digital version of the chapter, available at http://connect.springerpub.com/content/book/978-0-8261-5628-0/part/part02/chapter/ch11

CHAPTER 12

CANCER REHABILITATION
Samman Shahpar, Ishan Roy, Eric W. Villanueva, and Madeline Flores

EPIDEMIOLOGY

Cancer is one of the largest causes of morbidity and mortality across the United States and worldwide. On average, more than 1.6 million people are diagnosed with cancer each year in the United States.[1] Based on incidence rates, the leading cancers in the United States include breast, lung, prostate, colorectal, and melanoma. Over the next several decades, the number of new cases is projected to increase, and along with new scientific advancements and technologies so too will survival rates. In 2019, the estimated number of cancer survivors in the United States was 16.9 million, which is expected to increase to 22 million by 2030.[2] Despite improved survival rates, cancer survivors are often left with physical, cognitive, or psychological impairments, providing an opportunity for rehabilitation.

Cancer rehabilitation aims to improve function and promote physical, social, and emotional well-being to maximize one's quality of life related to cancer or its treatment. Cancer patients suffer from a wide variety of symptoms, including fatigue, pain, neuropathy, muscle wasting, cognitive dysfunction, mobility difficulties, lymphedema, dysphagia, bowel and bladder changes, and psychosocial distress.[3] Rehabilitation has been shown to be beneficial at all stages of cancer diagnosis and treatment and is available in clinical settings across the care continuum, including acute inpatient rehabilitation, acute consult services, subacute services, outpatient clinics, and hospice units. The most common cancers that may require care in inpatient rehabilitation facilities include those that affect the central nervous system, gastrointestinal, musculoskeletal, and hematologic systems. In one retrospective study surveying 70% of all inpatient rehabilitation facilities in the United States, most cancer patients admitted improved their function and were discharged to the community.[4] As more people survive and overcome their initial disease, the need for rehabilitation becomes paramount.

EFFECTS OF CANCER

Muscle Wasting

Muscle wasting disorders such as cachexia and sarcopenia are a significant source of impairment in patients with cancer. Cachexia is pathologically defined as muscle loss despite adequate nutrition in the setting of chronic disease-related inflammation.[5] Approximately half of all cancer patients will be affected by cachexia during the course of their disease and it can occur both at the early and late stages of the disease.[6] While cachexia is more closely associated with specific cancers,

TABLE 12.1 Consensus Cachexia Diagnostic Criteria[8]

Cachexia Categories	BMI Threshold	Weight Threshold in 6 Months
Cachexia	BMI ≥20 kg/m²	>5% weight loss
	BMI <20 kg/m²	>2% weight loss
Precachexia	–	0%–5% weight loss
No cachexia	–	No weight loss

BMI, body mass index.

including those of gastrointestinal, lung, or hematologic origin, it can affect patients with almost any type of cancer on an individual basis. It has historically been diagnosed using the weight of the patient in the prior 6 months (Table 12.1), although more modern screening tools that involve specific body mass index and weight deciles, as well as serum markers, are emerging.

Cachexia is often referred to as part of the cachexia-anorexia syndrome, which incorporates the multiple systemic effects of chronic inflammation seen along with weight loss, including loss of appetite, fatigue, change in sex endocrine function, and cardiovascular deconditioning. Screening for cachexia during functional assessment of cancer patients is recommended. Multidisciplinary inpatient and outpatient rehabilitation programs that also include nutritional guidance can help to not only reverse weight loss in cachectic patients, but almost improve muscle strength, physical function, fatigue, and quality of life.

By contrast, primary sarcopenia is defined as age-related muscle loss. The diagnostic criteria for sarcopenia have evolved over time to include strength/physical performance assessment and can now be diagnosed with cut-off points for grip strength, gait speed, and other physical performance tests, along with body composition evaluation via imaging (e.g., CT, MRI, DEXA, and bioimpedance).[7] While primary sarcopenia is not specifically due to a patient's cancer, it is a risk factor that should be screened for in cancer patients given its link to adverse outcomes related to cancer treatment. More broadly, sarcopenia is a significant source of disability in older adults and can be addressed with rehabilitation, exercise, and nutritional interventions.

Fatigue

While fatigue can occur due to muscle wasting disease in cancer patients, cancer-related fatigue (CRF) is a syndrome that can affect a much broader fraction of cancer patients. CRF is defined as persistent tiredness that is disproportionate to activity and prevents daily functioning.[9] Sources of fatigue include both the cancer itself and its treatments (see Effects of Cancer Treatments section) and affects between 70% and 100% of all cancer patients.[10] Importantly, fatigue manifests through physical, cognitive, or emotional symptoms, although the underlying etiology of these distinct presentations is unclear. Several studies have shown that exercise can be an effective intervention for CRF and most likely should include both aerobic and resistant modes. Recent studies have also suggested that patients with persistent or chronic fatigue with primarily cognitive or emotional symptoms may respond to multidisciplinary approaches that also include psychological assessment and intervention, such as cognitive behavioral therapy.[11]

Bone Metastases

As part of the evaluation prior to starting any exercise or rehabilitation intervention, the presence and status of any bony metastases need to be assessed in order to determine the risk of fracture and need for any precautions. Bony metastases may occur in the extremities or axial skeleton. They may be diagnosed on staging imaging without symptoms, although pain is often a presenting symptom. If a bony metastatic lesion is suspected, the patient should be placed on precautions to minimize stress on the area of concern. Precautions may include limiting weight-bearing, lifting, and/or range of motion depending on the location of the suspected lesion. In a patient with known malignancy, there should be a low threshold for imaging.

In 1989, Dr. Hilton Mirels published a scoring system to quantify the risk of sustaining a pathologic fracture from a metastatic lesion in the long bones. The scoring system is characterized by four categories, namely the site of the lesion, the type of the lesion, the size of the lesion, and the amount of pain. Each category is graded from 1 to 3, with a total score of 8 or higher indicating a higher risk of pathologic fracture and consideration of prophylactic fixation prior to radiation treatment.[12]

Axial metastatic lesions are assessed based on any neurologic compromise as well as spinal stability. Spinal stability should be assessed via the Spine Instability Neoplastic Score (SINS). The scoring system is characterized by six categories, namely the site of the lesion, amount of pain, type of the lesion, spinal alignment, amount of vertebral collapse and tumor involvement contributing to spinal instability, and invasion of the tumor of the posterior structures of the spine. A total score of 7 or higher indicates pending spinal instability, a total score of 13 or higher indicates spinal instability, while surgical stabilization should be considered with any score of 7 or higher.[13]

Hematologic Changes

Anemia, thrombocytopenia, and neutropenia are known common complications that can occur due to cancer and/or cancer treatments. Complications may be transient or persistent and thus need to be considered during any rehabilitation intervention or exercise recommendation. However, there is a limited amount of evidence to guide specific activities based on the hematologic issue.

Individuals with anemia generally tolerate most rehabilitation interventions and exercises without complications. While the absolute level is important, symptoms, such as fatigue and shortness of breath, and comorbidities, specifically cardiac and cardiovascular diseases, are often the most important factors and should be considered in any interventions or modifications in activity. In many institutions, the threshold for transfusion is a hemoglobin level of <7 g/dL if there are no symptoms, significant comorbidities, or recent bleeding complication, and <8 g/dL if symptomatic, with significant comorbidities, or had a recent bleeding complication. However, these guidelines often vary on a case-by-case basis. With regard to activity restrictions, if hemoglobin is <8 g/dL, limiting progressive and/or high-intensity aerobic activity or resistance exercises should be considered, but should also be evaluated on a case-by-case basis.

Thrombocytopenia tends to be the most activity-limiting hematologic complication due to the risk of bleeding. With progressively lower levels of platelets, the risk of spontaneous bleeding increases, even without any rehabilitation or activity intervention. There have been limited studies that have clearly linked rehabilitation or activity interventions with increased bleeding in patients with thrombocytopenia, but it is common knowledge that certain activities and rehabilitation interventions may have an increased risk of trauma or injury to soft and connective tissues, including muscles, which will increase the risk of bleeding. Consideration of activity restrictions and limitation of resistance exercises generally starts with platelet level <50,000/μL based off of historical guidelines and known risks of spontaneous bleeding. The risks of bleeding need to be balanced with delays in rehabilitation interventions that can compound the weakness and impairments experienced in this patient population, even when platelets drop below 20,000/μL.[14]

Neutropenia needs to be considered primarily when determining the appropriate rehabilitation or exercise setting. Group or public settings are generally avoided, if possible, and any interactions between rehabilitation or exercise professionals and a neutropenic patient should be undertaken with appropriate personal protective equipment, including masks and gloves. Medical interventions to avoid would include any rectal manipulation, including with suppositories or enemas.

EFFECTS OF CANCER TREATMENTS

Chemotherapy-Induced Peripheral Neuropathy

Chemotherapy-induced peripheral neuropathy (CIPN) is a common neurologic sequela of many treatment regimens contributing to morbidity and significantly affecting the quality of life of many cancer survivors. The incidence is approximately 30% to 40% for all cancer patients.[15] This side effect is dose-dependent, but the exact severity depends on the agent, dose, route of administration, and duration.[16] It can affect cancer outcomes by resulting in dose reduction or early discontinuation of treatment. CIPN is classically linked with drugs such as platinum-based agents, taxanes, and vinca alkaloids, and some immunotherapies such as bortezomib. Clinical presentation includes sensory-predominant symmetric distal numbness and tingling, pain, and difficulty with fine motor tasks. This occurs due to damage to the dorsal root ganglion, axons, or sensory nerve terminals. Motor and autonomic symptoms can occur depending on the agent, but are less common (Table 12.2). Typically, symptoms start in the

TABLE 12.2 Common Presentations of Chemotherapy-Induced Neuropathy[15,19,20]

Drug Class	Mechanism	Sensory	Motor	Autonomic	Additional Features
Platinum compounds (cisplatin, oxaliplatin)	Nuclear and mitochondrial DNA damage	Stocking glove LE>UE	Normal	Rare	Coasting phenomenon
Taxanes	Stabilization of microtubules	Stocking glove LE>UE	LE weakness	Rare	Rare optic neuropathy
Vinca alkaloids	Destabilization of microtubules	LE sensory loss, rare UE involvement	Symmetric LE weakness	Constipation, orthostatic hypotension	Occasional cranial nerve involvement
Proteasome inhibitors		Stocking glove distribution	LE weakness	GI effects (constipation/diarrhea), orthostatic hypotension	
Immunomodulating agents		Stocking glove distribution	Mild weakness of all extremities	Constipation	

GI, gastrointestinal; LE, lower extremity; UE, upper extremity.

first several months following initiation of chemotherapy, progress throughout treatment, and plateau following completion. However, in platinum-based regimens, CIPN symptoms may worsen following chemotherapy cessation, known as the "coasting phenomenon." Risk factors for developing CIPN include older age, diabetes, and preexisting peripheral neuropathies.[16] There is currently no preventive treatment; however, neuropathic agents such as duloxetine or gabapentin can be used for paresthesia. Multiple studies have demonstrated that exercise can also help mitigate symptoms related to CIPN.[17] Although data are limited, questionnaires such as the European Organization for Research and Treatment of Cancer (EORTC) and the CIPN Rasch-built Overall Disability Scale (R-ODS) have been developed to quantify the extent of disability and the impact on quality of life that CIPN has in these patients.[18]

Hormonal/Endocrine Therapy

Hormonal therapy is a form of cancer treatment which aims to target hormone production for a wide variety of tumors, including breast, prostate, endometrial, and adrenal cancers. Side effects depend on the agent but can include systemic symptoms such as fatigue, mood changes, hot flashes, or weight gain. For hormone receptor-positive breast cancer, aromatase inhibitors are often used. One common side effect is the aromatase inhibitor musculoskeletal syndrome (AIMSS). Prior studies indicate an incidence of at least 50% in women starting aromatase inhibitors.[21] Although there are no diagnostic criteria, AIMSS can present as symmetrical pain over widespread joints of the upper and lower extremities, including the shoulders, hands, knees, hips, lower back, and feet. Presentation can be associated with morning stiffness and extra-articular manifestations, including myalgia, tendinopathy, or neuropathy.[22] Symptoms arise in the first few of months of aromatase inhibitor treatment and are correlated with eventual disease progression and worsened quality of life. The pathophysiology of this syndrome is not completely understood but is believed to be associated with estrogen deprivation in the neurologic and musculoskeletal systems. Management of AIMSS includes analgesia with nonsteroidal anti-inflammatory drugs or duloxetine, aerobic and resistance-based exercise, vitamin D supplementation, and omega-3 fatty acid supplementation.[23]

Immunotherapy and Cellular Therapies

Immunotherapy aims to harness the body's immune system to prevent and control malignancy. The spectrum of immunotherapeutic modalities includes therapeutic cancer vaccines, immunostimulatory cytokines (interleukin [IL]-2, IFN-α, interferon [IL]-12, granulocyte macrophage-colony stimulating factor [GM-CSF], and tumor necrosis factor-α [TNF]-α), immunomodulator monoclonal antibodies, and more recently adoptive cell and gene therapies. Historically used in patients with end-stage cancer or patients who have failed other therapies, immunotherapy today is also considered a first-line treatment for a wide range of cancers (Box 12.1).[24,25] The two main strategies of cancer immunotherapy are to reduce tumor-mediated immunosuppression by blocking the negative regulators of the immune system to enhance antitumor response and to provide activated immune cells or materials to prime immune cells against tumor cells. These effects of immunotherapy offer a long-term adaptive immune response that can fight against established cancer, prevent cancer progression, and preclude new metastases. Side effects of immunotherapy in general include autoimmune manifestations, as well as rash, pruritus, colitis, nausea, vomiting, hepatotoxicity, adrenalitis, pancytopenia, isolated neutropenia, and respiratory or urinary tract infections. Many new immunotherapies are under development and investigation in clinical trials, and the list of cancers treated by immunotherapy is expanding.

Adoptive immunotherapy with genetically modified T cells is a relatively new and expanding immunotherapy modality. Chimeric antigen receptor (CAR) T cell therapy involves the harvesting of T cells from cancer patients, followed by manipulation and reintroduction of

> **BOX 12.1** Cancers Treated by Immunotherapies Approved by the Food and Drug Administration[25]
>
> Chronic lymphocytic leukemia
> Non-Hodgkin lymphoma
> Hodgkin lymphoma
> Acute leukemia
> Breast cancer
> Lung cancer
> Colorectal cancer
> Bladder cancer
> Prostate cancer
> Renal cell carcinoma
> Basal cell carcinoma
> Melanoma
> Cervical cancer
> Hepatocellular carcinoma
> Soft tissue tumors

> **BOX 12.2** Cancers Treated by Chimeric Antigen Receptor T Cell Therapy[25]
>
> Neuroblastoma
> Hepatocellular cancers
> Gastric cancer
> Metastatic melanoma
> Hematologic malignancies
> Colorectal cancer
> Breast cancer
> Ovarian cancer
> Renal cell carcinoma
> Advanced lung cancer
> Nasopharyngeal carcinoma

primed T cells into the patient. The T cells are engineered to express the T cell receptor necessary for tumor recognition or to express CAR, which directly binds to tumor antigens and activates an antitumor immune response.[26] Initially used in the treatment of lymphoma patients, CAR T cell therapy treats a growing list of cancers (Box 12.2). CAR T cell patients should be monitored for signs or symptoms of cytokine release syndrome (CRS), a dangerous systemic inflammatory response which manifests as fever with or without multiple organ dysfunction 1 to 14 days after CAR T cell therapy. Patients can also develop immune effector cell-associated neurotoxicity syndrome (ICANS), an encephalopathic syndrome often in conjunction with CRS. For both syndromes, patients may need an ICU level of care.[27,28]

Radiation Therapy

Radiation therapy (RT) is a cancer treatment modality that aims to maximize quality of life and tumor control while minimizing toxicity and preserving organs. RT may be used solely or concurrently with other treatment modalities. For example, RT before or after surgery in breast cancer can reduce local relapse and improve overall survival.[29] RT can be used as a single-modality definitive treatment for laryngeal, oropharyngeal, and prostate cancers. Additionally, RT can be used to relieve symptoms, such as painful bone metastases, in incurable disease.[30] The types of RT can be differentiated by source of radiation. External beam RT delivers radiation from a source outside the patient, while brachytherapy involves placing the radiation source inside or near a target area in the body. Other modalities include intraoperative RT and targeted radionucleotide therapy, which utilizes decaying radionucleotides in specific body locations. The mechanism of action involves damaging the double-stranded structure of DNA within cancer cells through ionization, which leads to cancer cell death. However, both tumor and normal cells in the area of treatment may be affected. Normal cells are generally able to repair damage from ionization, whereas cancerous cells, which disinhibit cell repair mechanisms to promote tumor growth, lack these repair mechanisms and are preferentially damaged by RT.

Patients can experience multiple acute side effects from RT in tissues having cells with high turnover rates, such as the gastrointestinal mucosa, bone marrow, skin, and oropharyngeal and esophageal mucosa. Side effects are often related to the location of treatment; for example, irradiating the head and neck can lead to mouth and throat sores. Adverse effects can include integumentary changes including alopecia and lymphedema; gastrointestinal changes including stomatitis, mucositis, enteritis, and esophagitis; neurologic changes including somnolence and short-term memory loss; and genitourinary changes including urinary or bowel changes. These side effects may occur during the course of therapy or within 1 to 2 months of completion and typically resolve as tissue swelling and irritation decrease after treatment.[31] Long-term sequelae of RT include cardiac toxicities such as pericarditis or myocarditis, as well as infertility if the therapy field includes the testicles or ovaries. Over time, radiation exposure can cause progressive tissue fibrosis, which leads to the clinical syndrome called radiation fibrosis syndrome (RFS). This syndrome can present as pain, weakness, rigidity, spasms, or skin changes such as hyperpigmentation. The most commonly affected anatomic regions include the breast, head and neck, and connective tissues. Treatment is targeted at symptoms. For example, neuropathic pain may be treated with pregabalin, gabapentin, or duloxetine, whereas orthoses can address weaknesses such as foot drop.[32]

Surgery

The oldest of the modalities of cancer treatment, oncologic surgery aims to excise the tumor while leaving a surrounding margin of healthy tissue. Local tumor excision of many major cancer types, including breast, colorectal, gastric, esophageal, lung, and neurologic cancers, is common. Technological advances in surgery, specifically with the introduction of robotic, laparoscopic, and reconstructive surgical procedures, have reduced morbidity and mortality in contemporary radical cancer resections.[33] In combination with surgery, neoadjuvant therapies before surgery or adjuvant therapies after surgery can reduce the extent of surgery or render an inoperable disease operable. For example, a breast conservation surgery rate of greater than 70% for unifocal breast cancer was achieved with neoadjuvant chemotherapy in a disease previously judged suitable only for mastectomy.[34] More recently, the focus of oncologic surgery has shifted toward maintenance of form and function of the viscera and preservation of quality of life. Modern breast conservation surgery enables the surgeon to excise breast tissue while maintaining shape, resulting in better cosmetic outcomes and reduced rates of margin involvement.[35] Oncologic surgery also includes performing potentially curative resections of metastatic disease, and for those with incurable disease palliative surgery can ameliorate symptoms.

Lymphedema

Lymphedema is simply defined as edema as a result of dysfunction of the lymphatic system.[19] Although not isolated to oncology population, it is recognized as one of the most common impairments seen in this population. Although a detailed discussion of lymphedema is outside the scope of this chapter, we present some general principles when evaluating for cancer-related lymphedema.

Based on history of cancer and cancer-related treatment, ensure thorough examination of all potential areas of lymphedema including the breast, chest wall, inguinal, and genital areas. Musculoskeletal structures and biomechanics surrounding the area of concern should be assessed for postural abnormalities, range of motion limitations, and weakness. These abnormalities may limit lymphedema management.

It is important to recognize that not all edema is lymphedema. The differential for acute edema includes deep vein thrombosis, superficial thrombophlebitis, cellulitis, trauma-related focal swelling, and recurrent malignancy. The differential for chronic edema includes venous insufficiency and recurrent malignancy. Additionally, lymphedema may present without significant increase in size but changes in the texture of the cutaneous and subcutaneous tissue. Red flags suggesting alternative diagnoses include erythema, acute pain, fever, chills, and new-onset nodules, papules, or lumps.

REFERENCES

The full complete reference list for this chapter appears in the digital version of the chapter, available at http://connect.springerpub.com/content/book/978-0-8261-5628-0/part/part02/chapter/ch12

CHAPTER 13

TRANSPLANT REHABILITATION

Laura Malmut

EPIDEMIOLOGY

Transplantation is a definitive treatment option for patients with end-organ dysfunction. The field of solid organ transplantation has made tremendous progress since the first successful kidney transplant in 1954, owing to advancements in surgical technique, organ allocation protocols, and immunosuppression therapy. Solid organ transplantation has transformed the survival and quality of life of patients with end-stage diseases.[1] According to the United Network for Organ Sharing database, 39,719 organ transplantations were performed in 2019, including 7,397 living donor organ donations.[2,3] Common indications for organ transplantation are depicted in Table 13.1.

An increasing need for transplantation in combination with relatively low organ availability has resulted in progressively extended waiting list times for patients seeking transplantation.[4] As of October 2021, there are over 100,000 candidates on the national organ transplantation waiting list in the United States, including 90,260 kidney, 11,739 liver, 3,481 heart, and 987 lung candidates.[5]

Transplantations may be performed with organs from living donors or deceased donors by brain death or by cardiac death. The current era of organ shortage has necessitated a widening of criteria for donation that includes an increase in higher risk or extended criteria donors, including older organs and those with positive serology for viral pathology.[4]

Solid organ transplant recipients benefit from both a reduction in morbidity and increased survival. According to a 2015 study that looked at 25 years of transplantation data, compared with patients who remained on the waiting list, the median survival of transplant recipients was an additional 7 years for kidney transplants, 8.5 years for liver transplants, 7.2 years for heart transplants, and 2.9 years for lung transplants.[1]

PRETRANSPLANT CONSIDERATIONS

The pretransplant process begins when a patient with end-stage organ failure is referred to a transplant specialist. Pretransplant testing can take place in an outpatient or inpatient setting and varies depending on the transplant center and individual patient factors. The transplant team typically includes a medical and surgical team, transplant coordinator, social worker, and other specialists based on the patient's needs and comorbidities.[6,7]

The initial pretransplant medical evaluation includes a general health assessment and a detailed history and physical examination.

TABLE 13.1 Common Indications for Organ Transplantation

Kidney	Liver
ESRD due to: • Diabetes • HTN • Glomerulonephritis • Obstructive nephropathy • Cystic kidney disease	• Acute liver failure • HCV • NASH • Alcohol-related liver disease • Cholestatic liver disease • HCC
Heart	**Lung**
• Nonischemic cardiomyopathy • Coronary artery disease • Cardiogenic shock requiring inotropic therapy or mechanical circulatory support • Other (restrictive cardiomyopathy, congenital heart disease, hypertrophic cardiomyopathy)	• IPF • COPD • CF • A1ATD • PAH

A1ATD, alpha-1 antitrypsin deficiency; CF, cystic fibrosis; COPD, chronic obstructive pulmonary disease; ESRD, end-stage renal disease; HCC, hepatocellular carcinoma; HCV, hepatitis C virus; HTN, hypertension; IPF, idiopathic pulmonary fibrosis; NASH, nonalcoholic steatohepatitis; PAH, pulmonary arterial hypertension.

Active or chronic medical conditions are treated or optimized prior to transplantation. Testing generally includes routine laboratory studies, compatibility studies, and infectious workup. Serological testing is routinely performed for hepatitis viruses (hepatitis A, hepatitis B, and hepatitis C viruses), HIV, Epstein–Barr virus (EBV), cytomegalovirus (CMV), syphilis, and tuberculosis. Additional tests may be performed based on individual risk factors. Other assessments include cardiac tolerance for surgery, age-appropriate cancer screening, dental evaluation, and nutritional assessment.[6,7]

All vaccines that are appropriate for age, exposure history, and immune status should be administered prior to transplantation. In addition to the usual vaccine schedule, there are further recommendations for patients awaiting solid organ transplantation, which include hepatitis A, herpes zoster, and pneumococcal vaccination. Live virus vaccines should be administered in advance of transplantation due to posttransplant immunosuppression and risk of disseminated infection.[6,7]

Extensive patient and family education is done to make sure the patient understands the complexity of the proposed surgery, potential complications, implications of having a transplanted organ, and the importance of strict adherence to immunosuppressive medications. All potential transplant recipients should undergo a psychosocial evaluation to identify behavioral, social, and/or financial issues that may influence adherence and outcomes after transplantation. Ongoing substance abuse or dependence is a contraindication to transplantation.[6,7]

Ideally, a partnership between the transplant team and the rehabilitation team should begin before transplantation to maximize benefits and limit complications.[8] Nutritional status, baseline level of function, and rehabilitation potential are important factors to consider prior to transplantation. Frailty and poor functional capacity are associated with pretransplant morbidity, waitlist mortality, and poor surgical outcomes.[9-13] Correction of malnutrition is indicated.[13] Special consideration should be taken for referral to physical therapy to optimize functional status preoperatively.[8] Prehabilitation is well-tolerated in transplant candidates, effective at improving physical fitness, and has promising implications on postoperative outcomes.[9,14]

TRANSPLANT PHARMACOLOGY

The goal of immunosuppression therapy is to optimize allograft survival and prevent rejection while limiting drug toxicities. Protocols for immunosuppression can be divided into three general categories: induction, maintenance, and treatment of rejection (Figure 13.1).[6] Induction agents include anti-interleukin-2 receptor antibodies (basiliximab) or anti-thymocyte globulins that are administered before or at the time of surgery. Transplant recipients are then maintained on lifelong therapy that is titrated according to each transplant center's protocol. Tacrolimus and cyclosporine are dosed by 12-hour trough whole blood levels.[4,6]

Transplant recipients are susceptible to opportunistic infections. The risk of infection is highest during the early posttransplant period with maximal effects of immunosuppression therapy. Antimicrobial agents are prescribed to provide prophylaxis against certain viral, fungal, and bacterial infections.[6]

Common maintenance immunosuppressants and antimicrobials are described in Table 13.2.[6,15-18] Additional medications may be prescribed depending on individual risk factors and serological testing. Aspirin is often prescribed as prophylaxis against graft thrombosis.[19,20]

MEDICAL COMPLICATIONS

Several medical problems are routinely encountered following solid organ transplantation. Patients may have complications related to the surgery or a prolonged hospital course. Additional concerns are rejection, recurrence of underlying disease, and complications of immunosuppression therapy, which can include hypertension, renal

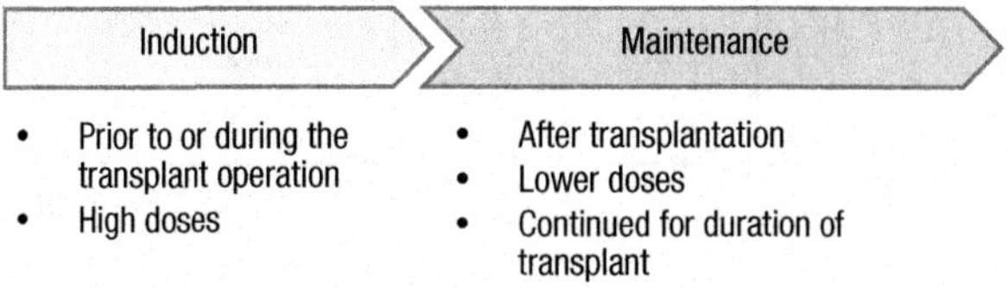

Induction	Maintenance
• Prior to or during the transplant operation • High doses	• After transplantation • Lower doses • Continued for duration of transplant

FIGURE 13.1 Phases of immunosuppression related to solid organ transplantation.

TABLE 13.2 Transplant Pharmacology

	Actions	Adverse Effects
Immunosuppression		
Calcineurin inhibitors • Tacrolimus • Cyclosporine	• Inhibitors of T cell activation (early) • Block IL-2 production	• Nephrotoxicity • Neurotoxicity • Posttransplant diabetes • Hyperkalemia • Hypomagnesemia • Hypertension • Hyperlipidemia
Antimetabolites • Mycophenolate • Azathioprine	• Inhibit purine synthesis required for T and B cell proliferation	• Diarrhea • Nausea • Leukopenia • Thrombocytopenia • Anemia • Hepatotoxicity and pancreatitis (azathioprine)
Corticosteroids • Prednisone • Methylprednisolone	• Nonspecific inhibitors of immune function • Block IL-1 production	• Hyperglycemia • Hypertension • Hyperlipidemia • Gastric ulcers • Osteoporosis • Suppression of HPA axis • Psychosis
mTOR inhibitors • Sirolimus • Everolimus	• Inhibitors of T cell activation (late) • Inhibit IL-2 activity and activation of cell cycle	• Hypertension • Hyperlipidemia • Peripheral edema • Anemia • Thrombocytopenia • Delayed wound healing • Interstitial lung disease • Headache • Mucositis • Proteinuria
Infection Prophylaxis		
Antibacterial • Trimethoprim-sulfamethoxazole • Atovaquone	• Pneumocystis pneumonia prophylaxis	• GI intolerance • Skin reactions • Cytopenias • Hyperkalemia • Sulfa allergy • *Clostridioides difficile* diarrhea • Dose adjustment in renal impairment

(continued)

TABLE 13.2 Transplant Pharmacology (*continued*)

	Actions	Adverse Effects
Antiviral • Valganciclovir • Acyclovir	• Valganciclovir: CMV and HSV prophylaxis • Acyclovir: HSV prophylaxis only	• GI intolerance • Cytopenias • Neurotoxicity • Dose adjustment in renal impairment
Antifungal • Fluconazole • Clotrimazole • Nystatin	• Systemic candidiasis prophylaxis (fluconazole) • Thrush prophylaxis (all three)	• Azoles inhibit CYP3A4 to reduce tacrolimus metabolism (and increase drug levels) • QTc prolongation • GI intolerance • Skin reactions

CMV, cytomegalovirus; GI, gastrointestinal; HPA, hypothalamicpituitary axis; HSV, herpes simplex virus; IL, interleukin; mTOR, mammalian target of rapamycin.

insufficiency, infection, malignancy, a variety of dermatologic conditions, avascular necrosis, osteoporosis, and metabolic derangements such as diabetes, obesity, and hyperlipidemia.[21]

Graft function surveillance is typically performed through serial laboratory monitoring, imaging, and other noninvasive tests. Heart transplants may additionally undergo interval right heart catheterization with endomyocardial biopsy to screen for rejection. Similarly, lung transplants may undergo interval bronchoscopies.[6] Protocols vary per transplant center.

SPECIAL CONSIDERATIONS FOR INPATIENT REHABILITATION

The inpatient rehabilitation unit offers an ideal setting for postoperative transplant recipient patients to receive therapies to improve functional status while allowing for close medical oversight.[8] Given the need for frequent medication titration, laboratory monitoring, the large number of potential interactions, and the high risk of complications, collaborative treatment between the rehabilitation physicians and the transplant team will help minimize adverse events and reduce readmissions to acute care.[22] Deconditioning and frailty due to end-stage disease prior to transplantation are compounded by the effects of major surgery and prolonged hospitalization, which may result in further weakness, myopathy, neuropathy, and other immobility-associated complications.[22] Postoperative restrictions, including sternotomy precautions after heart transplantation and thoracotomy precautions after lung transplantation, will further impact the recovery course.[6,23] After cardiac transplantation, patients develop chronotropic incompetence and diminished exercise capacity due to denervation of the transplanted heart. Resting tachycardia develops due to loss of parasympathetic input through the vagus nerve, which modulates the sinoatrial and atrioventricular nodes to slow the native heart rate. With the loss of sympathetic innervation, the donor heart is dependent on circulating catecholamines to increase heart rate, with a delayed heart rate peak and fall after exercise.[6]

A rehabilitation treatment plan should be devised with involvement of an interdisciplinary team of physicians, therapists, nurses, wound care specialists, social workers, and psychologists if available. A comprehensive rehabilitation program can significantly improve physical function, mobility, and independence of debilitated transplant recipients, with a high likelihood of achieving home discharge. Compared with a general rehabilitation inpatient population, transplant rehabilitation inpatients have higher rates of readmission to acute care and a longer mean length of stay. At discharge from inpatient rehabilitation, close follow-up with the transplant team and other necessary specialists should be scheduled.[22]

REFERENCES

The full complete reference list for this chapter appears in the digital version of the chapter, available at http://connect.springerpub.com/content/book/978-0-8261-5628-0/part/part02/chapter/ch13

CHAPTER 14

EFFECTS OF DEBILITY AND IMMOBILITY

Carley N. Sauter, Sarah Wineman, and Nethra S. Ankam

DEFINITIONS

Reduced mobility is commonly seen in patients cared for by physical medicine and rehabilitation physicians and is a contributor to debility and morbidity. The effects of immobility are widespread, affecting all systems of the body, and efforts to reduce immobility may result in better patient outcomes. Debility is commonly defined as weakness or infirmity due to illness or disease. A single concept of immobility for medical inpatients has not been clearly defined and varies by study. Immobility is considered to be on a continuum of fully bedridden to reduced mobility.[1] However, several frameworks to further delineate immobility and debility have been outlined.

Perhaps the most common definition of activity is through use of the metabolic equivalent unit (MET) framework. One MET is defined as the oxygen consumption of a 70-kg, 40-year-old man resting quietly. Using this framework, "sedentary activity" is defined as 1 to 1.5 METs or the energy expenditure of sitting and resting quietly. Examples of sedentary activity include sleeping, sitting quietly, and lying down, as well as most screen-based activities. Sedentary activity is known to increase morbidity and mortality.[2]

Frailty is a related measure of debility. Frailty is commonly defined as a condition characterized by loss of biological reserves across multiple organ systems, failure of homeostatic mechanisms, and vulnerability to physiologic decompensation after minor stressor events.[3] While frailty may be linked to the aging process, it can also be seen in chronic disease states in other patients. There are several commonly accepted ways of measuring frailty. The phenotype model identifies frailty based on five physical characteristics: weight loss, exhaustion, low energy expenditure, slow gait speed, and reduced grip strength. People without these characteristics are considered "fit," those with one or two of these characteristics are considered "pre-frail," and those with three or more are considered "frail." Another model is the cumulative deficit model, which identifies frailty based on a range of deficit variables, including clinical signs, symptoms, disease, disabilities, and abnormal labs leading to a frailty index score.[3] The syndrome of frailty, regardless of how it is measured, is a contributor to the systemic insults that occur with immobility.

EFFECT OF DEBILITY AND IMMOBILITY ON ORGAN SYSTEMS

Cardiopulmonary

Decreased activity can have numerous deleterious effects on the cardiopulmonary system. Prolonged bedrest results in deconditioning of the diaphragm and intercostal muscles. This leads to difficulty clearing secretions and a weakened cough, which can put patients at risk of a number of complications, including atelectasis and pneumonia.

Immobility decreases one's overall cardiopulmonary fitness. Over time, resting heart rate will increase while stroke volume will decrease.[4] Maximal oxygen consumption (VO_2) max is often considered an excellent indicator of fitness and aerobic endurance as it is the maximum oxygen that can be utilized by a person performing maximal activity. Multiple studies have found that 10 days of bedrest in healthy adults reduces VO_2 max by over 10%.[5,6]

Immobility results in multiple circulatory changes. Prolonged supine positioning increases renal blood flow and promotes diuresis, effectively decreasing circulating fluid volume. This can result in orthostatic hypotension as the remaining volume pools in the lower extremities and cardiac output is unable to adequately compensate.[7] Similarly, bedrest can cause an increased risk of venous thromboembolism (VTE). Patients with reduced mobility will often have elements of the Virchow triad, which includes endothelial dysfunction/damage, stasis of blood flow, and hypercoagulability. Prolonged bedrest (>14 days) leads to a fivefold increased risk of deep vein thrombosis and reduced mobility leads to a twofold to threefold increased risk of VTE.[1]

Musculoskeletal

Immobility can quickly lead to a significant weakening of the musculoskeletal system, with an estimated decrease in muscle mass of .5% to .6% per day[8] and loss of muscle strength of 2% to 10% per week.[9–11] Similarly, sarcopenia is defined as loss of skeletal muscle mass or function, and has traditionally been associated with aging but can also be seen in patients with other disease states, including acutely, such as with sudden immobility during hospitalization, or chronically associated with chronic disease.[12] Diagnosis requires measurement of muscle mass, muscle strength, and physical performance, and can be seen in obese as well as in normal- or low-weight patients. Sarcopenia is associated with adverse outcomes in patients, including falls, frailty, and mortality.[12] Bedrest tends to have greater deleterious effects as individuals age, and older adults can lose almost 1 kg of lean tissue from the lower extremities after 10 days of bedrest.[6]

In addition to decreased muscle mass and strength, immobility can put individuals at risk of joint contractures. Contractures are a complex phenomenon that involves both shortening of muscle sarcomeres and changes within the joint capsule itself, causing an irreversible decrease in range of motion.[13,14] For those who exclusively use bed or wheelchair, the hip flexors, knee flexors, and ankle plantar flexors are at particular risk.

Finally, prolonged bedrest decreases the stress on weight-bearing bones, leading to decreased osteoblast and increased osteoclast activity. Over time, this mismatch results in altered calcium homeostasis, decreased bone mineral density, and development of osteopenia.[10–15]

Gastrointestinal and Genitourinary

Bedrest and immobility can also cause gastrointestinal (GI) and genitourinary (GU) complications. Without the assistance of gravity, acid reflux can develop or become more problematic. Additionally, prolonged bedrest increases the risk of constipation.[16] Bedrest can have similar gravity-associated effects on the GU system. In nursing home residents, supine voiding may be associated with incomplete bladder emptying, putting individuals at risk of urinary tract infections.[17] However, positioning does not seem to have the same effect in healthy adult men.[18] Finally, as bone homeostasis changes and bone breakdown occurs, individuals become more at risk of kidney and bladder stones from hypercalciuria.[19]

Endocrine

Bedrest and immobility increase insulin resistance, an effect that is seen particularly in skeletal muscle tissue.[20,21] These changes occur quickly. Studies show a single day of sitting can reduce the effect of insulin even when calorie intake is limited to match decreased energy expenditure.[22] Additionally, fat metabolism changes significantly with bedrest. Adipose tissue accumulates centrally in the abdomen and liver, further predisposing sedentary individuals to metabolic syndrome and type 2 diabetes.[21]

Integumentary

The skin as an organ system is vulnerable to injury with immobility. Pressure injuries may result from prolonged immobility, with an incidence of over 20% in acute healthcare settings.[23] Pressure injuries are most common at bony prominences and sites of pressure or shear, such as the ischium, sacrum, greater trochanter, and heels. They are also more common in patients with reduced mobility, older adults, and individuals with motor, sensory, or cognitive impairments.[24] In patients with stroke, out-of-bed mobilization during hospitalization is shown to reduce pressure injury.[25]

REFERENCES

The full complete reference list for this chapter appears in the digital version of the chapter, available at http://connect.springerpub.com/content/book/978-0-8261-5628-0/part/part02/chapter/ch14

CHAPTER 15

MEDICAL COMPLICATIONS DURING REHABILITATION

Kim Barker and Martin Laguerre

INTRODUCTION

People who require admission to an inpatient rehabilitation facility are becoming more and more medically complex with various comorbidities. They are also being admitted at earlier points in their recovery. Despite the variety of medical comorbidities, there are certain complications that can inhibit the rehabilitation process and these are detailed in this chapter.

HETEROTOPIC OSSIFICATION

Heterotopic ossification (HO) is the formation of lamellar bone at an abnormal anatomic site, usually in the soft tissue, due to the metaplasia of mesenchymal cells into osteoblasts. No definitive pathogenesis has been established on the etiology of HO. Precipitating factors include musculoskeletal trauma (e.g., fracture, burn injury, or joint replacement surgery) and neurologic pathology (e.g., spinal cord injury [SCI], stroke, and traumatic brain injury [TBI]). Risk factors for HO include prolonged immobilization, degree of spasticity, completeness of injury (SCI), pressure injury in proximity of the joint, and presence of deep vein thrombosis (DVT).[1] With SCI, common HO sites include (in order of occurrence) the hip (anterior-medial aspects), knee, elbow, shoulder, and feet. With burn injury, common HO sites (in order of occurrence) include the elbow (posterior > anterior), shoulder, and hip. Interestingly, HO locations do not necessarily coincide with the area of the burn. Burns involving >20% of the body have a higher risk of HO.[1] Hip HO is commonly seen following total hip arthroplasty (THA). HO may occur at the distal end of amputated limbs. Overall, HO is typically seen around large joints and below the levels of the neurologic injury.

Symptoms of HO may include heat/warmth, edema, pain, and loss of joint mobility in the later stages. If HO is suspected, a plain x-ray or a three-phase bone scan may be obtained. The bone scan may be positive at least 1 week before the x-ray is positive; phases 1 and 2 (flow phase and blood pool phase) of the bone scan are highly sensitive. Some complications of HO include peripheral nerve entrapment, pressure ulcers, and functional impairment if joint ankylosis develops.

Heterotopic Ossification Treatment

Resting the acutely involved joint for up to 2 weeks is recommended to reduce inflammation and microscopic hemorrhage.[2] Ice may also be helpful. While still controversial, gentle and painless (passive and/or active) range of motion (ROM) exercises are recommended to maintain joint mobility.[3] More aggressive ROM may be initiated after the first 2 weeks, but must be curtailed if erythema or swelling increases.[2] Immobilization in a functional position is prudent, particularly if ankylosis is inevitable.

There is no definitive standard medical treatment for HO. Medical options include indomethacin at 75 mg/d if creatinine phosphokinase (CPK) is elevated (administered until CPK normalizes) or etidronate (dosing varies based on CPK) for 6 months. Nonsteroidal anti-inflammatory drugs (NSAIDs) inhibit prostaglandin E2, a major contributor of HO formation. Other NSAIDs can be used for prophylaxis (e.g., ibuprofen, meloicam, celecoxib, diclofenac), but indomethacin is still preferred for treatment.[4] Etidronate is thought to reduce further HO formation by reducing osteoblasticosteoclastic activity and calcium phosphate precipitation.[2] Medical therapy does not treat HO that has already formed; it is intended to prevent additional HO formation. Etidronate had previously been used for HO prophylaxis, but data are limited and it is not commonly used in this manner.

Radiation therapy has been used to prevent and/or treat HO in post-THA patients, although it is primarily used as prophylaxis in people with known prior HO.[3]

Surgical resection may be indicated to address significant functional limitations. The ideal surgical candidate has no joint pain or swelling, is 12 to 18 months post injury, and has a three-phase bone scan demonstrating mature HO. It is important to ensure that the HO has reached maturity before resection because resection of immature HO leads to recurrence rates of nearly 100%. Gentle, early (within 48 hours) postoperative ROM is recommended.[2]

DEEP VENOUS THROMBOSIS

DVT is a condition in which a blood clot forms in a vein. Risk factors for DVT include history of venous thromboembolism (VTE), major trauma, immobility, surgery lasting >2 hours, cancer, long-distance travel, paralysis, SCI, prolonged hospitalization, smoking, congestive heart failure, central venous access devices, increased estrogen states, pregnancy, brain injury, stroke, obesity, chronic obstructive pulmonary disease, and inherited coagulopathies.[5] Greater than 90% of DVTs occur in the lower limbs, with approximately 25% of distal DVTs propagating to the proximal veins. Most pulmonary embolisms are associated with proximal DVTs of the lower limbs that are located above the knee. Compression ultrasonography with Doppler is the gold standard imaging test in patients with suspected DVT.

Selected Prophylaxis and Treatment Options

Unfractionated heparin (UFH): UFH binds with antithrombin III to inhibit factor IIa (thrombin) and factors IXa, Xa, XIa, and XIIa (intrinsic clotting pathway). Initial treatment of a DVT in the absence of contraindications is typically intravenous (IV) UFH due to its quick onset, ease of reversibility (protamine sulfate), and ease of transitioning to other agents. UFH is also used subcutaneously prophylactically, particularly if the patient has end stage renal disease (ESRD) or is an older adult.[6]

Low-molecular-weight heparin (LMWH): The mechanism of action is similar to UFH, but the reduced binding with plasma proteins results in a longer and more predictable half-life. For prophylaxis, enoxaparin (Lovenox) 40 mg daily given subcutaneously is generally the standard dose for patients during the rehabilitation stay or until they are ambulating longer distances. LMWH is contraindicated in heparin-induced thrombocytopenia (HIT). LMWH is excreted renally and does require dosing adjustments based on creatinine clearance (in general its use is avoided in patients with ESRD).[6]

Warfarin (vitamin K antagonist): Warfarin inhibits the vitamin K-mediated production of procoagulant factors X, IX, VII, and II (extrinsic pathway) and anticoagulant proteins C and S. There is an initial paradoxical procoagulant effect since proteins C and S are depleted first; thus, patients are normally bridged when starting these medications. Warfarin and other vitamin K antagonists can be reversed with administration of vitamin K or prothrombin complex concentrate dosing depending on international normalized ratios (INR) and the presence of symptoms (bleeding or decreasing hemoglobin). These medications require regular monitoring of INR and dosing adjustments based on the patient's diet.[7]

Select direct oral anticoagulants (DOACs): Compared with heparin and warfarin, DOACs provide the advantage of lower risk of bleeding, less need for laboratory monitoring (due to wider therapeutic windows), and improved pharmacokinetic profiles. However, they do not have an accessible reversal agent and thus carry an increased risk of uncontrolled bleeding if a person falls or sustains another injury while on this medication. DOACs are generally more expensive than warfarin. Dabigatran (Pradaxa) is an active direct thrombin inhibitor which inhibits clot-bound and circulating thrombin. Dabigatran can be used if a patient is diagnosed with or suspected of having HIT. Rivaroxaban (Xarelto) and apixaban (Eliquis) are both factor Xa inhibitors. Both rivaroxaban and apixaban are generally used for DVT treatment (after transitioning from UFH). Both rivaroxaban and apixaban, like LMWH, are excreted renally and do require dosing adjustments based on creatinine clearance.[5]

Other: Inferior vena cava filters are used for pulmonary embolism (not DVT) prophylaxis in patients who have contraindications to anticoagulation.

Deep Vein Thrombosis Prophylaxis in Selected Conditions

Major orthopedic surgerytotal hip or knee arthroplasty (THA/TKA): The recommended options are LMWH, UFH, warfarin, or sequential compression devices (SCDs). LMWH is the preferred choice for THA, TKA, and hip fracture surgery. Dual prophylaxis with an antithrombotic

TABLE 15.1 Suggested Chemoprophylaxis Based on ASIA Grading

Complete SCI with other risk factors[a]	At least 12 weeks
Complete SCI without other risk factors[a]	At least 8 weeks
Incomplete SCI	During hospitalization

[a]Other risk factors include lower limb fracture, cancer, previous deep vein thrombosis, heart failure, obesity, and age >70 years.[6]

ASIA, American Spinal Injury Association; SCI, spinal cord injury.

Source: Hull RD, Garcia DA, Burnett AE. Heparin and LMW Heparin: Dosing and Adverse Effects. UpToDate; 2021. https://www.uptodate.com/contents/heparin-and-lmw-heparin-dosing-and-adverse-effects?search=unfractionated%20heparin&source=search_result&selectedTitle=1~150&usage_type=default&display_rank=1

agent and an SCD is recommended during hospitalization following major orthopedic surgery.[8]

SCI: Mechanical and anticoagulation treatment should be initiated as early as possible provided there is no active bleeding, coagulopathy, or other contraindications.[9] SCDs with or without graduated compression stockings plus LMWH are the prophylactic choice during the acute care phase following SCI. UFH and warfarin are not recommended unless there is contraindication to LMWH.

Suggested duration of chemoprophylaxis is based on the American Spinal Injury Association (ASIA) grading, which can be found in Table 15.1.[9]

PRESSURE INJURY

A pressure injury is defined by the National Pressure Injury Advisory Panel (NPIAP) as:

Localized damage to the skin and/or underlying soft tissue usually over a bony prominence or related to a medical or other device. The injury can present as intact skin or an open ulcer and may be painful. The injury occurs as a result of intense and/or prolonged pressure or pressure in combination with shear. The tolerance of soft tissue for pressure and shear may also be affected by microclimate, nutrition, perfusion, comorbidities and condition of the soft tissue.[10]

Pressure injury is currently staged according to the NPIAP as follows (photos can be accessed at https://npiap.com/):[11]

Stage 1 Pressure Injury

- This is characterized by nonblanchable erythema of an intact skin—intact skin with a localized area of nonblanchable erythema (may appear differently in darkly pigmented skin)
- Presence of blanchable erythema or changes in sensation, temperature, or firmness may precede visual changes.
- Color changes do not include purple or maroon discoloration, which may indicate deep tissue pressure injury.

Stage 2 Pressure Injury

- This is characterized by partial-thickness skin loss with exposed dermis—partial-thickness loss of skin with exposed dermis.
- The wound bed is viable (pink or red, moist). It may also be intact or a ruptured serum-filled blister.
- Adipose tissue and deeper tissues are not visible; granulation tissue, slough, and eschar are not present.
- These injuries commonly result from adverse microclimate and shear in the skin (e.g., over the pelvis or over the heel).
- This stage should not be used to describe moisture-associated skin damage that includes incontinence-associated dermatitis, intertriginous dermatitis, medical adhesive-related skin injury, or traumatic wounds (skin tears, burns, and abrasions).

Stage 3 Pressure Injury

- This is characterized by full-thickness skin loss—full-thickness loss of skin, in which the adipose is visible in the ulcer.
- Granulation tissue and epibole (rolled wound edges) are often present as well.
- Slough and/or eschar may be visible. The depth of tissue damage varies by anatomic location; areas of significant adiposity can develop deeper wounds.
- Undermining and tunneling may occur. The fascia, muscle, tendon, ligament, cartilage, and/or bone are not exposed.
- If slough or eschar obscures the extent of tissue loss, this is an unstageable pressure injury (UPI).

Stage 4 Pressure Injury

- This is characterized by full-thickness skin and tissue loss—full-thickness skin and tissue loss with exposed or palpable fascia, muscle, tendon, ligament, cartilage, or bone in the ulcer. Slough and/or eschar may be visible.
- Epibole, undermining, and/or tunneling often occur. The depth varies by anatomic location.
- If slough or eschar obscures the extent of tissue loss, this is a UPI.

Unstageable Pressure Injury

- This is characterized by obscured full-thickness skin and tissue loss—full-thickness skin and tissue loss in which the extent of tissue damage within the ulcer cannot be confirmed because it is obscured by slough or eschar.
- If slough or eschar is removed, a stage 3 or stage 4 pressure injury will be revealed. Stable eschar (i.e., dry, adherent, intact without erythema or fluctuance) on the heel or ischemic limb should not be softened or removed.

Deep Tissue Pressure Injury (DTPI)

- This is characterized by persistent nonblanchable deep red, maroon, or purple discoloration—intact or nonintact skin with localized area of persistent nonblanchable deep red, maroon, or purple discoloration, or epidermal separation revealing a dark wound bed or blood-filled blister.
- Discoloration may appear differently in darkly pigmented skin. Pain and temperature change often precede changes in skin color.
- This injury results from intense and/or prolonged pressure and shear forces at the bonemuscle interface. The wound may evolve rapidly to reveal the actual extent of tissue injury or it may resolve without tissue loss.
- If necrotic tissue, subcutaneous tissue, granulation tissue, fascia, muscle, or other underlying structures are visible, this indicates a full-thickness pressure injury (unstageable, stage 3, or stage 4).
- Do not use DTPI to describe vascular, traumatic, neuropathic, or dermatologic conditions.

Additional definitions of pressure injury include the following:

Medical Device-Related Pressure Injury

- This describes an etiology.
- Medical device-related pressure injuries result from the use of devices designed and applied for diagnostic or therapeutic purposes.
- The resultant pressure injury generally conforms to the pattern or shape of the device. The injury should be staged using the staging system.

Mucosal Membrane Pressure Injury

- Mucosal membrane pressure injury is found on the mucous membranes with a history of a medical device in use at the location of the injury.
- Due to the anatomy of the tissue, these injuries cannot be staged.

Prevention and Treatment

Pressure injury prevention should include appropriate seating/bed equipment, proper positioning, pressure relief (e.g., weight-shifting every 15–20 minutes for 30 seconds while sitting; turning in bed every 2 hours), education on pressure relief, and proper skin monitoring. Other issues that may need to be addressed include nutrition, tissue perfusion, oxygenation, local body heat management, and skin moisture management.

Treatment of pressure injuries includes pressure relief, addressing other etiologic factors, treatment of infections, debridement of necrotic tissue, regular wound cleansing, and use of appropriate wound dressings. A trial of topical antibiotics (e.g., silver sulfadiazine) may be helpful in wounds that are not healing with optimal debridement and cleansing. Wound cultures are not generally thought to be helpful because most wounds are colonized with bacteria. Systemic antibiotics should be reserved for cases with evidence of osteomyelitis, infectious cellulitis, or systemic infection.

Pressure injury wound care modalities include electrical stimulation, ultrasound, UV light, laser radiation, low-intensity vibration, wound vacuum-assisted (VAC) therapy, and hyperbaric oxygen therapy, and have been utilized clinically to accelerate wound repair. In particular, VAC therapy has become an increasingly popular treatment modality for pressure injuries.

Surgical flaps may expedite the healing of noninfected deep ulcers by filling the void with well-vascularized healthy tissue. The flaps, however, are themselves still vulnerable to pressure injury, particularly during the early healing stages, and generally require prolonged bedrest with timed pressure off-loading in the postoperative period.

Stages 1 and 2 pressure injuries are usually nonoperative. Stages 3 and 4 pressure injuries may benefit from surgical intervention.

INSOMNIA/SLEEPWAKE CYCLE DISTURBANCES

There is a wide array of literature documenting the importance of sleep to overall health. Sleep deprivation has been shown to cause hemodynamic instability (increased heart rate and blood pressure), increased inflammation, immune system dysregulation, and decreased pain tolerance.[12] In inpatient rehabilitation, sleep deprivation can lead to increased daytime drowsiness and inability to participate with therapies, resulting in delayed functional improvements. For patients undergoing neurorehabilitation, sleep is a particularly important tool for recovery and improved function.

Barriers to sleep while on inpatient rehabilitation include stress, noise, lights, alarms, hospital beds, awakening by healthcare staff, and unfamiliar surroundings. Certain medications, including corticosteroids and neurostimulants (e.g., methylphenidate), can potentially cause insomnia as a side effect. Sleep logs and diaries can be helpful tools to evaluate for insomnia or sleep deprivation. For patients with insomnia or sleepwake cycle disturbances, behavioral modification is generally the first-line treatment (reinforcing sleep hygiene, decreasing nighttime stimulation, limiting noise, and discouraging daytime sleeping/napping). After behavioral modification has been attempted, numerous medications can be used to treat insomnia.

Insomnia Medications

Melatonin receptor agonists (melatonin and ramelteon): Melatonin is a hormone secreted by the pineal gland in response to decreased light associated with control of the sleepwake cycle. Exogenous melatonin plasma levels generally peak 1 to 2 hours after administration. Melatonin receptor agonists are generally well-tolerated, but certain studies have found that exogenous melatonin can modulate the immune system, so use with caution in certain populations, for instance those on certain immunosuppressant medications.[13]

Nonbenzodiazepines so use with caution in certain populations, for instance those on certain immunosuppressant medications. receptor agonists (zolpidem [Ambien] and eszopiclone [Lunesta]): These are selective gamma-aminobutyric acid (GABA) type A receptor agonists. Because of this selectivity, they have less side effects than benzodiazepines (less anxiolytic action and less cardiopulmonary depression). Side effects include drowsiness, dizziness, complex sleep-related behaviors (e.g., sleep-walking), and dependence/habituation.[14]

Antidepressants (trazodone, mirtazapine, and amitriptyline): Antidepressants generally inhibit serotonin reuptake, but there is also significant histamine receptor antagonist action for antidepressants used to promote sleep. Trazodone, in particular, is widely used for insomnia; however, the American Academy of Sleep Medicine recommends against its use based on conflicting evidence.[14] Side effects of trazodone include drowsiness, prolonged QT interval, orthostatic hypotension, and priapism in male patients. Mirtazapine has a side effect of stimulating appetite and can be used for insomnia in patients with anorexia/poor appetite. Dosing of mirtazapine is unusual in that lower doses cause more somnolence.[15] Amitriptyline and other tricyclic antidepressants (TCAs) block reuptake of norepinephrine and have an antagonist action at acetylcholine receptors. TCAs can also be effective for neuropathic pain and can be used to promote sleep and serve as a multimodal pain adjunct. Side effects of amitriptyline include anticholinergic effects (altered mental status, tachycardia, and dry mouth), EKG changes, and arrythmias.[16]

Atypical antipsychotics (e.g., quetiapine [Seroquel]): These are dopamine and serotonin receptor antagonists. Like trazodone, Seroquel has widespread use for insomnia despite lack of cohesive evidence. It is useful in patients with comorbid psychiatric conditions. Side effects include metabolic abnormalities, drowsiness, and weight gain.[10]

FALLS

Falls are a major cause of morbidity in inpatient rehabilitation facilities, often increasing length of stay and readmission to acute care. The typical patient population admitted to inpatient rehabilitation has a variety of preexisting high-risk factors for falls, including weakness, unsteady gait, poor coordination, impaired sensation, wheelchair use, cognitive impairment and/or confusion, and advanced age. As patients are challenged to achieve a higher level of function in inpatient rehabilitation, fall prevention is a considerable challenge. Rates of falls in inpatient rehabilitation vary from 2.72 to 17.8 falls per 1,000 patient days compared with three to six falls per 1,000 patient days in acute hospital settings.[17] Falls are a significant source of injury to patients (13%–29% of injuries to stroke patients while on inpatient rehabilitation units) and contribute to increased length of stay, which in turn increases medical cost.[18] Factors that may influence falls are time of day (some studies note these are more frequent at night), number of days from time of admission to fall (more studies note the first week of admission is more common), and location (patient's room rather than the therapy gym).[19] As a potentially preventable cause of increased medical costs, falls are an impact factor of Centers for Medicare & Medicaid Services (CMS) reimbursement. Thusly, fall prevention is an important component of any inpatient rehabilitation facility's protocol. While specific fall prevention protocols are often individualized to each particular rehabilitation facility's case mix of patients, there are a number of general considerations that if implemented can reduce the rate of falls.

Fall Prevention Strategies

Minimizing altered sleepwake cycles: Poor sleep and altered sleepwake cycles can lead to daytime drowsiness and increased confusion in brain-injured patients, leading to increased falls.

Medication review of sedating or orthostatic hypotension causing drugs: A number of medications have been found to increase the risk of fall of patients. Some important classes of medications to review include pain, insomnia, anticholinergic, diuretic, and alpha-blocker medications.

Room/environmental modifications: Ensure the patient's bed is on the lowest position with the brakes on, the brakes on the wheelchair are set, frequently used items are within reach (e.g., call light, water, phone, and television remote), use of slip-resistant socks and footwear, and use of bed alarms for patients with poor safety awareness.

Clear communication: Multiple different providers and caregivers for a patient may lead to patient disorientation and unclear patient handoffs. Verbal handoffs from provider to provider can help reduce any miscommunication. Family education on the causes of falls as well as prevention strategies can be helpful.[15]

REFERENCES

The full complete reference list for this chapter appears in the digital version of the chapter, available at http://connect.springerpub.com/content/book/978-0-8261-5628-0/part/part02/chapter/ch15

CHAPTER 16

RHEUMATOLOGIC DISORDERS AND OSTEOPOROSIS

Theresa J. Lie-Nemeth, Kimberly J. Mercurio, and Artelio L. Watson

OSTEOARTHRITIS

Osteoarthritis (OA) is one of the leading causes of disability and the most common type of arthritis.[1] Nonmodifiable risk factors include increasing age, female gender, race or ethnicity, and genetics. Modifiable risk factors include obesity, muscle weakness, and trauma, in which obesity is the most important. Obesity is also associated with hand OA; as the hands are not weight-bearing joints, this demonstrates obesity is a systemic risk factor.

Clinical Manifestations

Joints frequently affected in OA are located in the axial spine (mostly in the cervical and lumbar apophyseal joints), hands (the proximal and distal interphalangeal [DIP] joints and the first carpometacarpal [CMC] joint), hips, and knees. OA is less common at the shoulders, ankles, feet, and hand metacarpophalangeal (MCP) joints. Symptoms of OA include pain during activity, stiffness lasting <30 minutes after inactivity, and functional limitations. On physical examination, patients may be noted to have crepitus, joint margin tenderness, restricted range of motion, bony enlargement, muscle weakness around the joints, and joint deformities. In the knee, patients may have genu varum from medial compartment OA or genu valgum from lateral compartment OA. Medial compartment knee OA is more common. Deformities in the fingers are called either Heberden (involving the DIP joints) or Bouchard (affecting the proximal interphalangeal joints) nodes. Squaring of the first CMC joint may also be seen.

Laboratory and Imaging Findings

On plain radiographs, the following findings are indicative of OA: nonuniform joint space narrowing, subchondral sclerosis, subchondral cysts, and osteophytes. There is no correlation between the severity of x-ray findings and symptoms.

Treatment

Education and self-management programs are key components of the conservative management of OA.[2] Further, weight loss improves the symptoms of knee OA.

- *Therapy and exercise:* Exercise is important in patients with OA, although no specific regimens have been shown to be more efficacious.[2,3] In general, aerobic exercises combined with strengthening exercises to stabilize the joints should be recommended.[4] Aquatic therapy can provide exercise while decreasing stress through the joints. Research has now shown that tai chi is also beneficial in OA.[2]
- *Medications:* The initial treatment regimen should incorporate topical nonsteroidal anti-inflammatory drugs (NSAIDs).[2,4] If topical agents are insufficient, patients may progress to oral NSAIDs. Acetaminophen, tramadol, and duloxetine may be considered in those unable to take NSAIDs. Lower doses from different classes can be combined for synergistic analgesia.
- *Complementary and alternative medicine:* Glucosamine and chondroitin have been investigated for years, but have not been shown to be efficacious.[2,5]
- *Injections:* Intra-articular corticosteroids can provide temporary symptom relief and have been shown to be superior to viscosupplementation.[4] Prolotherapy and platelet-rich plasma (PRP) are still being investigated as treatments for OA, but so far have not been consistently shown to be beneficial.[2]
- *Surgical:* When conservative management fails, patients can be referred for total joint replacements, most commonly total hip and total knee arthroplasties.[1,4]

RHEUMATOID ARTHRITIS

Clinical Manifestations

Rheumatoid arthritis (RA) is an autoimmune, inflammatory joint disease that can lead to significant disability.[5] The joints of the hands (excluding the DIP joints), wrists, and feet are the most affected.[6] Shoulders, elbows, hips, knees, ankles, and cervical spine may also become symptomatic. In contrast to OA, RA has symmetric involvement, with joint swelling and morning stiffness lasting more than 1 hour. Deformities can be seen in the later stages of RA, such as ulnar deviation of the fingers, boutonnière deformity, swan-neck deformity, ulnar deviation of the MCP joint, radial deviation of the radiocarpal joint, hallux valgus, hammer toes, and claw toes. Tenosynovitis is common in RA. Physicians should be aware of the potential neurologic complications resulting from atlantoaxial subluxation in the cervical spine, as well as median or ulnar neuropathy caused by tenosynovitis-related compression.[7]

Laboratory and Imaging Findings

Acute phase reactants such as erythrocyte sedimentation rate and C-reactive protein may be elevated. Autoantibodies develop in RA, resulting in positive rheumatoid factor or anticitrullinated protein antibodies in many, but not all, patients.[8]

On plain radiographs, patients may be noted to have soft tissue swelling, juxta-articular demineralization, marginal bone erosions, and uniform joint space narrowing. Synovial cysts and deformities may also be seen. MRI and ultrasound may be more sensitive in early disease and can assess for tenosynovitis and effusions.[8]

Treatment

Patient education and self-management should be considered for first-line treatment.[9,10] This includes joint protection, work simplification, energy conservation, and cognitive behavioral therapy.

- *Orthoses and assistive devices/adaptive equipment:* Orthoses can reduce pain, assist in positioning to increase function, and provide stability to attempt to prevent or correct deformities. For patients with hand and wrist symptoms, one may prescribe a wrist cock-up splint, resting hand splint, ulnar deviation splint, thumb spica orthosis, and finger splints.[1] Physical therapy (PT) and occupational therapy (OT) should issue assistive devices and adaptive equipment as appropriate.
- *Therapy and exercise:* Aerobic and strengthening exercises, along with aquatic therapy, have been shown to be beneficial, although less intensive exercises should be performed during acute exacerbations.[9]
- *Medications:* Oral medications for RA include early initiation of disease-modifying rheumatic drugs (DMARDs), with methotrexate being the most commonly used.[6,8] If needed, short-term NSAIDs and corticosteroids can provide immediate symptom relief on a temporary basis.
- *Surgery:* Synovectomy at the hand, wrist, elbow, or knee can be performed to relieve pain and inflammation.[5,11] Patients may also undergo arthrodesis at the hand and wrist, foot and ankle, or cervical spine.[1,5] As with OA, total joint arthroplasty can be performed in the hip or knee, but can also be done in the shoulder, elbow, wrist, MCP, or ankle joints.[5]

GOUT

Gout is a commonly seen crystal-associated arthropathy caused by monosodium urate crystal deposition precipitated by hyperuricemia.[12]

Clinical Manifestations

The most common joint involved is the first metatarsophalangeal joint, but gout can also affect the ankles, knees, hands, wrists, and elbows in an asymmetric fashion. Tophi (subcutaneous nodules) may be observed in patients with advanced gout. Gout may manifest as an acute, subacute, or chronic arthropathy. In an acute flare, patients will present with severe pain, redness, warmth, and swelling of the affected joint. Medications that may trigger a gout flare include diuretics, so physicians should be mindful to monitor for signs and symptoms of a flare when prescribing these medications.

Laboratory and Imaging Findings
Examination of the synovial fluid under polarized light microscopy will demonstrate negatively birefringent crystals. Radiographic findings include soft tissue swelling, tophi, overhanging edges, and bone erosions.

Treatment
Lifestyle modification includes reduced consumption of red meat, seafood, alcohol, and high-fructose corn syrup.

- *Medication:* For a gout flare, medications used include systemic and intra-articular glucocorticoids, NSAIDs, and colchicine. Urate-lowering medications include allopurinol, febuxostat, probenecid, and pegloticase.[12]

PSEUDOGOUT/CALCIUM PYROPHOSPHATE DEPOSITION DISEASE

Clinical Manifestations
Another major crystal deposition disorder is calcium pyrophosphate deposition disease (CPPD). Pseudogout refers to a symptomatic arthropathy resulting from CPPD.[13] The presentation may resemble that of acute gout, with monoarticular/oligoarticular warmth, swelling, and pain. The knee is the most commonly affected joint, and the wrist is the second. A chronic form of CPPD arthropathy may resemble OA and some patients may have both types of arthritis concurrently.

Laboratory and Imaging Findings
In contrast to gout, the crystals of CPPD are positively birefringent and rhomboid-shaped on polarized light microscopy. On radiographs, chondrocalcinosis, or calcification in the cartilage, is seen at the knee, wrist, and symphysis pubis. Ultrasonography can detect chondrocalcinosis earlier than radiographs.

Treatment
Treatment of acute calcium pyrophosphate (CPP) crystal arthritis includes intra-articular glucocorticoid injection, NSAIDs, and colchicine.

SERONEGATIVE SPONDYLOARTHROPATHIES

Seronegative spondyloarthropathies are a group of multisystem inflammatory disorders affecting the spine, peripheral joints, and periarticular structures, and are associated with distinguishing extra-articular manifestations.[14] The majority of patients are human leukocyte antigen (HLA) B27 positive and rheumatoid factor negative. The four major disorders are ankylosing spondylitis, reactive arthritis, psoriatic arthritis, and enteropathic arthritis/spondyloarthropathy associated with inflammatory bowel disease.

FIBROMYALGIA

Approximately four million American adults are affected by fibromyalgia, a chronic pain condition.[15] The female to male ratio is roughly 2:1 or 3:1.[16,17] Risk factors include female gender, older age (mean age 50), family history, preexisting rheumatologic condition (e.g., OA, RA, and systemic lupus erythematosus), trauma (physical or psychological), infections (especially viral), and obesity.[17]

Clinical Manifestations

The hallmark symptoms of this debilitating condition are chronic (>3 months) generalized pain, sleep disturbances, fatigue (physical or mental), and dyscognition. Other associated symptoms include stiffness, depression, anxiety, posttraumatic stress disorder, headaches (tension and migraine), temporomandibular joint syndrome, gastrointestinal complaints/irritable bowel syndrome, pelvic pain (e.g., dysmenorrhea and interstitial cystitis), autonomic symptoms/dizziness and lightheadedness, environmental sensitivities, restless legs, and paresthesias.[17]

The current diagnostic criteria are based on generalized pain ≥3 months, the Widespread Pain Index (WPI), which is the patient's self-report of generalized pain out of 19 body parts, and the Symptom Severity Score (SSS), which assesses associated symptoms such as sleep problems, impaired cognition, and fatigue, as well as somatic symptoms.[16,18]

Treatment

Multimodal approach is recommended with medications, exercise, and self-management strategies.[16,18] Because there is no cure, the treatment goals are to improve function, improve quality of life, and symptom control by decreasing pain, improving mood, and restoring sleep quality.[16]

- *Nonpharmacologic treatment:* Table 16.1 lists the interventions, exercises, and treatment modalities that have been proven to improve function and quality of life in fibromyalgia patients.[16,18,19] Fibromyalgia patients should avoid strenuous exercises which can exacerbate pain and avoid tender point injections, which are not efficacious.
- *Medications:* See Table 16.2 for pharmacologic treatments for fibromyalgia.

TABLE 16.1 Nonpharmacologic Treatments for Fibromyalgia

Exercises	Interventions	Psychotherapy	Avoid
Low-impact aerobics Tai chi or yoga Functional training program	Acupuncture Manual therapy Kinesio-taping Electrotherapy (TENS)	CBT Mindfulness Biofeedback Coping skills	Strenuous exercise Tender point injections

CBT, cognitive behavioral therapy; TENS, transcutaneous electrical nerve stimulation.

TABLE 16.2 Pharmacologic Treatments for Fibromyalgia[18]

FDA-Approved	Beneficial Off-Label Use	Avoid	Limited Data
Duloxetine Milnacipran Pregabalin	Amitriptyline Cyclobenzaprine Tramadol Gabapentin Venlafaxine Fluoxetine Vitamin D	NSAIDs Corticosteroids Opioids	Cannabis Lidocaine infusions Naloxone

FDA, Food and Drug Administration; NSAIDs, nonsteroidal anti-inflammatory drugs.

OSTEOPOROSIS

Osteoporosis (OP) is a skeletal disorder characterized by compromised bone strength which predisposes patients to an increased risk of fracture. Bone strength reflects the integration of two main features: bone density and bone quality.[20] OP is caused by an imbalance between bone resorption and bone formation, with resorption overtaking formation after peak bone mass is attained between the ages of 30 and 35.[21,22] Risk factors for OP include age, female sex, low body mass, smoking, excessive alcohol use, prior fracture, family history, use of glucocorticoids >3 months, RA, secondary OP, radiographic osteopenia, malabsorption syndromes including celiac disease and gastric bypass, anorexia nervosa, sedentary lifestyle, immobility, calcium and vitamin D deficiencies, early menopause, hyperthyroidism, diabetes, and anticonvulsant use.[21]

Laboratory and Imaging Findings

Bone mineral density (BMD), measured using dual-energy x-ray absorptiometry (DXA) scan, is a well-established predictor of risk of fracture. BMD is reported using T-scores and Z-scores, which are expressed in *SD* from the means of reference populations. T-scores use a reference population of young, healthy adults matched for gender. Z-scores use age, gender, and ethnicity matched reference populations. The World Health Organization (WHO) BMD criteria, which use T-scores at the lumbar spine and femoral neck, are

TABLE 16.3 WHO Criteria for Diagnosis of OP

Normal BMD	T-score −1 or above
Low bone mass (osteopenia)	T-score between −1 and −2.5
OP	T-score −2.5 or below
Severe osteoporosis	T-score −2.5 or below with fragility fracture

BMD, bone mineral density; OP, osteoporosis.

recommended for diagnosis of OP in postmenopausal women and men aged ≥50 years[21] (see Table 16.3).

The 2020 update of the American Association of Clinical Endocrinologists Guidelines for Diagnosis and Treatment of Postmenopausal OP emphasizes that OP can also be diagnosed clinically based on a low-trauma fracture of the hip or spine regardless of BMD *and* in patients with a T-score between −1.0 and −2.5 with a fragility fracture of the proximal humerus, pelvis, or distal forearm. OP may also be diagnosed in patients with osteopenia and increased fracture risk using the Fracture Risk Assessment Tool (FRAX™),[23] which is based on country-specific thresholds.[20,24,25] Using these criteria recognizes and addresses the fact that OP has been underdiagnosed and undertreated when only the WHO criteria are used.[20,24] Recent studies show a high and early risk of subsequent fracture after an initial fracture. Timely management with consideration of pharmacotherapy is warranted in older women following all fracture types.[26]

The WHO BMD criteria should not be used to diagnose OP in children, premenopausal women, or men aged <50 years. In these groups, the diagnosis of OP should not generally be made by the BMD criteria alone, and only Z-scores should be reported, not T-scores.[20] A Z-score greater than −2.0 is interpreted as within the expected range for age, and a Z-score of −2.0 or below is interpreted as below the expected range for age. Low Z-scores typically alert clinicians to the presence of secondary OP.

Screening

The Bone Health and Osteoporosis Foundation (BHOF) recommends BMD testing for all women aged ≥65 years and all men aged ≥70 years, and postmenopausal women and men aged 50 to 69 years based on risk factor profile.[27] Postmenopausal women and men aged ≥50 years who have had an adulthood fracture should also be tested to diagnose and determine the degree of OP at a DXA facility using accepted quality assurance measures.[28] Vertebral fracture assessment (VFA) can be done at the same time as DXA and is recommended in patients with low-trauma fracture, height loss >4 cm, women ≥70, men ≥80, glucocorticoid therapy >3 months, and kyphosis. Trabecular bone scoring (TBS), an analysis of the microarchitecture of the bone, is a newer modality available on DXA machines that improves assessment of fracture risk.[20]

Treatment

National Osteoporosis Foundation (NOF) guidelines recommend that men aged 50 to 70 years consume 1,000 mg of calcium daily. Women aged >50 years and men aged >70 years should consume 1,200 mg of calcium daily. Intake of higher amounts of calcium has not been shown to confer additional benefit and may increase the risk of kidney stones, cardiovascular diseases, and stroke.[28] Adults aged >50 years should consume 800 to 1,000 IU/d of vitamin D_3.[27]

Two types of medication are currently used as treatment for OP: antiresorptives and osteoanabolics. Common antiresorptives include oral (alendronate and risedronate) and intravenous (IV) bisphosphonates (zoledronic acid), which bind to the hydroxyapatite in the bone to prevent resorption, and denosumab. Denosumab (60 mg subcutaneously every 6 months) is a receptor activator of nuclear factor kappa-B ligand (RANKL) inhibiting osteoclast development and mitigating bone resorption. It has been shown to increase BMD and reduce fracture risk for >10 years. Selective estrogen receptor modulators (SERMS), including raloxifene, maximize the beneficial effect of estrogen on the bone while minimizing the deleterious effects on the breast and endometrium and reduce vertebral fracture risk by 30% in patients with prior vertebral fracture and by 55% in patients without vertebral fracture. Reduction of nonvertebral fractures has not been documented.[29] Estrogen is approved by the Food and Drug Administration (FDA) for prevention of postmenopausal OP with the added caveat: "when prescribing solely for the prevention of post-menopausal OP, therapy should only be considered for women at significant risk of OP and or whom non-estrogen medications are not considered to be appropriate."[20] Osteoanabolic medications include the parathyroid hormone (PTH) analogs teriparatide and abaloparatide and the antisclerostin monoclonal antibody romosozumab.[20,30] These medications build bone and lead to greater increases in BMD and reduced fracture risk and are used in patients at very high risk of fracture. Osteoanabolics can increase BMD by 6% to 12% at the lumbar spine and to a lesser degree at the total hip within 1 to 2 years of treatment[23] and reduce vertebral fracture risk up to 73%.[30]

Therapy and exercise: Bone responds to mechanical loading, so regular weight-bearing exercise should be advocated throughout life. Bone strengthening activities are those that are dynamic, moderate to high in load magnitude, short in load duration, odd or nonrepetitive in load direction, and applied quickly. In patients with OP, weight-bearing exercises, strength training, and balance and postural exercises are recommended. Interventions to reduce the risk and/or impact of falls, including appropriate assistive devices, exercise programs, and avoidance of medications affecting the central nervous system (CNS), may reduce the incidence of hip fracture. Poor back extensor strength has been reported to correlate with a higher incidence of vertebral fractures.[31-33] People with OP should avoid spinal flexion exercises and loading of the spine in a flexed posture.[31,32] The Spinal Proprioceptive Extension Exercise Dynamic (SPEED) program improves balance, gait, and risk of falls in women with OP kyphosis.[34]

REFERENCES

The full complete reference list for this chapter appears in the digital version of the chapter, available at http://connect.springerpub.com/content/book/978-0-8261-5628-0/part/part02/chapter/ch16

CHAPTER 17

COVID-19 REHABILITATION

Jacqueline Neal, Rachna Soriano, and Jessica Dangelmaier

INTRODUCTION

In December 2019, the first reports of a novel coronavirus were described in Wuhan, China. The virus evolved rapidly, spreading quickly in communities and soon across the globe, and on March 11, 2020 the World Health Organization declared the novel coronavirus (COVID-19) outbreak a global pandemic.[2] Many patients require prolonged hospitalizations, which frequently lead to severe debility and ultimately the need for physiatric intervention, including inpatient rehabilitation. Even in those who have not experienced severe acute illness, many continue to experience prolonged constellation of symptoms beyond the acute infectious stage of the illness, regardless of severity of the initial illness. Persistent symptoms are varied and extensive, involving essentially all organ systems. The most frequent symptoms reported are fatigue, breathlessness, postexertional malaise, and cognitive dysfunction.[1] Other common symptoms include muscle weakness (63%), sleep difficulties (26%), anxiety and depression (23%), with >20% of patients demonstrating abnormal 6-minute walk test results.[2,3] At this timepoint, it is unclear how long these symptoms may persist. Per the National Institutes of Health (NIH)/Centers for Disease Control and Prevention (CDC), these ongoing symptoms are called postacute sequelae of COVID-19 (PASC) if they persist beyond 4 weeks. This definition is evolving over time and there are many other terms describing these symptoms, such as "long COVID," "long-haulers," "Post-COVID syndrome," or "Post-COVID-19 conditions." The magnitude of PASC is emerging. Studies around the world have reported various incidence rates for PASC, ranging from 32% to 96%.[4-8] Given that millions of people worldwide have suffered from COVID-19, the societal impacts are expected to be profound, possibly causing long-lasting changes to the healthcare system.[4-8] The field of physiatry is aptly trained for management of these symptoms, particularly as they pertain to the impact on quality of life. This chapter includes a summary based on information available at the time of publishing. As this is a new and evolving topic, it is likely that these recommendations may change over time.

CONSIDERATIONS FOR INPATIENT REHABILITATION

Post-COVID-19 and PASC symptoms are often managed initially in an inpatient rehabilitation setting, although the majority of patients present with symptomatic complaints in the outpatient setting. Inpatient rehabilitation intervention poses many challenges to this population. Depending on timing, patients will require isolation for the safety of the healthcare workers and other patients admitted within the facility. Many facilities have developed specialized airborne isolation units for this population, requiring proper personal protective equipment (PPE) to minimize risk of transmission. Isolation poses challenges in that frequently therapy equipment could not be accessed. In addition, family training is difficult due to visitation policies in place, necessitating training to be performed in a virtual training environment.

DYSPNEA

Many PASC patients present with dyspnea, and this symptom frequently results in limited activity tolerance. The severity of postacute lung disease appears to be associated with the severity of acute COVID-19 illness, especially in patients who have experienced acute respiratory distress syndrome (ARDS). However, shortness of breath is also common in patients who experienced mild acute COVID-19.[9] Dyspnea has been attributed primarily to intrinsic lung diseases, such as pulmonary fibrosis, following COVID-19, but can also be related to pulmonary embolism (PE), muscular deconditioning, cardiac dysfunction, medication effects, manifestation of dysautonomia, and anxiety/depression/posttraumatic stress disorder (PTSD).

When initially evaluating persistent dyspnea, the goal is to measure the patient's perceived severity of symptoms, to determine the underlying etiology, and to decide whether pulmonology referral is warranted. It is recommended that a validated measure of breathing discomfort be performed, for example the modified Medical Research Council Dyspnea Scale, Multidimensional Dyspnea Profile, Modified Borg Dyspnea Scale, and Duke Activity Status Index. Additionally, vital signs including pulse oximetry at rest and with activity are recommended to evaluate for hypoxemia, tachycardia, and tachypnea. A 30-second sit-to-stand, a 2-minute step test, and a 6-minute walk test are examples of ways to evaluate for hypoxemia with activity. Pulmonary function tests typically demonstrate a restrictive pattern, and abnormalities on chest imaging (chest x-ray [CXR], chest CT) often demonstrate fibrosis. Depending on the history, polysomnography may also be appropriate as PASC patients have been noted to have new or worsening sleep apnea. If there are abnormal vital signs and/or abnormalities on pulmonary function testing/imaging 8 weeks or more after the initial COVID-19 infection, referral to pulmonology is recommended. Treatment modalities include oxygen, with the goal of maintaining oxygen saturation >90%,[10] airway clearance techniques, as well as inspiratory muscle rehabilitation.[11,12] Pharmacologic intervention may be prescribed by pulmonology, and recommendations for medication management have been evolving over time. If available, pulmonary rehabilitation, although not demonstrating improvement in mortality, has demonstrated improvement in quality of life and may be beneficial to patients with abnormal pulmonary function study findings. It is recommended that functional measures be monitored to evaluate progress with treatment interventions.

NEUROLOGIC SEQUELAE

Numerous neurologic sequelae of PASC have been noted, most commonly cognitive impairment, sleep disorder, pain including headaches, compression neuropathies, critical illness polyneuropathy/myopathy, and strokes.[13,14]

Peripheral Compression Neuropathies

There have been several reports of peripheral neuropathies associated with severe COVID-19. With the advent of prone positioning for patients with COVID-19 ARDS, intubated patients are put at risk of compressive neuropathies, especially brachial plexopathies. Peripheral nerve injury can also occur due to postinfectious inflammatory neuropathy, systemic neuropathy, or nerve entrapment from hematoma. Neuropathy-related diaphragmatic dysfunction has also been notable. Identification of these neuropathies is critical both for prognostication and for appropriate orthotic fabrication. Electrodiagnostic studies and imaging of peripheral nerves in patients with COVID-19 may help localize the lesion and determine the severity, thereby helping direct treatment options and rehabilitation approaches/planning.

Critical Illness Neuropathy and Myopathy

ICU-acquired weakness is common, in particular critical illness neuropathy (CIN) and myopathy (CIM), where patients present with flaccid limb muscle weakness and failure to wean from the ventilator.[15] One of the medical challenges of treating COVID-19 patients is the high number of patients requiring prolonged mechanical ventilation in the ICU in combination with unusually high sedation requirements, predisposing to higher likelihood of ICU-acquired weakness. CIN and CIM are important to identify since survivors often present with severe residual disability and persistent exercise limitation. There is a clear distinction between outcomes in CIN versus CIM. Patients with CIN have slower or incomplete recovery and higher mortality rate, as opposed to patients with CIM who often show complete recovery within 6 months.

Headache

A study of 100 patients demonstrated that approximately 38% had ongoing headaches after 6 weeks,[13] and a meta-analysis noted the prevalence of post-COVID-19 headache to be 8% to 15% in the first 6 months.[14] These headaches are often refractory to traditional over-the-counter analgesics, and treatment may need to be escalated to prescription medications and other modalities.

COGNITIVE IMPAIRMENT

Patients with PASC often complain of cognitive impairment. Complaints may include memory problems, attention impairment, word-finding difficulties, or a sense of "brain fog" with slower processing speed that lasts for weeks to months.[13] In one study, approximately 80% of PASC patients undergoing inpatient rehabilitation demonstrated abnormalities on neuropsychologic tests.[16] Neuropsychologic tests have revealed deficits predominantly in executive function, specifically impairment in processing speed, set-shifting, and divided attention.[17] Impaired cognition can be related to several problems that occur in PASC, such as ongoing inflammatory processes, vitamin deficiencies and malnutrition, endocrine disorders, dysautonomia, rheumatologic disorders, and postintensive care syndrome (PICS). As such, laboratory evaluation is recommended. Brain imaging is not initially recommended unless there is concern for a focal central process. Specifically quantifying which types of cognitive impairments and the severity is useful for initial evaluation and monitoring of treatment outcomes. Use of a validated instrument to guide the need for further workup is recommended, such as the Montreal Cognitive Assessment (MOCA), Saint Louis University Mental Status, Brief Memory and Executive Test (BMET), or other similar evaluation tools. If abnormalities are noted or if there is high clinical suspicion, further evaluation via a neuropsychologic test is useful. Treatment options may include speech therapy, occupational therapy, and if available executive functioning coaching. Evidence regarding pharmacotherapy will likely be forthcoming.

FATIGUE

Fatigue is a feeling of weariness, tiredness, or lack of energy.[18] Fatigue is one of the most common symptoms of PASC and can be described as a physical sensation, cognitive fatigue, and emotional fatigue, and negatively impacts quality of life.[19] Although fatigue likely improves over time, it can persist beyond 6 months. If fatigue persists beyond 4 weeks after the initial COVID-19 illness and is impairing function, further evaluation is prudent. It is important to consider fatigue and diminished activity tolerance as related but distinct conditions, potentially with different underlying etiologies. There are numerous causes of fatigue and an evaluation to rule out common causes is recommended, including laboratory evaluation and/or imaging tests.[18] Postviral fatigue has been documented with other viral illnesses, which can lead to chronic fatigue syndrome (CFS) and/or myalgic encephalomyelitis (ME).[19] Another potential contribution that must be considered is PICS, which can cause fatigue related to sleep disorder, mood disorder, and critical illness polyneuropathy or myopathy.[20-22] Evaluation of the severity of fatigue is recommended to direct workup and treatment planning and to track the trajectory of symptoms of fatigue over time. Recommendations for managing fatigue include removing causative medications, energy conservation strategies, a phased versus paced versus graded exercise/activity program, dietary planning and hydration, as well as pharmacologic therapy and supplements.[18] Pharmacologic interventions to date have been chosen based on fatigue management recommendations in other patient populations, such as in ME/CFS, brain injury, and Parkinson disease, and include amantadine, modafinil, and methylphenidate.[23–25] At the time of publication, there is no consensus as to which pharmacologic intervention is most helpful.

CARDIOVASCULAR AND AUTONOMIC DISORDERS

Cardiovascular complications include myocardial infarction, heart failure, persistent dysrhythmias, myocarditis and pericarditis, venous thrombosis, thromboembolic disease, and autonomic dysfunction.[26,27] Myocardial ischemia and acute nonischemic myocardial injury have been reported in 7% to 40% of patients with COVID-19, heart failure in 23% to 33% among those who were hospitalized, arrhythmias in 18% of cases, venous thromboembolism in 15% to 21%, ischemic stroke in 4%, and myocarditis in 60% of patients.[28,29] COVID-19-associated cardiac dysfunction should be managed based on the underlying cardiac diagnosis.

Autonomic dysfunction can cause numerous symptoms, including arrhythmias, palpitations, orthostatic intolerance, and so forth. Historically, viruses have been known to cause disruption in the autonomic nervous system. The true prevalence following COVID-19 is unclear. Common presenting symptoms include shortness of breath, fatigue, chest pain, palpitations, dizziness, syncope or presyncope, orthostatic intolerance, leg swelling, and impaired activity tolerance. Additionally, those with autonomic dysfunction may also complain of headache, cognitive impairment, gastrointestinal dysfunction, genitourinary symptoms, and/or sleep disturbance. In-clinic evaluation may include vital signs, particularly evaluation of blood pressure and heart rate, and orthostatic vital sign evaluation, and if normal a 10-minute stand test should be considered. Consider tilt-table testing in symptomatic patients with negative 10-minute stand test.

Initial autonomic dysfunction management includes initiating a high-salt diet (>4 g of sodium daily and increasing fluid intake to >3 L/d) and physical counterpressure maneuvers such as compression garments, in addition to holding superfluous medications that may have problematic side effects and contribute to symptoms. If conservative measures are not helpful, trialing a low-dose beta-blocker, fludrocortisone, or midodrine can be considered.

HYPERCOAGULABILITY

Hypercoagulability due to COVID-19, even in the absence of severe illness, can cause stroke, acute coronary syndrome, PE, and deep vein thrombosis (DVT). These problems can occur both during acute illness and as recovery progresses. Numerous patients are noted to develop new DVT and PE in the rehabilitation setting due to increased risk of coagulopathies despite use of prophylactic anticoagulation. Markers such as elevated D-dimers, C-reactive protein (CRP), fibrinogen, prothrombin time, and platelet counts may help assess the risk of thromboembolism, although risk stratification for the development of thrombotic events is challenging. Further, patients with a recent history of COVID-19 frequently have hypoxemia in the rehabilitation setting, making it difficult to distinguish whether the etiology is related to a new PE or an underlying lung pathology. Appropriate DVT prophylaxis is critical in this patient population.

DYSPHAGIA

Among patients in the ICU with ARDS, a frequent complication following intubation and extubation is oropharyngeal dysphagia. It may be characterized by difficulty initiating a swallow, nasal regurgitation, aspiration into the airway, presence of pharyngeal residue, or incoordination between swallowing and respiration. The duration of intubation can increase the incidence of dysphagia. Postextubation dysphagia has been associated with aspiration pneumonia, transient hypoxemia, dehydration, and malnutrition, and resultant extended hospitalization, increased mortality rates, and reduction in quality of life. Best-practice guidelines in patients with COVID-19 include a mandatory postextubation screening for dysphagia at the bedside by a speech language pathologist, often followed by instrumental evaluation. Early and intense dysphagia interventions can be highly beneficial to the outcome of this patient population.

PRESSURE ULCERS

Patients with severe COVID-19 are at risk of pressure injury (PI), particularly along the face in those requiring prone positioning while intubated. There is also a high incidence of wound infections and resultant osteomyelitis requiring antibiotic treatment, which may then lead to other sequelae such as *Clostridium difficile* colitis. Prevention of PI is key. It is recommended that pressure points, such as the face, sacrum, and heels, be assessed to ensure no PI is visualized, as well as to promote early mobilization. The presence of pressure ulcers can directly impact therapy intervention due to positioning needs and limitations in sitting tolerance. Off-loading pressure points with an appropriate mattress as well as wheelchair cushion is useful, as well as optimizing nutrition for wound healing and recommending cessation of tobacco usage.

PSYCHIATRIC DISORDERS/SLEEP

Individuals with PASC experience a range of psychiatric symptoms. At 6-month follow-up, approximately a quarter of patients who have had COVID-19, regardless of the severity of the initial illness, will experience psychiatric symptoms, including PTSD, depression, anxiety, insomnia, and obsessive-compulsive symptomatology.[13] It is recommended that all patients being evaluated for PASC be assessed with standard screening tools to identify those with anxiety, depression, and PTSD. Patients complaining of insomnia or poor sleep benefit from standard screening, such as the Insomnia Severity Scale, a sleep diary, or a smart watch that measures sleep, as well as utilization of a tool to screen for sleep apnea. Further management may include counseling regarding sleep hygiene techniques, polysomnography, biofeedback, or acupuncture. Acupuncture has shown some beneficial effects on sleep quality and cognition in patients with traumatic brain injury and insomnia. If pharmacotherapy is deemed appropriate, consider starting melatonin and progressing to trazodone, which have been shown to be beneficial based on brain injury literature. Veterans with PTSD with chronic sleep disturbances respond to prazosin and cognitive behavioral therapy in veterans.[1,30]

EXERCISE PRESCRIPTION AND THERAPY INTERVENTION[31-36]

Safe and effective rehabilitation and exercise are a fundamental part of recovery from illness. Currently, insufficient evidence exists to guide best practice for safe and effective rehabilitation in PASC patients, although comparisons have been made with those with PASC and other infectious illnesses, such as severe ARDS and PICS, and occasional overlap with ME/CFS has been noted. In the absence of evidence for best practice, expert consensus has been provided. Before recommending rehabilitation intervention and/or exercise, risk stratification is recommended. PASC patients may benefit from screening for postexertional symptom exacerbation. Additionally, screening for cardiac, pulmonary, and autonomic dysfunctions to direct goals and parameters for exercising is prudent. If the patient is experiencing exertional oxygen desaturation in clinic, evaluation for need of oxygen with exertion via a 6-minute walk test prior to initiating an exercise intervention is recommended. Providing oxygen with an SpO_2 goal of 90% or more is recommended. Ideally, return to exercise is recommended after a patient is at least 7 days free of symptoms, especially if pursuing strenuous physical activity, although it is noted that PASC patients by definition have a prolonged course of symptoms and therapeutic intervention and/or exercise may need to be initiated prior to symptom resolution. In this case, return to exercise is best managed with physiatric involvement. Approximately 80% of patients with PASC experience exacerbation of symptoms with exertion.[37] Mild to moderate postexertional fatigue or tiredness without exacerbation of other PASC symptoms lasting 12 to 48 hours can be expected in anyone who participates in unaccustomed exercise and is indicative of deconditioning. Reassurance can be provided that this type of fatigue is an expected typical response and will improve with time. However, if there is exacerbation of other PASC-related symptoms (brain fog, etc.), as well as fatigue out of proportion of the "dose" of exercise, lasting days to months, then this type of exacerbation is termed postexertional malaise and reducing the dosage of activity/exercise below the level which precipitated symptom exacerbation is recommended and maintained until the associated exacerbation has resolved. Subsequently, incremental activity may be implemented with close monitoring for repeat symptom exacerbation. Lastly, those who do not tolerate upright activity due to symptom exacerbation may benefit from recumbent exercises, lower intensity exercises, or shorter duration exercises. Exercise prescriptions may be based on the Borg level of perceived exertion or metabolic equivalent levels.[31-36]

REFERENCES

The full complete reference list for this chapter appears in the digital version of the chapter, available at http://connect.springerpub.com/content/book/978-0-8261-5628-0/part/part02/chapter/ch17

CHAPTER 18

SURGICAL ORTHOPEDICS
Mani Singh, Tracey Isidro, and Jennifer Soo Hoo

INTRODUCTION

The 2019 American Joint Replacement Registry Annual Report reported a 28.5% increase in orthopedic procedures between 2018 and 2019, with total knee arthroplasty (TKA, 55.1%) and primary total hip arthroplasty (THA, 33.1%) comprising the majority.[1] Similarly, the 2020 Shoulder and Elbow Registry illustrated an increasing number of reverse total shoulder arthroplasty (RTSA) procedures since 2015.[2] Lumbar spine surgeries consist of another increasing group of procedures, with an estimated prevalence of 4.5% (North America) for low back pain secondary to lumbar spondylosis.[3] A number of these patients are discharged to acute rehabilitation postoperatively, with studies illustrating shorter lengths of stay and lower overall costs without an increase in adverse events.[4]

REHABILITATION AFTER JOINT REPLACEMENT

Rehabilitation After Knee Replacement

Total Knee Arthroplasty

Indications for TKA include osteoarthritis (OA) and inflammatory arthritis (rheumatoid arthritis).

There are two types of TKAs that are generally used: cemented and cementless fixations. Cemented fixation may allow immediate weight-bearing as tolerated (WBAT), while cementless fixation may require several months of restricted weight-bearing (WB) for complete stability. Cemented TKA is currently the gold standard method of fixation and is more commonly performed, although cementless fixation may be considered in younger patients. It has been shown that cementless fixation does not necessarily decrease the rate of revision after TKA and that cemented fixation may be associated with significantly better long-term functional recovery.[5]

Although TKAs have a high success rate with a less than 5% revision rate a decade after knee replacement, it is important to be knowledgeable of the causes of prosthetic failure.[6] Microscopic wear debris can trigger an inflammatory response with ensuing osteolysis and component loosening. An infected joint or polyethylene liner wear from premature breakdown due to biomechanical loading can also lead to surgical revision.

In terms of postsurgical rehabilitation goals after a TKA, regaining functional knee range of motion (ROM) from 0° to 90° before discharge is important. Physical therapy has been shown to restore ROM quicker as well as reduce swelling and improve strength.[7] Pillows under the knee should be avoided to prevent knee flexion contractures. Regarding continuous passive motion, it may decrease the length of inpatient rehabilitation stay and improve ROM by 10° at 1-year postoperatively; however, most studies have not demonstrated long-term benefits in ROM or functional outcome. Additional components of the rehabilitation program include isometric strengthening of the hip and leg muscles, transfer training, and stair negotiation. Prior to discharge home, the patient should demonstrate the ability to ambulate. Ambulation following surgery generally begins with a rolling walker and the patient is advanced to crutches or a cane as tolerated (postoperative day 2).

Rehabilitation After Shoulder Replacement

Total Shoulder Arthroplasty

Indications for total shoulder arthroplasty (TSA) include OA, inflammatory arthritis (rheumatoid arthritis), complex humeral head fractures, and avascular necrosis (AVN) with glenoid chondral wear.

TSA, or anatomic TSA, is the third most common joint replacement surgery after total hip replacement (THA) and TKA. Most commonly, a deltopectoral or anterior approach is utilized to expose the glenohumeral joint. Less commonly, the deltoid is split in a lateral approach, giving better glenoid exposure. Special care is taken in preserving the subscapularis tendon to preserve ROM during postoperative rehabilitation.[8] The humeral head is removed, along with any pathologic bone or osteophytes, and the prosthesis is implanted. A new metal-backed glenoid is fixated and screwed to the existing glenoid to articulate with the prosthetic humeral head. Larger implants preserve stability but limit ROM, whereas smaller implants provide more ROM at the cost of stability. Titanium alloy stems/humeral heads are used in conjunction with polyethylene glenoid cups.[8]

Postoperatively, rehabilitation is largely dependent on subscapular tendon repair and preservation. This directly affects shoulder function and stability, with poor repairs placing the patient at risk of superior migration of the humeral head and resultant instability. A shoulder immobilizer or sling is generally used 4 to 6 weeks postoperatively to limit external rotation and allow for healing.[8] Some studies report limiting ROM to 30° to 40°, although there is no clear consensus.[9] Postoperative precautions, in addition to limited external rotation, include avoiding excess internal rotation (IR; generally up to 6 weeks) and limiting excessive flexion or abduction (no >130°–150°) for 6 to 12 weeks. Initial movements begin in the scapular plane, followed by isometric strengthening at 4 to 6 weeks and scapular stabilization exercises. Overhead activities are some of the last to be reintroduced in the rehabilitation stage.[8] Patients may be returned to full strength with activity as tolerated between 8 and 16 weeks.

It is important to monitor for postoperative complications during the rehabilitation course, including infection, rotator cuff injury or tear, prosthetic loosening, periprosthetic fractures, or injuries to neurologic structures. Infections are less common in the acute postoperative period, with the average time to infection following surgery being 3.5 years.[10] Glenoid component loosening is the most common complication and may present as worsening pain. CT or x-ray images should be obtained if these complications are suspected. Patients generally report improved pain relief, improved function, and improved ROM following TSA.[8]

Reverse Total Shoulder Arthroplasty

Indications for RTSA include glenohumeral joint degeneration (OA, inflammatory arthritis) with return to clinic (RTC) injury and rotator cuff arthropathy.

RTSA is utilized when TSA is contraindicated in cases of RTC injury or arthropathy, as the stabilizing and compressive forces of the rotator cuff muscles cannot be utilized to stabilize the prosthetic humeral head. RTSA uses a reverse ball and socket design, switching the glenoid and humeral components, thus shifting the center of rotation. This allows the deltoid to initiate shoulder abduction without relying on the supraspinatus tendon. Deltopectoral and superior approaches can be used in RTSA as well.[8]

RTSA has a higher risk of dislocation when compared with TSA. Postoperative rehabilitation focuses on minimizing this risk by limiting internal humeral rotation, adduction, and extension. Immobilization periods range from 2 to 6 weeks before passive ROM should be attempted. Similar to TSA, significant IR or reaching behind the back is not allowed until 12 weeks. Deltoid strengthening and scapular stabilization begin at approximately 6 weeks with concurrent ROM exercises. Care must be taken to gradually build up deltoid strength to avoid significant transmission of force through the acromion. Higher repetition with lighter weight is preferred, although there is limited consensus on these exact rehabilitation guidelines.[8,9]

Similar to TSA, the patient's shoulder should be monitored in the postoperative period for instability, periprosthetic fractures, infections, glenoid or humeral component loosening, neurologic injury, rotator cuff injury, or venous thromboembolism. Outcomes are generally better when RTSA is performed for primary OA or in younger patients compared with posttraumatic injuries or older patients.[8]

Humeral Head Replacement

Indications for humeral head replacement (HHR) include inadequate glenoid bone stock, AVN of the humeral head with normal glenoid articular cartilage, and irreparable RTC tears.

HHR was originally utilized for treatment of proximal humerus fractures and is now considered as treatment for glenohumeral OA by surgeons who wish to avoid glenoid resurfacing, as can be seen with TSA. HHR, while simpler, quicker, and less costly, may provide less pain relief without providing a significant advantage in terms of glenoid component loosening and revisions.[11]

Following surgery, the shoulder is generally protected with an immobilizer for up to 6 weeks. Rehabilitation begins with passive ROM exercises, with active range and strengthening components being introduced at 6 weeks. Precautions include limiting external ROM until subscapularis healing. Sports activities may be resumed at 6 months.[12]

Rehabilitation After Hip Replacement

Total Hip Arthroplasty

Indications for THA include unstable hip fractures, OA, osteonecrosis, inflammatory arthritis, posttraumatic arthritis, malignancy, hemoglobinopathies, and hip dysplasia.

Various surgical approaches for THA have been described in the literature, including the lateral, posterior, and anterior approach.

The lateral approach (occasionally referred to as anterolateral) was first utilized in order to avoid trochanteric nonunion.[13] To expose the acetabulum, the abductor mechanism must be neutralized via trochanteric ostomy or partial detachment of the anterior gluteus minimus and medius, as well as the vastus lateralis.[14, 15] However, given higher rates of gluteal dysfunction using the lateral approach, the posterior approach was popularized. The posterior approach splits the gluteus maximus and remains posterior to the gluteus medius and minimus. The hip capsule is divided and the external rotators such as the piriformis, the superior and inferior gemelli, and the obturator internus are necessarily detached.[14] One limitation to this approach is a higher rate of instability. Both approaches are routinely performed and debate continues as to the benefits and limitations of each.[16]

More recently, the anterior approach (Hueter approach) has been popularized and started to be used more commonly. It is considered a less invasive approach as dissection occurs between the sartorius and tensor fascia lata without detachment of the abductor muscles. Particular care must be taken to avoid lateral femoral cutaneous nerve damage. Fascial dissection allows visualization of the superior femoral neck. This approach is also considered to be more technically challenging but with improved stability and decreased risk of dislocation.[15] However, recent evidence suggests the anterior approach may be associated with a higher rate of early major revisions or femoral complications compared with the posterior or lateral approach.[13]

Minimally invasive techniques have been developed over the past decade for each of these approaches in order to decrease incision sizes, decrease tissue trauma, and improve time to recovery. There are still no definitive data illustrating its superiority to traditional hip arthroplasty.[17,18] In the case of bilateral hip OA requiring THA, one-stage bilateral THA may be performed, with current evidence demonstrating no significant increase in the rate of complications.[19]

Biologically fixed or "cementless" implants provide a more durable bioprosthetic interface, but require a longer period of protective WB (e.g., touchdown WB to partial WB [PWB] for 2–3 months) to allow for osseous integration into the porous prosthetic surface. Cement-fixed implants are cheaper and may offer immediate WBAT. They may be beneficial in osteopenic or osteoporotic bone (given deeper penetration and fixation), or following radiation therapy, in patients of any age.[20] The cement, however, can be prone to deterioration, which may result in component loosening and ultimately require revision.

Precautions following surgery using different approaches vary. For a posterior THA, patients may be out of bed to chair with assistance on postoperative day 1. A triangular hip abduction pillow in bed is highly recommended for the first 6 to 12 weeks. Hip precautions generally continue for up to 12 weeks postoperatively to allow for the formation of a pseudocapsule and minimize the chance of dislocation. Patients are allowed flexion up to 90°, passive abduction, and gentle (<30°) IR while extended. There should be no adduction past midline and no IR while flexed. Active abduction, hyperextension, and external rotation are allowed with a posterior approach (gluteus medius preserved), but avoided after an anterolateral approach (gluteus medius split open). Flexion past 90°, adduction past neutral, and hip IR past neutral are avoided following lateral THA as well as for 6 to 12 weeks.[21] Typical patient instructions are diagrammed in Figure 18.1. The risk of hip dislocation is generally decreased following anterior THA and precautions are not as strict.[21]

Other key issues include deep vein thrombosis (DVT) prophylaxis, monitoring for postoperative anemia and infection, and pain control. Patients may often complain of perceived leg length discrepancies during the first several months postoperatively; prothrombin time (PT) to address muscle imbalances and tight capsules may be helpful. In general, prognosis following THA is excellent, although being younger, male, obese, and highly active may adversely affect outcomes.

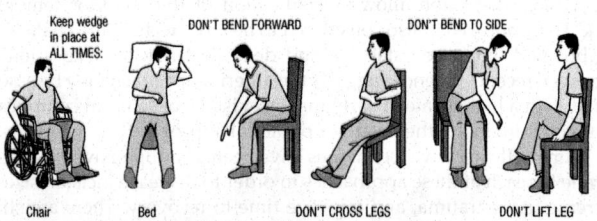

FIGURE 18.1 Rehabilitation after posterior total hip arthroplasty.

REHABILITATION AFTER HIP FRACTURE

The lifetime risk of hip fractures in industrialized countries is 18% for females and 6% for males.[22] Osteoporosis and falls are the primary risk factors. Mortality and morbidity following hip fractures are high: 20% are not alive 1 year after the fracture and 33% by 2 years.[23] Nearly one of three survivors are in institutionalized care within a year after the fracture, and as many as 66% of survivors do not regain their preoperative activity status.[24] Surgery is usually indicated for most hip fractures unless medically contraindicated or in nonambulatory patients.

Femoral Neck Fracture

Screw fixations (Figure 18.2) are typical for stable, nondisplaced fractures. Hemiarthroplasty (HA) may be performed in older patients at risk of AVN or with limited life expectancy and is noninferior to THA in these cases.[25,26] Ambulation with WBAT and an appropriate assistive device may be started during the first few days postoperatively. Bipolar endoprostheses (Figure 18.3) may be used for unstable, displaced fractures when satisfactory reduction cannot be achieved and the patient is over 65 years of age or has preexisting articular pathology (e.g., OA). Patients are usually mobilized quickly and allowed WBAT within the first few days postoperatively. Abduction pillows and short-term ROM restrictions (no adduction past midline, IR, or hip flexion past 90°) may be ordered to reduce the risk of prosthetic displacement. Precautions may be maintained for 6 to 12 weeks. Postoperatively, rehabilitation should focus on strengthening, gait training, and ROM exercises.[27]

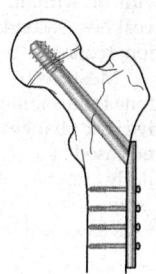

FIGURE 18.2
Screw fixation.

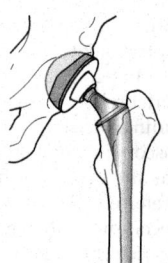

FIGURE 18.3
Bipolar endoprosthesis.

Intertrochanteric Fractures

Sliding hip screw fixation allows for early WBAT for stable fractures (intact posteromedial cortex) and provides dynamic compression of the fracture during WB. Intramedullary hip screws are another surgical option. A period of limited WB may be necessary following fixation of unstable fractures (Figure 18.4). Surgical management for *subtrochanteric fractures* also includes the use of sliding screw fixation and intramedullary nails/rods, although initial WB may be more limited.

Complications seen during rehabilitation and convalescence after hip fracture include

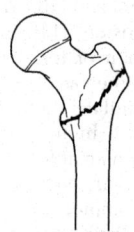

FIGURE 18.4
Intertrochanteric fracture.

atelectasis, pneumonia, anemia, fracture nonunion, AVN, surgical site infection, component loosening, leg length discrepancy, heterotopic ossification (HO), DVT, constipation, and skin breakdown.

REHABILITATION AFTER SPINE SURGERY

Indications include severe low back pain with functional impairments with or without radicular symptoms, including paresthesias, pain, weakness secondary to degenerative disc disease (DDD), disc herniation, scoliosis, spondylolisthesis, or spinal stenosis (or combination).

Most elective spine surgeries/procedures in the United States are done for disability from chronic low back pain secondary to degenerative disc changes or spondylosis. The number of lumbar fusions has increased at a significantly higher rate than even THA or TKA, particularly after the implementation of intervertebral fusion cages in 1996.[28] Laminotomy and laminectomy surgeries are often used in spinal stenosis as a means of spinal decompression.[29]

Lumbar Spinal Fusion

Spinal fusion surgeries are done to stabilize the spine, relieve pressure placed on vertebral discs or nerve roots, and treat low back pain. Outcomes are frequently better than decompression surgeries or disc replacements.[4]

In posterior or posterolateral lumbar interbody fusion (PLIF), the vertebral body and disc are accessed via a posterior incision. A longitudinal incision is made, the fascia and muscle are retracted, and fluoroscopic x-ray may be used to confirm appropriate spinal levels. PLIF has the benefit of better visualization of the neural elements and is preferred when one or two spinal levels are fused in conjunction with decompression. It generally involves bilateral partial laminectomies or discectomy, followed by insertion of interbody spacers or hardware (cortical screws, plates, and rods) to stabilize the spine. The intervertebral disc is removed by special instruments and bone spacers are placed in their stead. Bone graft is incorporated into the disc space itself to promote bony union. PLIF involves placing a bone graft spacer on both the right and left sides. Transforaminal lumbar interbody fusion (TLIF) is a more modern approach that avoids significant retraction of the spinal nerves and requires only one bone graft spacer. Whereas PLIF may involve bilateral partial facetectomy, TLIF involves unilateral facetectomy.

In anterior lumbar interbody fusion (ALIF), the disc is accessed via an anterior incision. ALIF approaches may be preferred in the cervical spine to avoid spinal cord injury or manipulation and are less commonly used in the lumbar spine and may be referred to as anterior cervical discectomy and fusion surgeries (ACDF). Care must be taken to avoid the esophagus or the carotid sheath (cervical) or abdominal organs (lumbar) during these surgeries.

Rehabilitation is an important part of postoperative care in these patients, although limited evidence is available on a formal rehabilitation protocol. Spine precautions include limiting bending, lifting, and twisting for approximately 6 to 12 weeks, although evidence is limited.[30] This involves restricting hip flexion past 90°, trunk rotation, and side bending to preserve spinal instrumentation and healing.[31] Critical to the efficacy of these surgeries is the success of bone grafting (autograft, allograft, or artificial—often from the iliac crest) in order to prevent bone nonunion.[32]

Patient education, cardiovascular exercise, motor control and strengthening, and early mobilization are important components of the rehabilitation program.[31] The rehabilitation program should include paravertebral muscle (extensors) strengthening, lumbopelvic mobility, and aerobic exercise (often on a treadmill or bike). Neural mobilization and myofascial release, when incorporated with core stabilization exercises, have been shown to be effective as well.[33]

REFERENCES

The full complete reference list for this chapter appears in the digital version of the chapter, available at http://connect.springerpub.com/content/book/978-0-8261-5628-0/part/part02/chapter/ch18

CHAPTER 19

ICU REHABILITATION

Julie Lanphere

INTRODUCTION

Intensive care unit (ICU) rehabilitation is a developing practice for critically ill patients. Survivors of critical illness frequently experience many long-term sequelae, including ICU-acquired muscle weakness (ICUAW), which can occur in a quarter to half of critically ill patients.[1,2] There is growing literature around the efficacy, safety, and quality of providing rehabilitation services in the ICU setting. Critically ill patients suffer from impairments that affect their cognitive and mental health, physical functioning, and quality of life.[3,4] Prolonged time in bed is associated with ICUAW and several factors contribute to this ongoing barrier,[1,3] including the patient themselves, their environment, the ICU culture, and other process-related issues. Multiple strategies exist for successful implementation, including therapy, nursing, and physician champions, safety criteria guidelines, and interdisciplinary team approach around coordination and communication to address perceived barriers.[2]

CLINICAL GUIDELINES

The Society of Critical Care Medicine (SSCM) 2018 Clinical Practice Guidelines for the Prevention and Management of Pain, Agitation/Sedation, Delirium, Immobility, and Sleep Disruption (PADIS) for adult patients in the ICU made a conditional recommendation suggesting performing rehabilitation or mobilization in critically ill adults; however, it has low quality of evidence given the lack of high-quality studies, evidence, and outcome measures.[5] The guidelines state: "For critically ill adults, rehabilitation is defined as a set of interventions (performed either in bed or out of bed) designed to optimize functioning and reduce disability in individuals with a health condition." Sixteen randomized controlled trials met the eligibility criteria and reported on five critical outcomes: muscle strength, duration of mechanical ventilation, health-related quality of life measure, hospital mortality, and short-term physical functioning measures. The safety, feasibility, and benefits of rehabilitation and mobilization delivered in the ICU setting have been evaluated as potential means to mitigate ICUAW, delirium, and impaired physical functioning. Important barriers to note within any ICU include sedation practices and pain management as these factors are associated with the ability of the patient to participate in rehabilitation.[5]

IMMOBILITY

ICU rehabilitation addresses the adverse effects of immobility and bedrest many experience due to illness. Bedrest is associated with multisystem involvement, including up to 30% muscle wasting in the first 10 days. There are consequences to many systems, including cardiac, renal, pulmonary, dermatologic, neurologic, musculoskeletal, metabolic, genitourinary, and gastrointestinal.[6] The most notable include delirium and neurocognitive/neuropsychologic impairments.

Critical illness renders patients bedbound due to several reasons out of their control, including clinical instability, need for life-saving interventions that require sedation, sedation practices in the ICU, complex medical management, airway protection, and coordination of care early in their course, among other things. There are hypotheses around nerve ischemia, disuse, and inflammatory processes leading to ICU-acquired weakness, including critical illness myopathy, critical illness polyneuropathy, isolated focal neuropathies, plexopathies, and delirium. Delirium is one of the most undertreated and underrecognized problems critically ill patients face. It is considered an acquired nontraumatic brain injury. Sasannejad et al. described 821 critically ill patients with a prevalence of delirium at 74%. The patients were of different ages and 40% were found to have global cognitive scores similar to a moderate traumatic brain injury and 26% with scores similar to Alzheimer disease up to 1 year post hospitalization.[7] There is long-term cognitive impairment after acute respiratory distress syndrome (ARDS), along with many factors that are centered around its clinical impact and the pathophysiologic mechanisms. These include inflammation, hypoxemia, cerebral autoregulation, bloodbrain barrier damage, amyloid beta, and cytokine accumulation. Neuroimaging comparisons in ARDS survivors within 1 year post discharge versus control patients demonstrate accelerated cerebral and hippocampal atrophy, and there are findings of hippocampal hypoxic ischemic lesions being the most commonly identified abnormality in ARDS patients.[8]

SAFETY

As ICU rehabilitation and mobilization implementation and feasibility studies have gained momentum, the ABCDEF bundle (Table 19.1) was created to guide and coordinate evidence-based care practices at the bedside.[9] With this bundle, there has been increased focus on providing evidence-based care to patients across the continuum of care. There is improved collaboration among clinical team members in ICU cultures. Mobility with the alignment of people, processes, and technology has been much more feasible. With regard to safety, serious events or harms do not commonly occur during physical rehabilitation or mobilization of adult patients in the ICU. Serious safety events or

TABLE 19.1 The ABCDEF Bundle

A—Assess, prevent, and manage pain
B—Both SAT and SBT
C—Choice of analgesia and sedation
D—Delirium assessment, prevention, and management
E—Early mobility and exercise
F—Family engagement and empowerment

SAT, spontaneous awakening trials; SBT, spontaneous breathing trials.

harm were rare (15 during >12,200 sessions of therapy/mobilization) and the majority of safety events were respiratory-related (four desaturations and three unplanned extubations).[5,10]

There are several studies that provide relative and absolute contraindications for mobilizing patients that were suggested to support safety criteria based on starting and stopping mobilization,[11] but these are not a substitute for clinical judgment. All thresholds should be interpreted or modified as needed around the patient's clinical picture, expected values, and recent trends that address the safety of patients.

FEASIBILITY, IMPLEMENTATION, AND CLINICAL PRACTICE

For a successful ICU rehabilitation, timing of therapy with sedation breaks coordinated with the nursing staff for patient participation, as well as proper identification and treatment of agitation, pain, and or delirium, as they limit successful mobilization, should be considered. Additional factors to take into account include rehabilitation equipment, chairs, and safety guidelines.[12]

Physical therapists (PTs) play the biggest role in ICU rehabilitation and provide early mobility, transfer training, exercise, and adaptive mobility devices.

Occupational therapists (OTs) can address delirium and cognitive and psychological impairments, promote orientation and executive function, and use assistive technology that allows active participation of patients during their ICU stay.[13]

Speech therapy can offer a number of opportunities to intubated patients in the ICU, including speaking valve trials for ventilated patients, and use of communication boards, assistive technology, and eye gaze, which allow social participation.[14] There are a fair number of cognitive assessments that can be used in the ICU by both the OT and the speech therapist, such as the complementary and alternative medicine (CAM)-ICU, the Glasgow Coma Scale, the Rancho Los Amigos Scale, the Coma Recovery Scale-Revised (CRS-R), and the Cognitive Assessment of Minnesota.

COST

ICU early rehabilitation program financial modeling demonstrated net cost savings based on actual experience, and published data showed that an early ICU rehabilitation program can generate net financial savings for U.S. hospitals.[15]

REFERENCES

The full complete reference list for this chapter appears in the digital version of the chapter, available at http://connect.springerpub.com/content/book/978-0-8261-5628-0/part/part02/chapter/ch19

CHAPTER 20

PEDIATRIC REHABILITATION

Sarah Macabales, Mary Keen, and Larissa Pavone

CEREBRAL PALSY

Definition

Cerebral palsy (CP) is a group of disorders of the development of movement and posture, causing activity limitations that are attributed to a nonprogressive disturbance that occurred in the developing fetal or infant brain.[1]

Etiology

CP is the most common pediatric physical disability, occurring in about 2 in 1,000 live births. The etiology of CP is often multifactorial. The greatest risk factor for CP is prematurity. Other major risk factors include low birth weight (<1,500 g), multiple gestation pregnancy, maternal infection, neonatal infection, and maternal substance use. Recently genetic factors have been implicated.[2]

Diagnosis

Children with CP may demonstrate unusual tone, unusual postures, and irritability. The Hammersmith Infant Neurologic Examination (HINE) and the General Movement Assessment (GMA) allow very early identification of children with CP. On examination, children may show signs of persistence of primitive reflexes after 6 months and delayed developmental milestones. Periventricular leukomalacia (PVL) is the most common finding on neuroimaging. MRI is the preferred imaging to evaluate for CP and should be used in conjunction with clinical evidence to diagnose CP.[3]

Classification

CP is classified according to body distribution, most commonly:

- *Hemiplegia:* one side of the body involved
- *Diplegia:* lower extremities involved
- *Quadriplegia:* full body involved

CP is also classified by tone abnormalities:

- Spastic (85%–91%)
- Dyskinetic, including dystonic and athetotic, hypotonic, and ataxic
- Spastic and dyskinetic mixed

CP is graded by the Gross Motor Function Classification System (GMFCS) as follows:

- *Level 1:* walks without limitations
- *Level 2:* walks with limitations
- *Level 3:* walks using a handheld mobility device
- *Level 4:* may walk short distances with assistive device but rely on power mobility
- *Level 5:* severely limited mobility

Associated Disorders

CP may be associated with intellectual disability, hearing and visual impairments, sensory impairments, communication difficulties, behavior problems, pain, epilepsy, autism, and neurogenic bowel and bladder.

Many children may have musculoskeletal issues such as hip uncovering, hip dislocations, scoliosis, osteopenia and osteoporosis, and muscle contractures (most commonly heel cord and hamstring contractures). Due to the many musculoskeletal issues outlined, gait abnormalities are common and can include scissoring, in-toeing, crouch gait, stiff knee, and toe gait.

Hip and spine surveillance should include regular clinical examination, with the addition of radiographic imaging depending on the GMFCS level. The risk of hip dislocations is correlated with increasing GMFCS levels. Patients may need referral to an orthopedic surgeon.[4]

Treatment

The treatment approach to CP is generally multimodal and includes occupational, physical, speech, and developmental therapies, in addition to orthotics, casting, pharmacologic management, and surgery. Spasticity is scored by the Modified Ashworth Scale (MAS). Management of spasticity focuses on encouraging developmental and pediatric milestones. Pharmacologic management for spasticity includes baclofen, diazepam, dantrolene, and tizanidine. Trihexyphenidyl has been used to treat dystonia. Focal treatment includes injectables such as botulinum toxin and phenol. Intrathecal baclofen is an option for difficult-to-control hypertonia that has not responded to oral medications or focal treatment.

Some children with spastic CP may be candidates for selective dorsal rhizotomy (SDR), a surgical procedure in which carefully chosen sensory nerve roots in the spinal canal are severed to decrease spasticity and preserve motor function. Candidates for SDR are children ideally of ages 3 to 7 years who have selective motor control and functional strength, with lack of significant contractures, and who will likely have good follow-up.[5]

Prognosis

Cerebral palsy can be diagnosed in infancy using the history, physical examination, and HINE score.[3] Generally, if toddlers are rolling supine to prone by 18 months, are reciprocal crawling by 1.5 to 2.5 years, or are sitting independently at 2 years of age, there is good prognosis for eventual ambulation. Total life expectancy depends on coexisting diagnoses.

Children with more severe CP are often diagnosed with global developmental delays, which applies to those with performance of at least 2 SD below the mean in two or more areas of development: motor (gross/fine), speech and language, cognition, personal-social, and/or daily living skills. Global developmental delay does not necessarily imply intellectual disability as 20% to 30% are not intellectually disabled at age 7. In general, the more severe the CP, the higher the likelihood of learning problems, but there is no direct correlation.

SPINA BIFIDA

Spina bifida and related disorders (spinal dysraphisms) occur as a result of disordered neurulation during embryologic development. Disordered neurulation can result in a variety of abnormalities of the brain, spinal cord, or both. It is commonly divided into three types: spina bifida occulta (a small opening with no neurologic sequelae), which is very common and usually asymptomatic; spina bifida aperta (placode open and flat); and spina bifida cystica (placode extruded within the sac). Spina bifida cystica can be further divided into meningocele (meninges only in the sac) and myelomeningocele (meninges and spinal cord extruded). The cause of these disorders is multifactorial and includes genetic/ethnic, environmental such as hyperthermia within the first 28 days, metabolic, toxic, and nutritional factors including maternal obesity. Folate deficiency is the most common risk factor.

The incidence of spina bifida in the United States has dramatically declined in the last 40 years and is now approximately 3:10,000 or 1,500 cases per year.[6] Even so, the incidence might be further reduced with improved maternal intake of folate of 400 mcg daily. While the incidence is decreasing, there is more prolonged survival, although morbidity is high due to complications such as skin breakdown, sleep disordered breathing, and neurogenic bladder.

Spina bifida is a multisystem disorder affecting neurocognitive function, with risk of attention deficit hyperactivity disorder (ADHD) and learning disabilities, variable motor impairments affecting gait and mobility as well as bowel and bladder function, and variable sensory impairments predisposing to pressure sores if wheelchair-reliant and other injuries especially to the feet and ankles if ambulatory. Therefore, individuals with spina bifida require lifelong neurosurgical, urologic, and rehabilitation management.

Neurosurgical Issues

Fetal surgery for spina bifida has led to better outcomes for many children.

In a study by Farmer et al. looking at the management of myelomeningocele, they found that in patients who underwent prenatal surgery, the presence of in utero ankle, knee, and hip movement, absence of a sac over the lesion, and a myelomeningocele lesion of L3 or lower than L3 were significantly associated with independent ambulation. Motor function post birth did not show a correlation with prenatal ventricular size or postnatal shunt placement.[7]

Chiari malformations are often associated with obstructive hydrocephalus and most often present early in life, but can present semiacutely with shunt malfunction or tethered cord.

Orthopedic Issues

Limb deformities present at birth can worsen over time as a result of progressive ongoing abnormal muscle pull. Examples of deformities that can progress include hip dysplasia and clubfoot. Acquired bone deformities can also occur, such as tibial torsion and hip dislocations. Treatment of dislocated hips is controversial. In nonambulatory patients, hip dislocations are not treated; in ambulatory patients, hips may be surgically treated to maximize gait. Scoliosis can be congenital or acquired. Progression of scoliosis can be a sign of tethered cord.

Most children with spina bifida have a neurogenic bladder of various types in association with renal/urinary tract anomalies, leading to a high risk of recurrent urinary tract infections and ultimately renal failure. Urologic management is critical and intermittent catheterization is the mainstay of treatment. Children may be taught intermittent catheterization in early childhood. Medications such as oxybutynin and imipramine may be helpful. Prophylactic antibiotics remain controversial. The Mitrofanoff procedure, which uses the appendix as a conduit from the bladder to the umbilicus, and bladder augmentation may be helpful for ease of bladder management. A nephrostomy or vesicostomy allows free drainage to prevent back pressure into the kidneys.

Rehabilitation Issues

Various brain anomalies such as dysgenesis of the corpus callosum and heterotopias often lead to ADHD and other learning disabilities; neuropsychologic testing is important to identify cognitive strengths and weaknesses, identify learning disabilities, and optimize the individualized education program (IEP) at school.

Children with spina bifida may need to be taught how to walk; they will be wheelchair-reliant if L3–L4 or above is affected. Orthotics management is critical for effective gait.

Insensate skin leads to a very high risk of pressure sores and tissue injury. Teaching families and patients to inspect the skin and care for the skin in insensate areas is critical.

Most children with spina bifida also have neurogenic bowel with incontinence; scheduled bowel programs are needed to optimize social participation.

All children should be referred to an interdisciplinary or multidisciplinary clinic if available. Frequent health supervision visits are essential to monitor bowel, bladder, skin, and neurocognitive status.

PEDIATRIC NEUROMUSCULAR DISORDERS

Neuromuscular disorders are disorders that affect the lower motor neuron. They can be classified anatomically to disorders of the anterior horn cell, disorders of the nerve fiber, disorders of the neuromuscular junction, and disorders of the muscles (Table 20.1).

Disorders of the Anterior Horn Cell
- *Inherited:* spinal muscular atrophy
- *Acquired:* polio, postinfectious myelitis

Disorders of the Nerve Fiber
- *Inherited:* hereditary motor and sensory neuropathy (HMSN), including Charcot Marie Tooth (CMT)
- *Acquired:* metabolic, postinfectious

Disorders of the Neuromuscular Junction
- *Inherited:* myasthenia gravis
- *Acquired:* botulism

Disorders of the Muscles
- *Inherited:* congenital myopathies, muscular dystrophies (MD), genetic myopathies
- *Acquired:* metabolic myopathies, postinfectious, inflammatory

TABLE 20.1 Epidemiology

Spinal muscular atrophy	1 in 6,000–10,000
Hereditary sensory neuropathy	1 in 3,300
Duchene muscular dystrophy	1 in 3,500
Myotonic dystrophy	1 in 8,000

Source: Data from National Institutes of Health. *Spinal Muscular Atrophy.* www.ninds.nih.gov/Disorders/All-Disorders/Spinal-Muscular-Atrophy-Information-Page; National Institutes of Health. *Hereditary Sensory Neuropathy.* www.ninds.nih.gov/Disorders/All-Disorders/Hereditary-Neuropathies-Information-Page; National Institutes of Health. *Duchenne Muscular Dystrophy.* www.ninds.nih.gov/Disorders/All-Disorders/Muscular-Dystrophy-Information-Page; National Institutes of Health. *Myotonic Dystrophy.* https://rarediseases.info.nih.gov/diseases/10419/myotonic-dystrophy.

DISORDERS OF THE ANTERIOR HORN IN CHILDREN

Spinal Muscular Atrophy

Spinal muscular atrophy (SMA) is a progressive, symmetrical hereditary proximal muscle atrophy. It is inherited in an autosomal recessive manner affecting the survival motor neuron gene (SMN) and affecting 1 in 10,000 children. Cognition is not affected.

There are three subtypes in children:

SMA type I (WerdnigHoffmann disease, infantile onset): This type presents before 6 months of age and may be apparent in utero. Most severely affected infants will be born with contractures, flaccid hypotonia, and have difficulty breathing. Other clinical signs include weak cry, tongue fasciculations, bell-shaped chest, frog leg posture, and feeding difficulty. They will never achieve sitting. If untreated, death will occur in the first year of life.

SMA type II (intermediate form): The first symptoms typically appear between 6 and 18 months. Children are able to sit unassisted but unable to stand or walk. Fine tremor may be present. Children will often have progressive kyphoscoliosis, with progressive lung disease. Hip dislocations may be present, as well as muscle contracture.

SMA type III (Kugelberg–Welander syndrome): Children develop symptoms after 18 months and can walk independently but may have difficulty with stairs or rising from a chair. Most have a normal life span.

Diagnostic Workup

At least 95% of deletions or mutations of the *SMN1* gene can be identified with genetic screening tests. Electromyography (EMG)/nerve conduction studies (NCS) may be considered.

Treatment

Treatment involves a multidisciplinary treatment team to improve posture, prevent joint immobility, and slow weakness while supporting function throughout the life span with stretching, strengthening, and equipment. Disease-modifying therapy is now available.

Disorders of the Nerve Fiber

Hereditary neuropathies are divided into four major subcategories: HMSN, hereditary sensory neuropathy, hereditary motor neuropathy, and hereditary sensory and autonomic neuropathy. Symptoms of hereditary neuropathies may be apparent at birth or appear in middle or late life. They can vary among different family members, with some family members being more severely affected than others.

CMT is the most common inherited chronic polyneuropathy that affects both the motor and sensory nerves in the upper and lower limbs. There are many subtypes of CMT indicating different genetic causes. There are over 100 genes that have been identified to cause CMT neuropathies. It typically becomes apparent in adulthood but can present in early childhood as well.

The most common forms are CMT1A and CMT1B and are characterized by abnormalities of the myelin and most often inherited in an autosomal dominant pattern. CMT2 is characterized by abnormality of the axon and demonstrates an autosomal dominant inheritance pattern.

Motor signs tend to present before sensory signs. Classic clinical findings include distal muscle weakness and atrophy and high-arched feet (cavus foot) with hammertoes. Individuals will also demonstrate abnormalities in sensation and scoliosis may also be present. Patients may have gait abnormalities, including loss of heeltoe gait pattern and a steppage-type gait. More severely affected individuals may develop hand weakness.

Genetic testing is recommended to determine the type of HMSN. Electrodiagnostic testing should be performed prior to genetic testing if suspected and no family history of HMSN.

There is no cure for congenital neuropathies and treatment involves therapy focusing on maintaining range of motion, strengthening, and avoiding overexertion, and therapeutic interventions to assist with function.

Postinfectious and Metabolic Polyneuropathies

Acute inflammatory demyelinating polyradiculopathy, also known as Guillain–Barré syndrome (GBS), is the most common cause of acute flaccid paralysis in children. Classic presentation begins with paresthesia in the toes and fingertips, followed by ascending symmetric weakness. In children, it will commonly present with pain and difficulty or refusal to walk. The main treatment includes intravenous immunoglobulin and plasmapheresis. In general, recovery is better in children than in adults.

Metabolic neuropathies that are not genetic often affect children and adolescents, especially children with renal disease and diabetes mellitus. Neuropathies may be caused by vitamin deficiencies through malnutrition, resorption disorders, or insufficient parental feeding.

Disorders of the Neuromuscular Junction

These disorders are rare and include botulism and myasthenia gravis. The infant with botulism may have history of constipation, followed by weakness, poor suck, weak cry, and descending paralysis with involvement of the cranial nerves.

Disorders of the Muscles

These disorders include inherited and acquired myopathies and muscular dystrophy (MD). Muscle weakness is the primary symptom of myopathy. Congenital myopathies are a group of disorders that are often evident at birth and children will demonstrate developmental delay. MDs are characterized by progressive weakness in voluntary muscles. Mitochondrial disorders are caused not only by mitochondrial genes but by thousands of nuclear genes needed for normal mitochondrial function.

Muscular Dystrophy

MD refers to a group of more than 30 genetic diseases that cause progressive weakness and degeneration of skeletal muscles. Some forms of MD are seen in infancy or childhood and others may not appear until adulthood. The most common form is Duchenne muscular dystrophy (DMD). It primarily affects males and is caused by an absence of dystrophin. Becker muscular dystrophy typically has milder symptoms due to abnormal or insufficient quantities of dystrophin Table 20.2.

TABLE 20.2 Comparison of Duchenne Muscular Dystrophy With Becker Muscular Dystrophy

	Duchenne Muscular Dystrophy	Becker Muscular Dystrophy
U.S. prevalence (estimate)	15,000	2,200
Incidence rate	1 in 3,500 male births	Unknown
Inheritance	X-linked	X-linked
Gene location	Xp21 (reading frame shifted)	Xp21 (reading frame maintained)
Protein	Dystrophin	Dystrophin
Onset	2–6 years	4–12 years (severe Becker muscular dystrophy) Late teenage to adulthood (mild Becker muscular dystrophy)
Severity and course	Relentlessly progressive Reduced motor function by 2–3 years Steady decline in strength Life span <35 years	Slowly progressive Severity and onset correlate with muscle dystrophin levels
Ambulation status	Loss of ambulation: 7–13 years (no corticosteroids) Loss of ambulation: 9–15 years (corticosteroids)	Loss of ambulation >16 years
Weakness	Proximal > distal Symmetric legs and arms	Proximal > distal Symmetric legs and arms

(continued)

TABLE 20.2 Comparison of Duchenne Muscular Dystrophy With Becker Muscular Dystrophy (*continued*)

Cardiac	Dilated cardiomyopathy in first to second decade Onset of signs in second decade	Cardiomyopathy (may occur before weakness) Frequent in third to fourth decade
Respiratory	Profoundly reduced vital capacity in second decade Ventilatory dependency in second decade	Respiratory involvement in a subset of patients Ventilatory dependency in severe patients
Muscle size	Calf hypertrophy	Calf hypertrophy
Musculoskeletal	Contractures: ankles, hips, and knees Scoliosis: onset after loss of ambulation	Contractures: ankles and others in adulthood
CNS	Reduced cognitive ability (reduced verbal ability)	Some patients with reduced cognitive ability
Muscle pathology	Endomysial fibrosis and fatty infiltration Variable fiber size and myopathic grouping Fiber degeneration/regeneration Dystrophin: absent Sarcoglycans: secondary reduction	Variable fiber size Endomysial connective tissue and fatty infiltration Fiber degeneration Fiber regeneration Dystrophin: reduced (usually 10%–60% of normal)
Blood chemistry and hematology	CK: very high (10,000–50,000) High AST and ALT (normal GGT) High aldolase	CK: 5,000–20,000 Lower levels with increasing age

ALT, alanine transaminase; AST, aspartate transaminase; CK, creatine kinase; CNS, central nervous system; GGT, gamma-glutamyl transferase.

Use of oral steroids early in Duchenne dystrophy substantially prolongs walking, which subsequently decreases the incidence of scoliosis. Steroids are thought to reduce fibrosis, inflammation, and muscle atrophy. There are other options for drug therapy to treat but not cure DMD.[8]

Facioscapulohumeral muscular dystrophy (FSHD) is one of the most common forms of MD in the United States, occurring in 4 in 100,000. Men and women are equally affected. It typically begins in the teenage years, causing variable progressive weakness in the face and shoulder girdle.

Emery Dreifuss muscular dystrophy (EDMD) is a hereditary myopathy with variable inheritance patterns. It occurs in 1 in 100,000. EDMD1 is the most common and has an X-linked recessive inheritance. Classic clinical findings include contractures of the elbow flexors, ankle plantarflexors, and posterior neck, as well as weakness. Cardiac diseases including arrhythmia and cardiomyopathy are associated.

Myotonic muscular dystrophy is the most common adult form of MD, occurring in 8 in 100,000. Congenital MD1 features include profound hypotonia, facial diplegia, poor feeding, arthrogryposis, and respiratory failure. It is often with associated clubfoot deformity.

Childhood inflammatory myopathies are rare, poorly understood disorders that typically affect children ages 2 to 15 years. Symptoms include proximal muscle weakness and inflammation, with muscle pain, edema, fatigue, and skin rashes. They may also experience difficulty swallowing, abdominal pain, fever, and contractures.

SPECIAL CONSIDERATIONS IN PEDIATRIC SPINAL CORD INJURY

Pediatric spinal cord injuries (SCIs) are relatively rare. Approximately 20% of all SCIs occur in individuals less than 20 years old and 3% to 5% occur in children less than 15 years old. Motor vehicle crashes (MVCs) are the most common cause of pediatric SCI. Other common causes include sports and violence (adolescents), in addition to falls (children <9 years old). In adolescence, males are four times as likely to have SCI. As age of onset of injury approaches 3 years of age, the incidence of SCI in males and females is nearly equal.[9]

The location of SCI varies in children compared with adults. Younger children have a larger head to body ratio, which places a larger force on the cervical region. Pediatric spinal trauma is more likely to involve the cervical region (60%–80%) compared with adults (30%–40%).[10] As children grow, injuries to the spinal cord may present lower. In pediatric patients, the elastic nature of the spinal cord ligaments and the immaturity of the spine contribute to the higher degree of motion at the spinal cord. Pediatric injuries are more likely to be stretch injuries rather than fractures and there is an increased incidence of spinal cord injury without radiographic abnormality (SCIWORA) in children compared with adults. Of note, children with Down syndrome are especially susceptible to atlantoaxial instability and are predisposed to high cervical SCI.

Due to skeletal immaturity at onset of pediatric SCI, children and adolescents are at a higher risk of scoliosis and hip subluxation and dislocation. Many patients with pediatric SCI require surgery for scoliosis. Thoracic lumbar sacral orthosis (TLSO) has been shown to decrease the rate of curvature progression and may delay the need for surgery. As such, proper monitoring of these complications is important.

In contrast to adult SCI guidelines on venous thromboembolism (VTE) prophylaxis, there are currently no universally accepted guidelines for length of VTE treatment and indication for VTE prophylaxis in pediatric SCI.[11] Studies have shown that risk factors for VTE in children with SCI include moderate to severe Glasgow Coma Scale (GCS) scores at presentation, abdominal injury, lower extremity injury, and obesity.[12] Routine chemical prophylaxis for VTE is typically not recommended in children less than 12 years of age as the risk of VTE in this age group is low unless risk factors are present.

Depending on the age of onset of SCI in children, certain skills, including bowel and bladder continence, may be considered habilitation rather than rehabilitation as children may not have learned these skills previously. Care of pediatric SCI patients should be family-centered and developmentally appropriate in order to promote proper development, independence, and a successful transition to adulthood.

SCOLIOSIS

Scoliosis is a three-dimensional deformity. The term refers to lateral bending of the spine with associated rotation of the vertebral bodies over five to ten segments. It is the most common spinal deformity affecting adolescents 10 to 16 years of age.

It is idiopathic in 70% of cases and almost all (97%) patients presenting with adolescent idiopathic scoliosis (AIS) have a positive familial history. After skeletal maturity, it is not likely to progress beyond 25°. Scoliosis can affect balance and gait.

Bracing is effective in controlling the curve if used at least 13 hours per day. There is a significant positive association between hours of brace wear and rate of treatment success.[13]

Neuromuscular Scoliosis

The likelihood and severity of the curve tend to increase with the degree of neuromuscular involvement. The incidence of scoliosis in CP with two limbs involved is 25%, with four limbs involved 80%, and in myelodysplasia lower lumbar 60% and thoracic level 100%. In SMA, the incidence is 67%.[14]

Symptoms

Children with neuromuscular scoliosis usually do not experience any pain from the condition.

Most children with neuromuscular scoliosis have poor balance and poor coordination of their trunk, neck, and head, contributing to ongoing asymmetry of posture during growth.

Prognosis

Compared with idiopathic scoliosis, neuromuscular scoliosis is much more likely to progress and continue progressing into adulthood. Curve progression and trunk imbalances are more severe in patients who are not able to walk. Neuromuscular scoliosis can lead to thoracic insufficiency syndrome (TIS), which is the inability of the thorax (chest) to support normal breathing and lung growth.

Bracing has been shown to have a positive effect on sitting function in children with neuromuscular scoliosis but does not alter the progression of the curve. Exercise alone is not effective.

Bracing is more effective with flexible curves, smaller curves, and sensate skin.[15]

CONGENITAL BRACHIAL PLEXUS PALSY

Brachial plexus injuries at birth result in weakness and sensory deficits of the involved upper limb. The incidence is between 1.6 and 2.6 in 1,000 births.[16] Common risk factors include large infants and shoulder dystocia. Mild injuries with significant recovery by 1 month do not require surgical repair. If no motor recovery by 3 months, surgical intervention may provide the best outcome.

There are characteristic patterns to upper and lower brachial plexus injuries. The most common presentation is injury to C5, C6, and C7 (Erb palsy), in which the proximal upper extremity is most affected. The shoulder will be adducted, arm internally rotated, elbow extended, forearm pronated, and wrist flexed. This is also called the waiter tip deformity. Injury to C8 and T1 (Klumpke palsy) results in the distal limb being affected and is infrequent. If the entire brachial plexus is involved, the arm will be flaccid and may be associated with Horner syndrome.

SPECIAL CONSIDERATIONS IN PEDIATRIC TRAUMATIC BRAIN INJURY

Traumatic brain injuries (TBIs) affect children differently compared with adults. The etiology of brain injuries in children varies by age. In children less than 5 years of age, falls are the most common etiology of TBI, followed by inflicted injuries and MVCs. In children ages 5 to 14 years assessed in the emergency department, falls remain the leading cause of TBI, followed by sports and MVC. The leading cause of TBI in children older than 15 years old is MVC.[17]

Survival and neurologic outcomes are generally worse for inflicted injuries than for accidental causes of TBI. Children who have had a TBI may have cognitive problems, including speech and language abnormalities, behavior problems, motor deficits, and less commonly epilepsy. Pediatric TBI can lead to neuroendocrine dysfunction, most commonly growth hormone deficiency, hypogonadism and, unique to children, precocious puberty. Thus, in pediatric TBI, it is important to monitor for neuroendocrine dysfunction immediately and as children develop. Pediatric endocrinology should be consulted early in their care if there is concern for neuroendocrine dysfunction.

Pediatric TBI may become more apparent during development as children "grow into their deficits." Damaged parts of the brain, such as the particularly vulnerable frontal lobes, may not be able to mature normally. Developmental delays from TBI can contribute to declines in academic performance or emotional and behavioral disorders.

PEDIATRIC CANCER

The most common pediatric cancer in children ages 0 to 14 years is leukemia, followed by brain and nervous system tumors, then lymphoma and reticuloendothelial neoplasms. In the adolescent age group 15 to 19 years, brain and nervous system tumors and lymphoma are the most common and leukemia is the third most common.

Treatment of leukemia can lead to neuromuscular and musculoskeletal complications, including myopathy, peripheral neuropathy, pain, avascular necrosis, and decreased bone mineral density. Steroid use is associated with myopathy, hyperglycemia, and osteonecrosis.[18]

Brain tumors are the second most common childhood malignancy behind leukemia and are the most common solid tumor in children and adolescents. The most common brain tumors are astrocytoma, medulloblastoma, and ependymoma.[19] Medulloblastoma is the most common malignant brain tumor in children.[20] Children may have impairments due to the tumor, resection, chemotherapy, and/or radiation.[21]

Osteosarcoma is the most common malignant bone tumor in children and adolescents. Ewing sarcoma is the second most common malignant bone tumor in children and adolescents. The incidence is higher in males and Caucasians. For both osteosarcoma and Ewing sarcoma, the most common presenting symptom is pain.[22]

Based on treatment for each type of cancer in children and adolescents, it is important to anticipate side effects and potential for long-term sequelae.

There are physical impacts from treatment, such as neuropathy and poor endurance, but also cognitive and psychosocial challenges. Treatment of childhood cancers continues to evolve to limit the short- and long-term side effects of cancer treatment.

JUVENILE IDIOPATHIC ARTHRITIS

Juvenile idiopathic arthritis (JIA) is the most common chronic rheumatologic disease in children and usually presents with peripheral arthritis. According to the International League of Associations for Rheumatology (ILAR), the diagnosis of JIA requires the following criteria: onset before 16 years of age, symptoms persist for at least 6 weeks, and all other conditions have been excluded. JIA is categorized into seven types: systemic arthritis, oligoarthritis, polyarthritis including rheumatoid factor (RF)-positive and RF-negative types, enthesitis-related arthritis, psoriatic arthritis, and undifferentiated JIA.[23]

Systemic arthritis: Systemic arthritis is characterized by fever of at least 2 weeks, occurring daily for at least 3 days, accompanied by one or more of the following: salmon-colored rash, lymphadenopathy, hepatomegaly, splenomegaly, and/or serositis.

Polyarthritis: Polyarthritis is characterized by involvement of five or more joints and divided into RF-positive and RF-negative classifications. According to the criteria, in order to be classified as the RF-positive type, patients should have at least two positive RF tests within 6 months.

Oligoarthritis: Oligoarthritis is characterized by involvement of less than five joints on diagnosis and is categorized by persistent or extended types. In the extended type, less than five joints are affected in the first 6 months, but these individuals progress to five or more joints affected after the first 6 months. In the persistent type, involvement does not extend further than four joints.

Enthesitis-related arthritis: Enthesitis-related arthritis is characterized by arthritis alone, enthesitis alone, or both arthritis and enthesitis, in addition to at least two of the following: sacroiliac joint tenderness, positive (HLA)-B27, first-degree relative with acute anterior uveitis, ankylosing spondylitis, inflammatory bowel disease (IBD) with sacroiliitis, or reactive arthritis, anterior uveitis, and onset of arthritis in males greater than 6 years old.

Psoriatic arthritis: Psoriatic arthritis is characterized by the presence of arthritis and psoriatic rash or arthritis and at least two of the following: dactylitis, psoriasis in a first-degree relative, nail pitting, or onycholysis.

Undifferentiated JIA: Children meet the criteria for JIA but do not meet any of the above criteria, or meet the criteria for more than one subtype of JIA.[24,25]

Some anomalies seen with JIA include micrognathia, leg length discrepancy, and hip dysplasia. The knee joint is the most commonly involved joint. Quadricep weakness and contractures may be seen. Children and adolescents with JIA may have wrist involvement, temporomandibular joint involvement (polyarticular form), shoulder involvement (psoriatic or polyarticular form), and cervical involvement.

Treatment for JIA in the rehabilitation setting should use a multidisciplinary approach, involving pediatric rheumatology, ophthalmology, orthopedic surgery, physiatry, physical therapy, occupational therapy, and psychology. Common nonpharmacologic treatments include resting the joint, splinting, stretching, and use of adaptive equipment. Pharmacologic treatment includes nonsteroidal anti-inflammatory drugs (NSAIDs) such as naproxen, ibuprofen, meloxicam, and indomethacin, which have been approved for use in children. Use of NSAIDs as monotherapy for over 2 months is discouraged if arthritis is still active.[26] Other treatments include intra-articular steroids, of which triamcinolone hexacetonide is preferred in JIA. Methotrexate (MTX) is the most widely used conventional disease-modifying antirheumatic drug (DMARD) for treatment of JIA due to its disease control and acceptable toxic effects.[26] JIA refractory to MTX may be treated with biologic DMARDs.

THERAPY SERVICES

Therapy for children is available in multiple settings. It is based on age, impact of the diagnosis on function, and availability. Who can provide services is regulated by state law. Federal and state laws regulate school-based therapy services.

Early intervention, mandated by the federal law, provides services for children from birth to 3 years of age who have diagnoses known to cause delays or who have documented delays in function for age. Criteria for services vary from state to state and availability varies widely.

School-based therapy was established by the federal law through the Individuals with Disabilities Education Act (IDEA) in 1975. IDEA mandates a free and appropriate public education (FAPE) in the least restrictive environment (LRE), based on an appropriate evaluation, with parent and teacher participation and procedural safeguards to establish an appropriate IEP.

IEPs involve goal-directed academic accommodations and support for children within schools. An IEP may begin with early childhood services up to kindergarten, offering classroom experiences and various therapies to prepare children for kindergarten, or begin at any other time from kindergarten through age 22. 504 plans are different from IEPs and accommodate physical disabilities without academic accommodations.

Medically based therapy generally provided in clinics and hospital settings is delivered based on diagnosis or impairments affecting daily function at home and in the community. Medically based therapies should be goal- and not diagnosis-driven in order to help the child achieve or maintain developmentally appropriate functional skills for home and the community. Goals can be habilitative, rehabilitative, preventive, or compensatory/adaptive.

REFERENCES

The full complete reference list for this chapter appears in the digital version of the chapter, available at http://connect.springerpub.com/content/book/978-0-8261-5628-0/part/part02/chapter/ch20

PART III

NEUROLOGIC REHABILITATION

CHAPTER 21

SPINAL CORD INJURY

Allison Kessler and Natasha Bhatia

EPIDEMIOLOGY OF TRAUMATIC SPINAL CORD INJURY

There are nearly 18,000 new spinal cord injury (SCI) cases in the United States each year.[1] Since 2015, the mean age has been 43 years old, up from 29 in the 1970s. The male to female ratio remains roughly 4:1. Incomplete tetraplegia is the most frequent neurologic category (47%), followed by incomplete and complete paraplegia (each ~20%) and complete tetraplegia (12%). Since 2010, the most common etiologies of SCI have been vehicular crashes (38%), followed by falls (32%), acts of violence (14%), sports/recreation (8%), medical/surgical (4%), and other causes (3%). Falls are the leading cause of traumatic SCI in people over the age of 65.[1,2]

SELECTED TRACTS

The major tracts of the spinal cord are depicted in Figure 21.1. The majority of the descending motor fibers from the motor cortex cross at the medulla to become the *lateral corticospinal tract* (CST). A small number of CST fibers do not decussate at the medulla and descend via the anterior CST before crossing at the level of the anterior white commissure.

The ascending dorsal columns, made up of the *fasciculus gracilis* and the *fasciculus cuneatus*, cross in the medulla via the medial lemniscus, then ascend to the thalamus. These fibers carry proprioception, vibration, and light touch (LT) sensation. The ascending *spinothalamic*

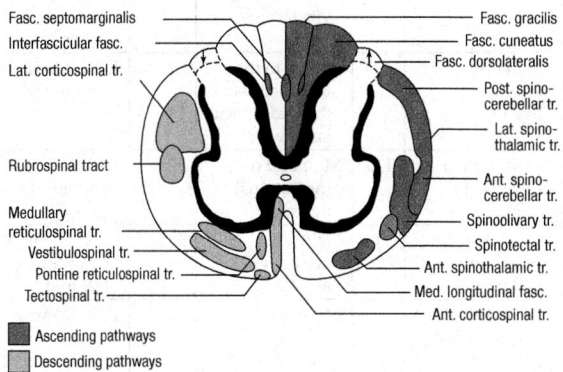

FIGURE 21.1 Ascending and descending pathways of the spinal cord.
Source: Ropper AH, Victor M. Adams and Victor's Principles of Neurology, 7th ed. McGraw Hill; 2000.

tracts, which carry pain, temperature, and nondiscriminative tactile sensations, cross to the contralateral side of the spinal cord shortly after entry in the ventral white commissure of the cord.

CLASSIFICATION OF SPINAL CORD INJURY

As per the International Standards for Neurological Classification of Spinal Cord Injury (ISNCSCI), the patient should be examined in the supine position in the following order[4]:

1. Perform a sensory examination of the 28 dermatomes at key sensory points (Table 21.1) on each side for pinprick (PP; poke once, not repeatedly) and LT (use a cotton-tipped applicator, stroke ~1 cm). Sensory levels are scored as 0 (absent), 1 (impaired, including hyperesthesia), 2 (normal), or not testable (NT). When scoring PP, the inability to discriminate PP from LT is scored 0.

   The sensory examination also includes evaluation of deep anal pressure, as determined by a reliable ability to feel the examiner's finger applying gentle pressure to the anorectal wall (graded as present or absent). The sensory level for each side is the most

TABLE 21.1 Selected American Spinal Injury Association Key Sensory Points

C2	At least 1 cm lateral to the occipital protuberance	T1	Medial epicondyle elbow	L3	Medial femoral condyle above the knee
C3	Supraclavicular fossa at the midclavicular line	T2	Apex of the axilla	L4	Medial malleolus
C4	Over the acromioclavicular joint	T4	Medial to nipple at the midclavicular line	L5	Dorsum of the foot at the third metatarsophalangeal joint
C5	Lateral antecubital fossa	T10	Lateral to the umbilicus at the midclavicular line	S1	Lateral heel (calcaneus)
C6	Dorsal thumb (proximal phalanx)	T12	Midpoint of the inguinal ligament	S2	Midpoint of the popliteal fossa
C7	Dorsal middle finger (proximal phalanx)	L1	Halfway between T12 and L2	S3	Ischial tuberosity or infragluteal fold
C8	Dorsal little finger (proximal phalanx)	L2	Midpoint between T12 and L3 (anteromedial thigh)	S4–S5	Perineal area <1 cm from the anal mucocutaneous junction

Source: American Spinal Injury Association. *International Standards for Neurological Classification of SCI (ISNCSCI) ISCOS Worksheet.* ASIA; 2019.

TABLE 21.2 American Spinal Injury Association Key Muscles

C5	Elbow flexors	L2	Hip flexors
C6	Wrist extensors	L3	Knee extensors
C7	Elbow extensors	L4	Ankle dorsiflexors
C8	Flexor digitorum profundus of the third digit	L5	Extensor hallucis longus
T1	Little finger abductors	S1	Ankle plantar flexors

Source: American Spinal Injury Association. *International Standards for Neurological Classification of SCI (ISNCSCI) ISCOS Worksheet.* ASIA; 2019.

caudal level with intact sensation for both PP and LT, where all rostral sensory levels are also intact.

2. Perform a motor examination of the 10 key muscle groups (Table 21.2) on each side, as well as voluntary anal contraction (instruct the patient to squeeze the examiner's finger as if holding back a bowel movement). Muscles are graded from 0 (total paralysis) to 5 (full active range of motion [ROM] against full resistance), or NT. A palpable or visible contraction is graded 1. Muscles limited by a non-SCI condition (such as peripheral nerve injury, fracture, burns, or pain) are documented with the actual (not normal) examination score and tagged with an asterisk '*'.[5] Plus and minus designations are not used in the ISNCSCI. If contracture limits more than 50% of the expected ROM, the muscle is NT. Voluntary anal contraction is graded as present or absent and must be distinguished from reflex contraction (e.g., due to Valsalva maneuver). The motor level for each side is the most caudal myotome with grade 3 or more, where all muscles rostral to it are grade 5.

3. Determine the single neurologic level of injury (NLI), which is the most caudal level with normal sensory and at least antigravity (3/5) motor function bilaterally, provided there is normal sensory and motor function rostrally.

4. Classify the injury as complete or incomplete. Complete injuries have no motor or sensory function, including deep anal sensation, preserved in segments S4 and S5. Somatosensory evoked potentials (SSEPs) may be useful in differentiating complete versus incomplete SCI in patients who are unconscious or unable to participate in the examination.

5. Categorize the injury using the American Spinal Injury Association (ASIA) Impairment Scale (AIS) A to E.[4]

    o *A. Complete:* No sensory or motor function is preserved in segments S4 and S5.
    o *B. Sensory incomplete:* Sensory function is preserved below the single NLI and *must* include segments S4 and S5. No motor function is preserved on either side of the body more than three levels below the motor level.

- C. *Motor incomplete:* Motor function is preserved more than three levels below the motor level on either side, and more than half of the key muscles below the NLI have a muscle grade less than 3/5.
- D. *Motor incomplete:* Motor function is preserved more than three levels below the motor level on either side, and at least half the key muscles below the NLI have a muscle grade greater than 3/5.
- E. *Normal:* Sensory and motor function of the key dermatomes and myotomes per the ISNCSCI is normal in all segments.

Note: To receive a grade of AIS C or D, there must be voluntary anal contraction *or* sensory sparing at the S4 and S5 level, with sparing of motor function more than three levels below the motor level on either side. According to the ISNCSCI, preservation of motor control of non-key muscles below the motor level may be used to determine sensory versus motor incomplete status (e.g., AIS B vs. C).

6. The ISNCSCI 2019 revision[5] defines the zone of partial preservation (ZPP) for all AIS grades, not just complete injuries. The ZPP is defined as the most caudal partially innervated sensory and motor segments below the sensory and motor levels, respectively (documented as four distinct levels: R-sensory, L-sensory, R-motor, and L-motor).

SPINAL CORD INJURY CLINICAL SYNDROMES

Central Cord

Central cord syndrome is an incomplete SCI syndrome usually seen in persons with preexisting cervical spondylosis who experience neck hyperextension injuries, typically due to falls. There is inward bulging of the ligamentum flavum into a stenotic canal, resulting in cord compression. Clinically, the arms are weaker than the legs, with variable sensory loss and with effects on bowel, bladder, and sexual function. Studies have shown significantly improved ambulation, self-care, and bowel/bladder function in patients aged less than 50 years compared with their older counterparts at the time of discharge from rehabilitation.[6]

Brown-Séquard

Brown-Séquard syndrome occurs with hemisection of the spinal cord resulting in ipsilateral paralysis (CST, spastic below the lesion and flaccid at the lesion level) and ipsilateral loss of fine touch, vibration, and proprioception (dorsal columns) at and below the lesion. Contralateral loss of pain and temperature sensation (spinothalamic tracts) starts one to two levels below the lesion. Brown-Séquard syndrome has the best prognosis for ambulation when compared with other incomplete SCI syndromes.[7] If the lesion is at or above T1, ipsilateral Horner syndrome may occur. Pure Brown-Séquard syndrome is rare; clinically mixed injuries may also have features of central cord syndrome.

Anterior Cord

The etiology of anterior cord syndrome is typically a vascular lesion in the territory of the anterior spinal artery. Other causes include retropulsed discs/vertebral fragments and radiation myelopathy. Intraoperative SSEPs, which primarily monitor the posterior column pathways, may miss the development of an anterior cord syndrome. There is variable loss of motor function and PP sensation, with relative preservation of proprioception and LT. Bladder and bowel functions are usually affected because the descending autonomic tracts to the sacral centers are typically involved. The prognosis for motor recovery is generally poor.

Cauda Equina

Cauda equina syndrome (CES) occurs from compression of the lumbosacral nerve roots within the spinal canal after the spinal cord has ended, resulting in lower motor neuron (LMN) injury. Sequelae depend on the roots involved. Clinical characteristics include urinary retention (with resulting overflow incontinence), bowel dysfunction, sexual dysfunction, flaccid lower limb weakness, and saddle anesthesia. Radicular neuropathic pain is common. CES is considered an emergency and urgent surgical consultation is indicated.

Conus Medullaris

A pure conus medullaris lesion results in saddle anesthesia and bowel, bladder, and sexual dysfunctions due to cord injury at the S2–S4 segments. While this syndrome may appear similar to CES, anal cutaneous and bulbocavernosus reflexes (S2–S4) and ankle deep tendon reflexes (S1–S2) may be preserved if the lesion is "high" in the conus. Conus lesions due to trauma (e.g., L1 vertebral body fracture) are typically accompanied by injury to some of the lumbosacral nerve roots, resulting in a mixed upper and lower motor neuron lesion presentation. The prognosis for recovery is poorer than for CES.

ACUTE TREATMENT OF SPINAL CORD INJURY

Multiple interventions in the acute care setting have been explored or are currently being studied; however, there is currently no cure for SCI. High-dose steroids are the most extensively studied: three large-scale studies (National Acute Spinal Cord Injury Study [NASCIS] 1, 2, and 3) showed the best effect if IV methylprednisolone was given within 8 hours of nonpenetrating injury, but was associated with increased infections in the acute care setting. The methods of these studies have been questioned and a 2012 Cochrane review failed to show enough data to recommend routine use of steroids after SCI. Currently, there is insufficient evidence to recommend corticosteroids as standard of care, but they are an option for treatment in acute SCI.[8–13]

Although there are no large-scale, randomized controlled trials for the timing of decompression for acute traumatic SCI, new clinical guidelines recommend early decompression (within 24 hours) when possible.[14] The Surgical Timing in Acute Spinal Cord Injury Study (STASCIS) showed early surgical intervention (<24 hours) was associated with higher total motor score and neurologic improvement compared with the late group.[15] Additional studies looking at acute traumatic central cord syndrome are less clear on the timing/need for surgical decompression; however, currently, the presence of mechanical instability, ongoing cord compression, fracture-dislocation type injuries, or focal and anterior cord compression favor surgical intervention.[9,15]

Maintenance of a mean arterial blood pressure (BP) of greater than 85 to 90 mmHg for the first week after SCI is recommended for spinal cord perfusion and has shown improved motor outcome scores.[16–18] In the acute setting, comprehensive medical treatment also includes cardiac, hemodynamic, and respiratory monitoring and support.[19,20]

PROGNOSIS AND RECOVERY IN TRAUMATIC SPINAL CORD INJURY

Complete Spinal Cord Injury

- 95% of persons with AIS A SCI at 1 month will remain AIS A at 1 year.[21]
- 73% of persons with AIS A paraplegia at 1 week post-SCI will remain AIS A at 1 year, 18% improve one level, and 9% improve two or more levels.[23]
- 5% of persons with complete paraplegia achieve community ambulation.[24]
- In persons with complete tetraplegia, more than 95% of key muscles in the ZPP with strength of 1 or 2 at 1 month post-SCI will reach grade 3 (antigravity) at 1 year.[22]
- About 25% of the most cephalad grade 0 muscles at 1 month will recover to at least grade 3 at 1 year,[21] with those having PP sensation being the most likely to recover motor function.
- Upper limb recovery has the greatest rate of change during the first 3 months, with potential improvement up to 12 to 18 months from injury.
- Motor level is superior to the neurologic or sensory level in correlating with function.

Incomplete Spinal Cord Injury

- Persons with incomplete tetraplegia often recover multiple levels below the initial level, with the majority of recovery occurring within the first 6 months.
- 46% of persons with incomplete tetraplegia can ambulate at 1 year.[24]

- As many as 80% of persons with incomplete paraplegia regain hip flexors and knee extensors (grade ≥3) by 1 year, resulting in a higher likelihood of community ambulation.[21]
- For persons with incomplete paraplegia, preservation of sacral PP has better prognosis for motor recovery and ambulation.[22]

Miscellaneous

- The 72-hour post-SCI neurologic examination may predict recovery more reliably than an examination performed on the day of injury.
- Absence of the bulbocavernosus reflex beyond the first few days can signify a LMN lesion and has implications on bowel, bladder, and sexual function.
- On MRI, the presence of hemorrhage and increased length of cord edema are independent negative predictors of motor function at 1 year.[21]
- Strength of 3/5 or more in the bilateral hip flexors and knee extensors on at least one side correlates with community ambulation.[25]

EXPECTED FUNCTIONAL OUTCOMES

The following are the expected functional outcomes in an average-age individual with SCI. Factors such as increased age, morbid obesity, cardiopulmonary disease, rotator cuff disorders, and concomitant injuries, among others, can negatively affect functional outcomes (I, independent; A, assist; D, dependent).

C1–C3: I with power wheelchair (PWC) mobility and pressure relief with enhanced equipment (e.g., sip-and-puff or head control); environmental control with assistive technology; D for all other self-care; goal for I for direction of care; ventilator-dependent.

C4: same as C1–C3, except variable ventilator status.

C5: usually no ventilator; I for feeding after setup and with adaptive equipment (e.g., a long opponens orthosis with utensil slots and mobile arm support); may be able to use a manual wheelchair (WC) with handrim projections on level, noncarpeted, indoor surfaces; may be able to drive adapted vans; A for other activities of daily living (ADLs).

C6: I with feeding with setup (may use tenodesis orthosis and short opponens orthosis with utensil slots); I for most upper body ADLs after setup with modifications (e.g., Velcro straps on clothing); A to D for most lower body ADLs, including bowel care; some male patients may be I with self-intermittent catheterization (IC) after setup; female patients are usually D; some patients may be I for transfers using a sliding board and heel loops, but many will require A; may be I with manual WC, but PWCs are often used, especially for longer distances and outdoors; may drive an adapted van.

C7: I for most ADLs, often using a short opponens splint and universal cuff; may require A for some lower body ADLs; women may have difficulty with IC; bowel care may be I with suppository inserter; I for mobility at a manual WC level, except for uneven transfers; patients may be I with a nonvan automobile with hand controls if they can transfer and load/unload the WC.

C8: I for ADLs including bowel and bladder care and mobility using manual WC; may drive adapted car.

Paraplegia: I for all ADLs from a wheelchair level with variable ambulation; trunk stability improves with lower lesions; those with upper and midthoracic injuries may stand and ambulate with bilateral knee ankle foot orthosis (KAFOs) and Lofstrand crutches (i.e., using swing-through or swing-to gait), but the intent is usually exercise, not functional mobility; patients with lower thoracic or L1 SCI may be able to ambulate at home using orthoses and gait-assistive devices, but rarely in the community; patients with L2 to S5 SCI may be community ambulators with or without orthoses (e.g., KAFOs or anklefoot orthosis [AFOs]) and/or assistive devices; driving with hand controls.

SELECTED ISSUES IN SPINAL CORD INJURY

Venous Thromboembolism

The incidence of venous thromboembolism (VTE) in the absence of chemoprophylaxis is 45% to 100%. Prior to routine use of chemoprophylaxis, pulmonary embolism (PE) was the leading cause of death after SCI. The highest risk is between 72 hours and 2 weeks post-SCI but remains high for at least 2 to 3 months. Guidelines recommend initiation of chemoprophylaxis as soon as no active bleeding is present and ideally within 72 hours of injury. Low-molecular-weight heparin is preferred. Direct oral anticoagulants can be considered in the rehabilitation setting but have not been extensively studied to make them a recommendation. VTE prophylaxis should be continued for at least 8 weeks, and up to 12 weeks in higher risk individuals.[26]

Autonomic Dysreflexia

Autonomic dysreflexia (AD) can occur in 48% to 85% of patients with SCI at T6 or above.[27] AD is defined as an increase in systolic blood pressure (SBP) greater than 20 to 40 mmHg above the person's baseline in response to a noxious stimulus below the level of injury.[27] Other symptoms may include diaphoresis above the injury level, piloerection, pounding headache, nasal congestion, cold extremities below the injury level, facial flushing, and a feeling of "impending doom." Figure 21.2 describes the mechanism by which AD occurs.

It is important to recognize AD early and begin treatment in order to prevent secondary injuries such as stroke, seizure, or death. The primary treatment of AD is removal of the noxious stimulus, which is most commonly due to bladder or bowel distension. Other causes can

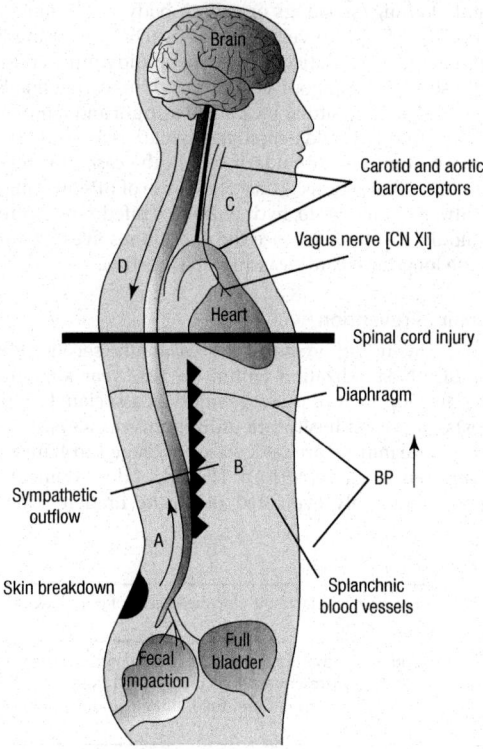

FIGURE 21.2 (A) A strong sensory input/noxious stimulus is carried into the spinal cord through intact peripheral nerves. (B) This sensory input evokes a massive reflex sympathetic surge from the thoracolumbar sympathetic nerves. This sympathetic surge causes widespread vasoconstriction, most significantly in the subdiaphragmatic (or splanchnic) vasculature, resulting in hypertension. (C) The brain detects this hypertensive crisis through intact baroreceptors in the neck delivered to the brain through cranial nerves (CN) IX and X (vagus). (D) The brain attempts two maneuvers to halt the progression of this hypertensive crisis. First, the brain attempts to shut down the sympathetic surge by sending descending inhibitory impulses. These inhibitory impulses do not reach most sympathetic outflow levels due to the spinal cord injury at T6 or above. Therefore, inhibitory impulses are blocked in the injured spinal cord. The second maneuver slows the heart rate through an intact vagus (parasympathetic) nerve. This may result in a compensatory bradycardia but is inadequate in reducing the hypertension. In summary, the sympathetic nerves prevail below the level of neurologic injury, and the parasympathetic nerves prevail above the level of injury. Once the inciting stimulus is removed, the reflex hypertension resolves.

BP, blood pressure.
Source: American Spinal Injury Association. Standards for Neurological and Functional Classification of SCI. 3rd ed. American Spinal Injury Association; 1990.

include tight clothing/stockings or splints, body positioning, urinary tract infections (UTIs), deep vein thrombosis (DVT), pressure injuries, abdominal emergencies, testicular torsion, epididymitis, endometriosis, undiagnosed fractures, gout, cellulitis, and ingrown toenails. Strategies to lower BP, such as sitting the patient upright and removing tight or restrictive clothing, should be initiated while workup and treatment for the noxious stimulus are undertaken. In the case of symptomatic AD without immediate source, consider the use of BP-lowering agents, including nitroglycerine paste, hydralazine, or nifedipine. Nitroglycerine paste should be removed once the episode resolves.[29,30] Recurrent AD can cause long-term cardiovascular dysfunction.

Pressure Injury Prevention

Skin disorders, including pressure injuries, are the second most common cause of rehospitalization within the first year after traumatic SCI.[31,32] The development of pressure injury is associated with higher medical costs, increased healthcare utilization, and worsened quality of life.[33–35] Pressure injuries are categorized as Stage 1 to 4, unstageable, or deep tissue injury (see Table 21.3). The risk of development of pressure injury is commonly evaluated using the Braden Scale, which

TABLE 21.3 Pressure Injury Staging

Stage 1	The skin is intact, with localized area of nonblanchable erythema.
Stage 2	There is partial-thickness loss of skin with exposed dermis and may present as intact or ruptured fluid-filled blister. Adipose, granulation tissue, slough, and eschar are *not* present.
Stage 3	There is full-thickness loss of skin. Fat and granulation tissue may be visible. Slough or eschar may be visible, but if they obscure the extent of tissue loss it is an unstageable wound.
Stage 4	There is full-thickness skin and tissue loss with exposed or directly palpable fascia, muscle, or bone. Tunnelling may occur. Slough and eschar are often present, but if they obscure the extent of tissue loss it is an unstageable wound.
Unstageable	There is obscured full-thickness skin and soft tissue loss due to eschar or slough. If the slough or eschar is removed, a stage 3 or 4 wound may be revealed.
Deep tissue injury	There is persistent, nonblanchable, deep red, purple, or maroon discoloration over intact or nonintact skin, or blood-filled blister. The wound may evolve to reveal the true extent of tissue loss or may heal.

Source: National Pressure Injury Advisory Panel. NPIAP Pressure Injury Stages. https://cdn.ymaws.com/npiap.com/resource/resmgr/online_store/npiap_pressure_injury_stages.pdf

assesses six categories (activity, mobility, sensory perception, nutritional status, skin moisture, and friction and shear) to determine the level of risk. Intrinsic risk factors for development of pressure injury after SCI include impaired sensation, immobility, greater injury severity (AIS A), mechanical ventilation, malnutrition, and medical comorbidities such as diabetes and renal disease.[36,37] Extrinsic risk factors include prolonged pressure, friction, excessive moisture due to urinary and fecal incontinence, and shearing forces.[38] Clinical guidelines recommend performing pressure relief every 15 to 30 minutes for a duration of at least 30 to 90 seconds when sitting and turning every 2 hours when lying in bed.[39,40] Management of fecal and urinary incontinence is also of utmost importance.

Treatment of pressure injuries depends on severity and underlying contributing factors. In general, a multidisciplinary approach should be implemented, with a focus on relieving pressure at the affected site, optimizing nutritional status, removing necrotic or infected tissue, and providing local wound care. Stage 4 pressure injuries may require surgical closure if nonsurgical methods fail.

Bone Metabolism

The risk of osteoporosis and fractures is increased below the level of injury following SCI, especially in the long bones. A new steady state is achieved between bone resorption and formation about 2 years following SCI. Clinical management can include treatment with calcium phosphate, vitamin D, calcitonin, and bisphosphonates, as well as functional stimulated exercises.[42]

Heterotopic ossification (HO) is an extraskeletal formation of bone, typically near the large joints. HO is common after SCI, affecting up to half of patients and beginning at approximately 12 weeks following injury. Patients with complete lesions and those who experience other complications such as spasticity, UTIs, and pneumonia have a higher risk of developing HO.[43] The hip is the most common site of HO in SCI. Symptoms occur in less than 20% of patients and can include pain, decreased ROM, and inflammation. A triple-phase bone scan is highly sensitive and may be positive well before plain radiographs. Initial treatment includes gentle passive ROM of the affected joint and nonsteroidal anti-inflammatory drugs (NSAIDs). Some studies have shown bisphosphonates may also be useful. Surgical excision is an option (after HO maturation), but recurrence rates are high.[44]

Cardiovascular Disease

As long-term survival has improved, cardiovascular disease (CVD) is an increasingly common complication of SCI. Risk factors such as obesity, abnormal lipid profiles, and impaired glucose metabolism are more prevalent in people with chronic SCI compared with the general population. Morbidity and mortality from CVD exceed those caused by pulmonary or renal conditions in the chronic SCI population.[45] Preventive measures and regular screening for CVD are warranted.

Urinary Tract Surveillance

Upper tract follow-up can include renal scan with glomerular filtration rate (GFR) or renal scan with 24-hour creatinine clearance annually to follow renal function. Renal and bladder ultrasound can be done annually to detect hydronephrosis and stones. Lower tract evaluation can include urodynamics once the bladder starts exhibiting uninhibited contractions (or at around 3–6 months postinjury) and then as determined by the clinician. Routine cystoscopy to potentially diagnose neoplasm at an earlier rather than a later stage should be performed annually as patients approach 10 years of chronic indwelling (urethral or suprapubic) catheter use, or sooner (e.g., after 5 years) if there are additional risk factors (heavy smoker, age greater than 40 years, and history of many UTIs).

Posttraumatic Syringomyelia

Posttraumatic syringomyelia (PTS) may be clinically significant in 3% to 8% of posttraumatic SCI patients and present in up to 20% on autopsy. Symptoms can include pain (often worsened by coughing or straining, but not by lying supine) and worsening neurologic function (e.g., ascending sensory loss, progressive weakness including the bulbar muscles, increased sweating, orthostasis, and Horner syndrome). Treatment is usually observational, with surgical interventions considered for large, progressive lesions with associated functional and neurologic decline.

Sexual Function and Fertility

Females

About 44% to 55% of women with SCI can achieve orgasm.[24] Menses may temporarily cease after SCI, but typically returns within 6 months postinjury, and reproductive function is preserved. In pregnancy, there are increased rates of UTI and cesarean sections compared with non-SCI pregnancies. The incidence of prematurity and small-for-gestational-age infants is higher, but there is no increase in spontaneous abortions or increase in long-term impairments in children born to women with SCI.[46] Spinal anesthesia is recommended during delivery in patients with SCI at T6 or above to prevent AD, as 85% of patients with SCI at these levels have been observed to develop AD during labor.[47]

Males

With complete upper motor neuron SCI, reflexogenic erections can usually be achieved, although ejaculation is rare. With incomplete SCI, reflexogenic erections are usually attainable; ejaculation is less rare than for those with complete SCI and some patients can achieve psychogenic erections. Complete or incomplete injuries below T11 may result in erections of poor quality and duration. Treatment options for erectile dysfunction (ED) can include medications, assistive devices, and surgical prosthetic implants. Phosphodiesterase-5 (PDE-5) inhibitors (e.g., sildenafil, tadalafil, and vardenafil) have been shown to improve ED and patient satisfaction. While PDE-5 inhibitors are well-tolerated in general, contraindications include the use of organic nitrates and some alpha-blockers. Direct self-injection of alprostadil (prostaglandin E1) into the corpus cavernosum is highly effective for ED, but is invasive and carries risks of priapism and penile fibrosis. Infertility after SCI is common due to factors such as retrograde ejaculation, poor sperm quantity and motility, and anejaculation. Penile vibratory stimulation for ejaculation requires resolution of spinal shock and an intact ejaculatory reflex (sympathetic fibers from the superior hypogastric plexus/T10-L2 for emission; and somatic fibers from the pudendal nerve/S2–S4 for expulsion). Electroejaculation (seminal vesicle and prostatic stimulation through the rectum) is another option and requires general anesthesia in those without complete SCI. The ejaculate is collected and processed for intrauterine or in vitro fertilization.

Tendon Transfer Surgery in Tetraplegia

Triceps function can be restored in patients with C5 or C6 SCI using a posterior deltoid-to-triceps or a biceps-to-triceps transfer. Lateral key grip can be restored in patients with C6 SCI via the modified Moberg procedure, which involves attachment of the brachioradialis (C5, C6) to the flexor pollicis longus (C8, T1) and stabilization of the thumb carpometacarpal and interphalangeal (IP) joints. Surgery is generally not undertaken until at least 1 year from injury.

Nerve Transfer Surgery in Tetraplegia

A newer technique than tendon transfers aimed at restoring upper extremity function after SCI is nerve transfer. Nerve transfers have a more variable outcome but do not require immobilization after surgery. The selection of nerves is dependent on the level of injury and concomitant LMN damage, requiring careful evaluation for selection prior to surgery.

REFERENCES

The full complete reference list for this chapter appears in the digital version of the chapter, available at http://connect.springerpub.com/content/book/978-0-8261-5628-0/part/part03/chapter/ch21

CHAPTER 22

TRAUMATIC BRAIN INJURY

Sangeeta Driver and Jamie Ott

EPIDEMIOLOGY

Traumatic brain injury (TBI) is a serious public health problem. Globally, 69 million individuals are estimated to suffer from TBI.[1] In the United States, there were approximately 223,135 TBI-related hospitalizations in 2019 and 64,362 TBI-related deaths in 2020.[2] Per the most recent surveillance report of the Centers for Disease Control and Prevention, the most common causes of TBI-related civilian hospitalizations are falls (59%), motor vehicle accidents (29%), assaults (8%), and unintentional blunt trauma (3%). In a survey of post-9/11 veterans, the most common mechanisms of TBI were blast (33.1%), object hitting the head (31.7%), and fall (13.5%).[3]

PATHOPHYSIOLOGY AND FUNCTIONAL IMPAIRMENTS

Injury pattern should be classified broadly between diffuse and focal with correlation to functional impairments. The primary injury occurs on impact and within the first few hours of the injury. *Diffuse axonal injury* (DAI) is the shearing of axons secondary to acceleration-deceleration, rotational forces, and differences in tissue density between the white and gray matter on impact. DAI is graded on MRI of the brain by the location of the associated petechial hemorrhages: 1-cortical-subcortical, 2-corpus callosum, and 3-midbrain.[4] Widespread injury to the axons and the ascending reticular activating system (RAS) is likely to cause impairments in consciousness, processing speed, and attention.

Focal injuries include contusions, bleeds, penetrating injuries, and ischemia due to arterial dissections. A *cerebral contusion* is the result of coup–contrecoup injury involving rapid acceleration-deceleration. It primarily affects the orbital/inferior frontal and the anterior temporal lobes due to the sharp inner skull ridges. Contusions typically resolve over months and may impair executive functions, behavioral regulation, mood, and communication. *Subdural hemorrhages* (SDHs) are crescent-shaped and are the most common bleed in TBI. SDHs may be due to shearing of bridging veins or arterial vessel damage. An *epidural hemorrhage* is elliptical in shape and commonly due to injury of the middle meningeal artery and a related temporal fracture. An enlarging SDH or epidural bleed can cause a midline shift and subsequent herniation syndromes that become surgical emergencies. Functional impairment correlates with the amount of focal ischemia due to compression from the bleed. A *subarachnoid hemorrhage* (SAH) occurs between the pia and the arachnoid space and can lead to communicating hydrocephalus due to damage of the arachnoid granulations that reabsorb cerebral spinal fluid. *Penetrating or "open" injuries* are usually due to trauma such as gunshot wounds, with functional impairments that correlate with the anatomic area of damage. Significant risks of seizures and infection occur in these patients due to exposure of the brain tissue to the external environment.

Secondary injury occurs in response to the primary injury in hours to days after the TBI. There may be biochemical changes, inflammatory changes, ischemia, hypoxia, or anoxia related to hypoperfusion. Vasogenic (extracellular) and cytogenic (intracellular) edema may be a result of disruption of the blood–brain barrier, damaged blood vessels, and cytoskeletal membrane integrity. These secondary injury processes are interrelated, each exacerbating the other. Biomarkers are currently being developed to identify the presence or extent of brain injury.

CLASSIFICATION OF TRAUMATIC BRAIN INJURY SEVERITY

TBI severity can be classified using various scales (see Tables 22.1 and 22.2).[5,6]

Posttraumatic amnesia (PTA) is the inability to retain memory after TBI, such as day-to-day information or ongoing events. It is measured using the Galveston Orientation and Amnesia Test (GOAT) or the Orientation Log (O-Log). GOAT is a series of questions related to orientation and recall of recent events. O-Log was developed as an alternative to GOAT and appears to be a better predictor of outcome. The end of PTA is marked by a score of 75 on GOAT or 25 on O-Log on two consecutive days. Severe disability is unlikely when PTA is less than 2 months and good recovery is unlikely when greater than 3 months.

The *Rancho Los Amigos Cognitive Functioning Scale* (Table 22.3) helps provide generalized descriptions of behaviors commonly seen during recovery in diffuse TBI patients.[7]

DISORDERS OF CONSCIOUSNESS

Consciousness is the state of being awake and aware of one's surroundings and requires intact function of both the cerebral hemispheres and

TABLE 22.1 Classification of Traumatic Brain Injury Severity

	Mild	Moderate	Severe
Loss of consciousness[a]	<30 min	30 min–24 hr	>24 hr
Glasgow Coma Scale (best in 24 hours)	13–15	8–12	3–8
Posttraumatic amnesia	0–1 d	1–7 d	>7 d

[a]Loss of consciousness not required to diagnose concussion.

Source: Adapted from Brasure M, Lamberty GJ, Sayer NA, et al. *Multidisciplinary Postacute Rehabilitation for Moderate to Severe Traumatic Brain Injury in Adults.* Agency for Healthcare Research and Quality (US); 2012.

TABLE 22.2 Glasgow Coma Scale

	Response	Score
Eye opening	Spontaneously	4
	To speech	3
	To pain	2
	None	1
Verbal response	Oriented	5
	Confused	4
	Inappropriate	3
	Incomprehensible	2
	None	1
Motor response	Obeys commands	6
	Localizes to pain	5
	Withdraws from pain	4
	Flexion to pain (decorticate posturing)	3
	Extension to pain (decerebrate posturing)	2
	None	1

Source: Adapted from Teasdale G, Jennett B. Assessment of coma and impaired consciousness. A practical scale. *Lancet*. 1974;2(7872):81–84.

TABLE 22.3 Rancho Los Amigos Cognitive Functioning Scale[a]

Rancho Level	Clinical Correlate
I	No response
II	Generalized response
III	Localized response
IV	Confused, agitated response
V	Confused, inappropriate response
VI	Confused, appropriate response
VII	Automatic, appropriate response
VIII	Purposeful, appropriate response

[a]Extended version exists.

Source: Adapted from Hagen C, Malkmus D, Durham P. *Levels of Cognitive Functioning*. Rancho Los Amigos Hospital; 1972.

the RAS. Severe brain injuries can result in disorders of consciousness (DOC), in which there is disruption of arousal and/or awareness. The different states of DOC exist on a continuum and include coma, the vegetative state/unresponsive wakefulness syndrome (VS/UWS), and the minimally conscious state (MCS). Coma is a pathologic state of unconsciousness in which the patient has no arousal or self/environmental awareness, characterized by no eye opening and absence of sleepwake cycles on EEG. Longer duration of coma is associated with worse outcome. Severe disability is unlikely when coma lasts less than 2 weeks. Good recovery is unlikely when coma lasts longer than 4 weeks.

Spontaneous eye opening and restoration of sleep–wake cycles on EEG mark progression into VS/UWS. Important prognostic classifications include persistent VS/UWS if this state continues 1 month postinjury and chronic VS/UWS if this state continues 3 months postinjury for a nontraumatic brain injury (nTBI) and 1 year for a TBI.

Progression to MCS requires minimal but definite behavioral evidence of self and environmental awareness. This may include the intermittent presence of at least one of the following: visual tracking, following a command, communication (verbal or gestural responses), and nonreflexive behavior triggered by external stimuli (e.g., functional object use or emotion). The JFK Coma Recovery Scale-Revised (CRS-R) is a standardized neurobehavioral assessment designed to help differentiate between VS/UWS and MCS. Emergence from MCS requires demonstration of reliable functional communication or functional object use.

Treatment of DOC generally focuses on sensory stimulation, physical rehabilitation including prevention of secondary complications, and neuromodulation through both pharmacologic and brain stimulation interventions. While there is a dearth of high-grade evidence demonstrating efficacy in the use of neurostimulants, many are used off-label and current practice guidelines recommend trialing amantadine for traumatic VS/UWS or MCS patients between 4 and 16 weeks postinjury to hasten functional recovery.[8]

ACUTE CARE MANAGEMENT OF TRAUMATIC BRAIN INJURY

Intracranial pressure (ICP) monitoring may play a role in early TBI care, although there is a lack of high-quality data indicating that routine ICP monitoring in TBI improves clinical outcomes. The rationale for ICP monitoring is that increased ICP causes decreased cerebral perfusion pressure (CPP = mean arterial pressure − ICP). ICP may be increased by temperature, stress, stimuli, elevated blood pressure, lying supine, suctioning, or aggressive physical therapy. An external ventricular drain is placed in the setting of severe brain injury (e.g., Glasgow Coma Scale [GCS] ≤8) when accompanied by edema, compressed basilar cisterns, or clinical decline. Increased ICP (>20 mmHg; normal is 2–5 mmHg) can be managed by elevating the head, using diuretics (mannitol) or hypertonic saline, barbiturates/sedatives, neurosurgical decompression with a craniectomy/craniotomy, or hyperventilation.

TRAUMATIC BRAIN INJURY REHABILITATION HISTORY AND PHYSICAL

In addition to a general rehabilitation examination, TBI-specific elements include the following:

- History
  - Mechanism of injury (fall, motor vehicle collision, blunt/bullet, blast)
  - *Psychiatric history:* history of mood, substance abuse, trauma exposure
  - *Cognitive baseline:* educational level and work, history of developmental disorder (e.g., attention deficit hyperactivity disorder [ADHD])
  - Premorbid personality
- Functional examination
  - Cranial nerves (CN) with focus on CN I (olfactory), which is the most commonly injured, as well as CN VII (facial) and CN VIII (vestibulocochlear), often associated with temporal bone and skull base fractures
  - Behavior, mood, emotional lability, agitation
  - *Cognition:* arousal, processing speed, attention, memory, executive function, spatial neglect
  - *Communication:* verbal and nonverbal (non-dominant), speech
  - Vision, hearing, smell
  - Vestibular function

TREATMENT OF TRAUMATIC BRAIN INJURY SYMPTOMS AND MEDICAL COMPLICATIONS

Impairments in Sleep, Cognition, and Behavior

Sleepwake disturbances (SWD) usually require a multifactorial approach. First-line treatment should focus on nonpharmacologic interventions such as sleep hygiene techniques, including establishing a regular bedtime routine, optimizing the bedroom environment with minimal light and ideal ambient temperature, minimizing daytime napping, limiting evening caffeine and alcohol intake, and avoiding late-night screen time. In addition to sleep hygiene, other evidence-based nonpharmacologic treatments include cognitive behavioral therapy (CBT), acupuncture, bright light therapy, and addressing sleep-related breathing disorders such as obstructive sleep apnea (OSA). Second-line treatment is pharmacologic management. Medications such as benzodiazepines and anticholinergic medications should generally be avoided given their adverse effects on cognition. Treatment options include over-the-counter (OTC) melatonin (3–10 mg), melatonin receptor agonist ramelteon (8 mg), and atypical antidepressant trazodone (25–150 mg). Other nonbenzodiazepine agents such as zolpidem and eszopiclone have been utilized, although there are few data describing its effectiveness in this patient population.

Poor arousal, attention, and memory can be addressed with pharmacologic agents such as amantadine, bromocriptine, levodopa/carbidopa, modafinil, methylphenidate, and donepezil. Stimulants such as amantadine may lower the seizure threshold and should be used cautiously in patients at risk of seizure.

Posttraumatic agitation is defined as "a subtype of delirium unique to survivors of a TBI in which the survivor is in a state of PTA and there are excesses of behavior that include some combination of aggression, akathisia or inner restlessness that may manifest in motor activity, disinhibition, and/or emotional lability."[10] Agitation can be measured and tracked using the Agitated Behavior Scale (ABS). Management focuses on environmental and behavioral modifications (e.g., minimizing sensory stimulation) and ruling out underlying causes of agitation (e.g., pain, infection, seizure, metabolic derangements, endocrine dysfunction, and alcohol/drug withdrawal). Physical restraints should be restricted to situations where there is risk of injury to self or others. Pharmacotherapy is second-line intervention and may include use of mood stabilizers (valproic acid, lamotrigine, and carbamazepine), atypical antipsychotics (risperidone, ziprasidone, olanzapine, and quetiapine), antidepressants (selective serotonin reuptake inhibitors [SSRIs], buspirone), and lipophilic beta-blockers (propranolol). Medications should be initiated at low dosages and uptitrated slowly while monitoring for side effects. Neurostimulants such as amantadine may improve agitation by improving confusion and frustration related to poor attention and executive function. In general, benzodiazepines and typical antipsychotics should be avoided given their adverse effects on neurorecovery.

Posttraumatic Seizures

Posttraumatic seizures can be subclinical (nonconvulsive), simple partial (localized with no loss of consciousness [LOC]), complex partial (localized with LOC), or generalized tonic-clonic/grand mal. Postinjury classification includes immediate seizures (occur within 24 hours after injury), early seizures (occur <1 week after injury), and late seizures (occur more than 1 week after injury). Increased risk of seizures can be seen with factors such as bilateral contusion (especially parietal and temporal), penetrating injury, focal hemorrhage, foreign bodies, dural tear, compressed skull fracture, midline shift >5 mm, and severe injury measured by GCS. An anticonvulsant such as phenytoin or levetiracetam is recommended for prophylaxis for 1 week after moderate-to-severe TBI to prevent seizures.[11] Prophylaxis beyond 1 week is not recommended and can negatively impact neurologic function and recovery. Management of immediate seizures is similar to prophylaxis guidelines given this type of seizure is not predictive of future seizures. The optimal management of early posttraumatic seizures has yet to be established, but typically patients are treated with anticonvulsants for a period of 6 months. About 25% of patients who experience an early posttraumatic seizure will have a subsequent seizure.

Late seizures should be managed with long-term anticonvulsants (at least 2 years). Carbamazepine and valproic acid are recommended anticonvulsant medications due to their preferable side effect profile, including their mood-stabilizing effects in the setting of TBI. Other commonly used medications include levetiracetam, lacosamide, phenobarbital, phenytoin, lamotrigine, and gabapentin. Anticonvulsants are used as long as seizures persist, and medication weaning may be considered if seizure-free for at least 2 years. EEGs are often performed prior to cessation of anticonvulsants.

Hydrocephalus

Posttraumatic hydrocephalus (PTH) is a common complication occurring in up to 45% of severe TBI patients.[12] PTH is characterized by accumulation of cerebrospinal fluid (CSF) and ventriculomegaly, most commonly caused by impaired CSF resorption. PTH should be considered if an unexpected functional plateau or deterioration is observed during rehabilitation. Treatment includes ventriculoperitoneal (VP) shunt placement.

Paroxysmal Sympathetic Hyperactivity

Paroxysmal sympathetic hyperactivity (PSH) is a widespread autonomic system disorder. While the mechanism is not fully understood, PSH is thought to result from loss of cortical inhibition on sensory afferent information activating the sympathetic nervous system.[13] It can occur in up to one-third of TBI patients and presents as a constellation of symptoms that can include six core features: tachycardia, hypertension, tachypnea, fever, diaphoresis, and dystonia. Treatment includes minimizing stressors (e.g., pain or noise), environmental measures (e.g., cooling blankets), and pharmacologic interventions. Common medication treatments include propranolol, clonidine, benzodiazepines, bromocriptine, morphine, gabapentin, dantrolene, and intrathecal baclofen.

Heterotopic Ossification

Heterotopic ossification (HO) is the formation of bone in soft tissue structures and can occur following TBI due to stimulation of osteoprogenitor cells. It can affect up to 10% to 20% of TBI patients and most commonly affects the hips, knees, elbows, and shoulders. Common risk factors include long bone fractures, coma of more than 2 months, and immobility. See Chapter 15 for further details.

Neuroendocrine Dysfunction

An estimated 30% to 50% of patients who survive TBI have endocrine abnormalities. Screening is recommended at 3 to 6 months and 1 year postinjury (morning cortisol, follicle-stimulating hormone [FSH], luteinizing hormone [LH], testosterone, prolactin, insulin-like growth factor 1 [IGF-1], estradiol, thyroid panel, and prolactin). Treatment generally involves hormone replacement.

Sodium abnormalities are common and may be secondary to the syndrome of inappropriate antidiuretic hormone (SIADH), cerebral salt wasting (CSW), or diabetes insipidus (DI). SIADH results in euvolemic hyponatremia (low serum osmolality, high urine osmolality, and increased urine output). Treatment includes free water restriction. In more severe cases, hypertonic saline infusion may be required (risk of pontine myelinolysis, if corrected too quickly). Chronic SIADH can be treated with demeclocycline, an antidiuretic hormone (ADH) inhibitor. CSW results in hypovolemic hyponatremia (low serum osmolality, high urine osmolality). The key distinguishing feature between SIADH and CSW is the dehydration/hypovolemia seen in CSW. Treatment for CSW is hydration with isotonic saline. DI is caused by severe damage to the pituitary, with ADH deficiency resulting in hypernatremia (high serum osmolality, low urine osmolality). Treatment includes fluid replacement and vasopressin.

RECOVERY AND OUTCOMES

Neuroplasticity, the physiologic mechanism of learning, may influence recovery through processes such as long-term potentiation and depression, axonal and dendritic sprouting, and synaptogenesis.[9] Restoration of function after neurologic injury can occur through recovery, restitution, substitution, and compensation.[14] Restitution is the internal, biologic recovery of the injured neural networks. Substitution is the external, functional adaptation of spared neural networks. Alternative strategies, home equipment, and technology are examples of behavioral and environmental compensations.

Outcomes following TBI can be measured by return of function and independence, as well as quality of life measures. Functional recovery is commonly measured using the Disability Rating Scale (DRS). The DRS is intended to measure general functional changes over the course of recovery. It is a 30-point scale that scores impairment, disability, and handicap. Other functional outcome measures include the Functional Independence Measure and the Glasgow Outcome Scale-Extended.

A physiatrist should provide education to the patient and family regarding the type and severity of brain injury, the expected impairments, and the time frame for recovery. Recovery from DAI is a gradual process that may occur over 2 to 3 years, with common long-term impairments such as cognitive fatigue and slowed processing speed. In contrast, focal injuries such as contusions and intracranial hemorrhages typically improve over approximately 1 year and can result in long-term impairments similar to stroke patients. While neurologic recovery plateaus, there may be continued functional improvements over the lifetime.

REFERENCES

The full complete reference list for this chapter appears in the digital version of the chapter, available at http://connect.springerpub.com/content/book/978-0-8261-5628-0/part/part03/chapter/ch22

CHAPTER 23

CONCUSSION

Deena Hassaballa

DEFINITION

A concussion represents a low-velocity injury caused by brain "shaking" resulting in clinical symptoms that are not necessarily related to a pathologic injury.[1] This clinical syndrome of biomechanically induced alteration of brain function typically affects memory and orientation, which may involve loss of consciousness (LOC).[2] The Centers for Disease Control and Prevention (CDC) defines concussion as a type of traumatic brain injury (TBI) caused by a bump, blow, or jolt to the head or by a hit to the body that causes the head and brain to move rapidly back and forth.[3] This can result in a range of clinical symptoms that vary from individual to individual and that may or may not include LOC.[3] Symptoms that arise may include posttraumatic headaches, vision issues, sleep disturbances, mood changes, cognitive changes, and an overall change in a person's quality of life.

EPIDEMIOLOGY

Over 18 years ago, the CDC presented a report to the U.S. Congress reporting mild TBI as a "silent epidemic" and the numbers have since increased.[4] Evidence shows that data sources may only capture one out of every nine concussions sustained in the United States.[3] For all sports combined, there are more concussions in males than in females.[2,3] The risk of concussion is greater in female athletes participating in soccer or basketball.[2,3] The numbers vary when discussing work-related injuries, trauma in the workplace, and domestic violence/intimate partner violence (IPV).

MOLECULAR BASIS OF CONCUSSION

Within seconds after the trauma to the brain, a complex cascade of neurochemical and neurometabolic events occur.[5] These events ultimately lead to a disruption in brain function (Figure 23.1).

HISTORY

The diagnosis of concussion is made based on history and physical, including assessment of the biomechanics of the injury and acute injury characteristics, and an evaluation of the clinical signs and symptoms.[6] The history should include details surrounding the event.

History of details surrounding the event:

- Mechanism of injury
- Timeline of symptom appearance

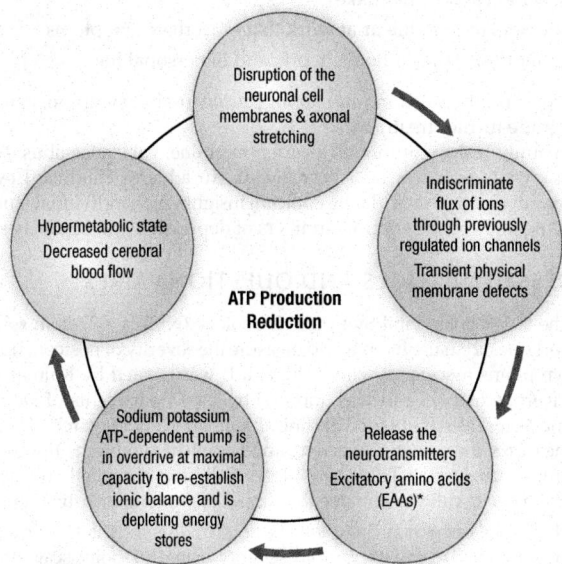

*which result in further ionic flux

FIGURE 23.1 A complex cascade of neurochemical and neurometabolic events occurs that results in a decrease in ATP production and cerebral blood flow, and puts the cerebrum in a hypermetabolic state.

ATP, adenosine triphosphate.

- Whether there was LOC and the length of LOC
- Litigation planned or pending
- Presentation to the emergency department
- Imaging findings
- If mechanism is motor vehicle collision: were seatbelts worn? airbags deployed?
- Witnesses
- Intoxication, with note of specific substances
- Previous concussions, duration of symptoms, how long ago, medically diagnosed and treated

Symptom history:

- Headache
- Dizziness
- Sleep (including questions related to sleep hygiene and medications being utilized)

- Nutrition and fluid intake
- Stressors in their life or at work that exacerbate symptoms
- Premorbid status at home, work, and in personal life

It is important to also inquire about preconcussion symptoms as this will guide further treatment.

Family history of mood disorder, migraine, substance abuse, and chronic pain disorders may be relevant. An adverse childhood event questionnaire may provide the clinician insight given individual studies showing higher self-reported numbers of depression and headaches.[7]

ASSESSMENT TOOLS AND QUESTIONNAIRES

- The Neurobehavioral Symptom Inventory (NSI) is a 22-item self-report questionnaire intended to measure the severity of postconcussion symptoms associated with mild TBI. It was created by Kalmar and Cicerone in 1995 and was adopted by the Departments of Defense and Veterans Affairs for TBI clinical evaluation and research.[8] The NSI measures the somatic, affective, and cognitive symptoms that sometimes present post-TBI. The NSI generally has acceptable reliability, although its validity remains the subject of ongoing investigations.[8]
- The Post-Concussion Symptom Scale (PCSS) is a 21-item self-report measure that records symptom severity using a 7-point scale. It has moderate test–retest reliability[9] and identifies concussion in athletes involved in an event with high specificity.[3] The PCSS has also been shown to discriminate between concussed and nonconcussed athletes.[9]
- The Graded Symptom Checklist (GSC) is an additional self-report measure of concussion symptoms and is a separate tool to identify concussion in athletes involved in an event with high specificity.[2,9]
- The Patient Health Questionnaire-9 is used to evaluate depression and generalized anxiety disorder.

PHYSICAL EXAMINATION

Vital signs: Evaluate for autonomic dysregulation with abnormal blood pressure and elevated heart rate.[9] Dysautonomia can delay clinical recovery as well as decrease exercise tolerance, which can limit return to previous activities, sports, and premorbid quality of life.[10]

Cervical/neck: Evaluate for trigger points, occipital tenderness, and thoracic spinal origins of pain. Assess passive and active range of motion.

Mood and cognition: Although the Mini-Mental State Examination can provide insight, a formal neuropsychological consultation with testing is recommended to diagnose true cognitive deficits.

Vision: Include pupillary light examination and examine smooth pursuits, saccades, gaze stability, and convergence. Extraocular motor function has gained attention with concussion assessments due to data showing that fiber tracts that connect the frontal cortex with the cerebellum may suffer shear damage from TBI.[10] This results in difficulty with eye-target synchronization that is worsened by cognitive strain.[10] Examination findings of abnormalities in saccades, smooth pursuits, convergence insufficiency, and nystagmus may not only be indicators of concussion but also poor prognostic indicators.[10]

Balance: Concussion can cause changes in static or dynamic balance.[10] The Balance Error Scoring System (BESS), which is used to evaluate a concussed patient, is an assessment tool that is likely to identify concussion with low to moderate diagnostic accuracy (sensitivity 34%–64%, specificity 91%).[2] Poor balance and postural instability have been reported in many studies after concussion and have been correlated with dysfunction in sensory integration.[2]

SYMPTOMS

Headache: Posttraumatic headache is a general umbrella term for the many diverse types of headaches that are seen after injury. Occipital headaches, tension headaches, cervicogenic headaches, and medication overuse headaches need to be differentiated as patients may display more than one. Cervicogenic headaches can develop with the onset of cervical disorders, such as biomechanical forces occurring during mild TBI; these secondary headaches may be targets for symptom management[11] and cervical injuries can cause persistent dizziness and balance difficulties, resulting in continuing headaches.[5] There is also evidence to suggest that temporomandibular joint disorders and thoracic abnormalities have been seen in conjunction with concussion with overlapping symptoms and should be considered.[10]

Mood: In adults, preinjury mental health problem and postinjury psychological distress are predictors of prolonged recovery.[9] Symptoms such as anxiety, irritability, and depression may be new symptoms or exacerbated after sustaining a concussion. Patients' significant others may also report changes in mood.

Sleep: Sleep disturbances can include hypersomnolence, insomnia, and further disruptions to the sleepwake cycle. It has long been recognized that sleep has both provoked and relieved headaches; the convergence of sleep and headache disorder is generally believed to have its basis in neuroanatomic connections and neurophysiologic mechanisms involving especially the hypothalamus.[6]

Vestibular: Patients may report changes in balance with increased falls, clumsiness, nausea, dizziness, and associated visual symptoms that may accompany vestibular changes, including photophobia, double vision, and blurry vision.

DIAGNOSTIC WORKUP

In sports-related concussion, CT imaging is not recommended to diagnose concussion, but rather used to evaluate for more serious intracranial injuries.[2] Blood-based biomarkers may have a role in preventing unnecessary CT imaging. The Scandinavian Neurotrauma Committee guidelines for adults recommend that S-100B values of <.10 µg/L, if sampled within 6 hours of injury, can help rule out the need for CT of the brain in patients younger than 65 years with a Glasgow Coma Scale (GCS) score of 14 or a GCS score of 15 with LOC or repeated vomiting.[9] In early 2018, the U.S. Food and Drug Administration approved the Banyan Brain Trauma Indicator (BTI) for adults with suspected mild TBI, but it has not yet been incorporated into published clinical practice guidelines.[9] The BTI is the first brain-specific biomarker blood screen to evaluate for TBI and aims to reduce the number of CT scans by stratifying the incidence of an intracranial lesion in patients with TBI by measuring two proteins that are released into the bloodstream and detected within hours after head injury.[7]

MANAGEMENT

Education and counseling: It is essential to provide enough time at the end of the physical examination to discuss the exact time frames for rest, expected symptoms, reassurance of recovery, proper hydration, and self-care. Reassurance is an important piece of education and counseling as many patients fear they will not recover. Approximately 10% to 15% of patients with concussion will present to clinic with persistence of symptoms.[10]

Rest: For patients being seen immediately after the event, relative rest is recommended for the first 24 to 48 hours. Complete rest without sensory stimuli does not accelerate recovery and is not advisable.[9]

Posttraumatic headache: Some supplements have been shown to be beneficial in posttraumatic headaches, including riboflavin 400 mg daily and magnesium oxide for headache/migraine prophylaxis. Studies have revealed decreased levels of micronutrients, such as riboflavin and magnesium, in the plasma and brain of migraine patients.[11] At the core of their effectiveness is their role in mitochondrial energy production and electron transport in the mitochondrial membrane.[12] Studies on use of riboflavin show a significant reduction in headache attack frequency with effective treatment compliance and even better tolerability.[13] Both intravenous and oral magnesium have evidence that demonstrates significant reduction in migraine frequency and intensity.[11] Magnesium is needed as a cofactor for proper functioning of the adenosine triphosphate (ATP) synthase, which produces ATP and is needed in various physiologic processes which influence the pathophysiology of migraine, such as vasoconstriction, platelet inhibition, and secretion of serotonin.[11] Magnesium deficiency is also associated with multiple conditions that are risk factors for migraine, such as caffeine overuse, metabolic syndrome, and obesity.[12]

Sleep: Sleep management should include sleep hygiene methods such as limiting screens 1 to 2 hours before bedtime, winding down before bedtime, and creating a sleep-supporting environment. Other sleep hygiene methods include limiting caffeine after 12 p.m. and limiting the duration and frequency of naps during the day so that sleep at night can be optimized. Utilization of evidence-based pharmacologic agents, such as melatonin, trazodone, and dual-use headache and sleep medications such as tricyclic antidepressants, is also recommended if sleep continues to be an issue after sleep hygiene modifications have been trialed.

Exercise: Exercise with supervision and guidance from physical therapy and occupational therapy is recommended. Exercise can improve brain function through favorable effects on brain neuroplasticity. Aerobic exercise has been shown to improve cortical connectivity and activation as demonstrated with functional MRI (fMRI).[14] Moderate aerobic exercise (60% of maximum heart rate performed for 150 min/wk) is cognitively protective.

REFERENCES

The full complete reference list for this chapter appears in the digital version of the chapter, available at http://connect.springerpub.com/content/book/978-0-8261-5628-0/part/part03/chapter/ch23

CHAPTER 24

STROKE

Joseph Burris

EPIDEMIOLOGY AND RISK FACTORS

Stroke is classically characterized as a neurologic deficit attributed to an acute focal injury of the central nervous system (CNS) by a vascular cause, including cerebral infarction, intracerebral hemorrhage (ICH), and subarachnoid hemorrhage (SAH).[1] The two major types of stroke are ischemic (87%) and hemorrhagic (13%).[2] Of ischemic strokes, 32% are embolic, 31% large vessel thrombotic, 20% small vessel thrombotic, 10% ICH, and 3% SAH.[2]

Risk factors for stroke are classified as modifiable and nonmodifiable. Nonmodifiable factors include age, race (African American > Caucasian), and family history. The strongest modifiable risk factors include hypertension (HTN), diabetes mellitus (DM), and smoking, followed by transient ischemic attack (TIA) or prior stroke, heart disease, atrial fibrillation, hyperlipidemia, carotid disease, hypercoagulable states, substance abuse, and physical inactivity. The risk of stroke is higher in men compared with women in those younger than 75 years of age, but becomes more common in women over the age of 75. Stroke remains the leading cause of severe long-term disability in the United States.

SELECTED ISCHEMIC STROKE SYNDROMES

Middle Cerebral Artery

Deficits can include contralateral (c/l) hemiplegia, c/l hypoesthesia (face and arm worse than the leg), c/l homonymous hemianopia, and ipsilateral (i/l) gaze preference. With *dominant* hemisphere involvement, receptive aphasia (inferior division of the middle cerebral artery [MCA] to the Wernicke area) and/or expressive aphasia (superior division of MCA to the Broca area) can occur. With *nondominant* hemisphere involvement, visuospatial impairment and hemi-inattention/neglect syndrome may be seen. Common *nondominant* hemisphere stroke-related impairments are anosognosia, a lack of awareness or insight; aprosody, blunted emotional inflection of speech output; and affective agnosia, inability to understand others' emotional component of speech context.

Anterior Cerebral Artery

Deficits can include c/l hemiplegia, c/l hypesthesia (leg worse than the arm, with the face and hands spared), alien arm/hand syndrome, urinary incontinence, gait apraxia, abulia (lack of will or initiative), perseveration, amnesia, paratonic rigidity (*Gegenhalten*, progressive resistance to passive range of motion [ROM]), and transcortical motor aphasia (with a dominant hemisphere anterior cerebral artery [ACA] lesion).

Posterior Cerebral Artery

Deficits can include c/l homonymous hemianopia, c/l hemianesthesia, c/l hemiplegia, c/l hemiataxia, and vertical gaze palsy. *Dominant-sided* lesions can lead to amnesia, color anomia, alexia without agraphia, and simultagnosia. *Nondominant-sided* lesions can lead to prosopagnosia (cannot recognize familiar faces). A bilateral (b/l) posterior cerebral artery (PCA) stroke can cause *Anton syndrome* (cortical blindness, with denial) or *Balint syndrome*, which consists of optic ataxia, loss of voluntary but not reflex eye movements, and an inability to understand visual objects (simultagnosia). *Central poststroke pain (DéjerineRoussy or thalamic pain) syndrome* can occur with involvement of the thalamogeniculate branch. *Weber syndrome* (penetrating branches to the midbrain) consists of i/l cranial nerve III palsy and c/l limb weakness.

Brainstem

Lateral medullary (Wallenberg) syndrome (posterior inferior cerebellar artery) consists of vertigo, nystagmus, dysphagia, dysarthria, dysphonia, i/l Horner syndrome, i/l facial pain or numbness, i/l limb ataxia, and c/l pain and temporary sensory loss. The *"locked-in" syndrome* (basilar artery) is due to b/l pontine infarcts affecting the corticospinal and bulbar tracts, but sparing the reticular activating system. Patients are awake and sensate, but paralyzed and unable to speak. Voluntary blinking and vertical gaze may be intact. *MillardGubler syndrome* is a unilateral lesion of the ventrocaudal pons that may involve the basis pontis and the fascicles of cranial nerves VI and VII. Symptoms include c/l hemiplegia, i/l lateral rectus palsy, and i/l peripheral facial paresis.

Lacunar

The more common syndromes include *pure motor hemiplegia* (posterior limb internal capsule [IC]), *pure sensory stroke* (thalamus or parietal white matter), *dysarthria-clumsy hand syndrome* (basis pontis), and *hemiparesis-hemiataxia syndrome* (pons, midbrain, IC, or parietal white matter). "Pseudobulbar palsy" is caused by anterior IC and corticobulbar pathway lacunes (loss of volitional bulbar motor control [e.g., dysarthria, dysphagia, dysphonia, and face weakness], but involuntary motor control of the same muscles is intact [e.g., can yawn or cough]). Emotional lability may be seen.

ISCHEMIC STROKE PHARMACOTHERAPY AND INTERVENTIONS

Guidelines for Acute Stroke Pharmacotherapy

Intravenous (IV) *tissue plasminogen activator* (tPA) is indicated for acute ischemic stroke within 3 hours of symptom onset. In 2009 and 2013, the American Heart Association (AHA)/American Stroke Association

(ASA) guidelines for administration of tPA following acute stroke were revised to expand the window of treatment from 3 hours to 4.5 hours to give more patients an opportunity to benefit from tPA, albeit with additional exclusion criteria. Intra-arterial fibrinolysis is also considered in a highly selective group of patients with major ischemic strokes of less than 6 hours in duration caused by occlusion of the MCA.

Absolute contraindications to use of tPA are head CT positive for blood; severe uncontrolled HTN, blood pressure (BP) greater than 185/110; head trauma or stroke in the previous 3 months; thrombocytopenia, platelet count less than 100,000; coagulopathy, international normalized ratio (INR) greater than 1.7 or protime (PT) greater than 15 seconds; treatment with therapeutic dose of low-molecular-weight heparin (LMWH), direct thrombin inhibitors, or factor Xa inhibitors within the past 24 hours; and blood sugar less than 50 or greater than 400. Relative contraindications are age greater than 80 years, mild/improving stroke symptoms, severe stroke/coma, major surgery within the past 14 days, gastrointestinal (GI) or genitourinary (GU) bleed within the past 21 days, seizure at the time of stroke onset, myocardial infarction (MI) within the past 3 months, and history of CNS structural lesion, for example intracranial neoplasm, arteriovenous malformation (AVM), or aneurysm.

Endovascular interventions, including mechanical thrombectomies, in addition to tPA, showed improved functional outcomes compared with tPA alone and may extend the window of interventions beyond the limitations of tPA alone or in combination treatments.[3]

Aspirin is recommended within 24 to 48 hours in patients with acute ischemic stroke not receiving thrombolytics or anticoagulation.[4] Administration of acetylsalicylic acid or other antiplatelet agents as an adjunctive therapy within 24 hours of IV thrombolysis is not recommended. Aspirin can be safely used with low-dose sternoclavicular (SC) heparin or LMWH for deep vein thrombosis (DVT) prophylaxis. Anticoagulation is considered in appropriate clinical settings. However, it is not recommended within 24 hours after administration of tPA.[4]

Elevated BPs may have a protective role initially after a stroke by improving perfusion to the ischemic but not infarcted penumbra. The goal of "permissive hypertension" is to optimize blood flow during this period.[5] Per the AHA/ASA guidelines, antihypertensive therapy within the first 24 hours after symptom onset is not recommended unless systolic blood pressure (SBP) is greater than 220 and/or diastolic blood pressure (DBP) is greater than 120 for this reason.[4] After this 24-hour period, however, AHA/ASA guidelines recommend that antihypertensive therapy be resumed or started, but an ideal BP goal has not been established.[4] The literature (e.g., the PROGRESS trial)[6] generally indicates that tighter BP control after the initial 24-hour period prevents recurrent stroke.

Recommendations for Secondary Prevention

Education on applicable lifestyle and risk factor modifications is critical. For noncardioembolic cerebral ischemic events, antiplatelet agents including acetylsalicylic acid, clopidogrel or ticagrelor, or a combination of acetylsalicylic acid and dipyridamole (Aggrenox) are considered. Dual antiplatelet therapy (DAPT) algorithms short term after stroke have been developed, but bleeding risk is elevated in DAPT and not recommended long term. For cardioembolic cerebral ischemic events, warfarin oral anticoagulation with a target INR of 2.5 (range 2.0–3.0) versus novel oral anticoagulants (NOACs) is recommended for secondary stroke prophylaxis.[7] Statins are considered as first-line treatment in secondary stroke prophylaxis, with high-dose statin therapy recommended for select populations based on overall risk profile, and not solely on serum lipid results.[8]

The North American Symptomatic Carotid Endarterectomy Trial (NASCET)[9] demonstrated a 6 to 10 times reduction in the long-term risk of stroke following carotid endarterectomy (CEA) versus medical management alone in patients with recent stroke or TIA with extracranial internal carotid artery stenosis of 70% to 99%. The benefit, however, was largely dependent on the skill of the surgeon. CEA for stenosis less than 70% was not supported. Guidelines for incidentally discovered asymptomatic carotid stenosis are less clear.

Patent foramen ovale (PFO) is relatively common in the general population, but its prevalence is higher in patients with cryptogenic stroke (i.e., stroke with no identifiable cause). Importantly, paradoxical embolism through a PFO should be strongly considered in young patients with cryptogenic stroke. There is no consensus on the optimal management strategy, but treatment options include antiplatelet agents, warfarin, percutaneous device closure, and surgical closure.

POSTACUTE MEDICAL COMPLICATIONS

The major causes of death after stroke are the stroke itself (e.g., recurrent stroke, progressive cerebral edema, and herniation), pneumonia, cardiac disease, and pulmonary embolism (PE). Complications can arise due to the stroke itself or from the ensuing disability or immobility. Complications noted during the postacute stroke rehabilitation period include pneumonia and pulmonary aspiration, falls, urinary incontinence, DVT, musculoskeletal pain, and central poststroke pain. *Urinary incontinence* typically improves but may still be present in 15% to 20% after 6 months.[10] Treatment can include timed voiding, fluid intake regulation, and treatment of urinary tract infections (UTIs). *Glenohumeral subluxation,* seen in 30% to 50% of patients, may play a role in poststroke shoulder pain. Arm trough or lapboard use while sitting, stretching of the shoulder depressors/internal rotators, Kinesio tape, functional electrical stimulation (FES), and avoidance of pulling on the affected arm during transfers can be key aspects of management during the early rehabilitation phase.

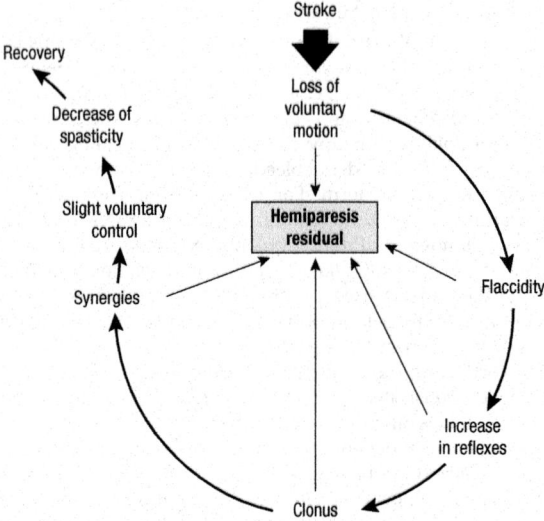

FIGURE 24.1 Stroke recovery pattern, per Cailliet.
Source: Stein J. Stroke Recovery and Rehabilitation. Demos Medical Publishing; 2009.

MOTOR RECOVERY FOLLOWING STROKE

Twitchell gave the first systematic clinical description of motor recovery following stroke.[11] In particular, tone and "stereotypic" movements, characterized by a tight coupling of movement at adjacent joints (later termed "synergy" by Brunnstrom), were noted to develop before isolated voluntary motor control was reestablished. In addition, it was noted that motor control returned proximally before distally and lower limb function recovered earlier and more completely than upper limb function. Full recovery, when it occurred, was usually complete within 12 weeks (Figure 24.1).

THERAPY APPROACHES

Traditional physiotherapeutic approaches (e.g., neurodevelopmental treatment [NDT]/Bobath approach, proprioceptive neuromuscular facilitation [PNF], and the Brunnstrom approach) have been in use for decades and are still commonly used in practice today. Using "hands on" techniques, these approaches focus on stimulating movement when there is weakness/inactivity, inhibiting excessive tone/primitive patterns of movement, and facilitating functional movement patterns. Systematic reviews, however, do not favor one approach over another.[12] For gait training, traditional approaches may be accompanied by neuromuscular reeducation, functional training, and body weight-supported treadmill training.[12] The strongest therapy recommendations in the 2016 AHA/ASA Guidelines for Adult Stroke Rehabilitation and Recovery are for intensive, repetitive, *task-specific training*; activities of daily living (ADL) and instrumental activities of daily living (IADL) training tailored to individual needs; and implementation of appropriate orthoses and other adaptive equipment.[12] Strengthening exercises complement task-specific training. *Constraint-induced movement therapy* (CIMT), which forces the patient to use the affected limb by restraining the unaffected one, and *neuromuscular electrical stimulation* (NMES) training use elements of task-specific training and are generally recommended. High-intensity interval training may improve cardiorespiratory fitness and mobility after stroke.[13]

FUNCTIONAL OUTCOMES FOLLOWING STROKE

The prognosis for a stroke survivor, overall, is generally good. Approximately 80% of stroke survivors walk within a year following stroke, 85% recover normal swallowing, 40% are able to return to work, and 90% are able to return home. The *Auckland Stroke Outcomes Study* showed that of 418 five-year stroke survivors, two-thirds had good functional outcome (defined as a modified Rankin Scale [MRS] score <3).[14] The MRS is a commonly used outcomes measure for neurologic conditions. It is a 7-point (0–6) ordinal scale, where 0 means no symptoms; 1 some symptoms but no significant disability; 2 a "slight disability" but independent; 3 a moderate disability requiring some help but able to walk independently; 4 a moderately severe disability; 5 a severe disability requiring constant nursing care; and 6 dead. The Auckland study did demonstrate that 22.5% had cognitive impairment indicative of dementia, 20% had experienced a recurrent stroke, almost 15% were institutionalized, and 29.6% had symptoms suggesting depression.[14] Stroke does remain the leading cause of long-term disability among adults.

In the Trial of Org 10172 in Acute Stroke Treatment (TOAST), the National Institutes of Health Stroke Scale (NIHSS) score strongly predicted outcomes after stroke.[15] An initial NIHSS score greater or equal to 16 forecasts a high probability of death or severe disability, whereas a score of less than or equal to 6 forecasts good recovery. The best neurologic recovery is seen by 11 weeks in 95% of patients; most ADL recoveries (by Barthel Index) are by 12.5 weeks with therapy.[16] The greatest proportion of recovery in ischemic strokes occurs in 3 to 6 months, although a proportion of patients may experience improvement for up to 18 months.[17] Prognosticating the recovery of specific neurologic deficits, such as weakness, aphasia, dysphagia, sensory loss, spatial neglect, and hemianopsia, is challenging. The time course and amount of improvement vary, but as a general rule mild deficits improve more rapidly and completely than severe deficits.

A number of factors affect outcomes after stroke, including age, stroke location, stroke type/severity, comorbidities, complications, acute interventions received (e.g., tPA), and whether an individual received stroke unit care and rehabilitation. Paolucci et al. reported better functional prognosis in stroke survivors with hemorrhagic stroke versus ischemic stroke.[18] *The Copenhagen Stroke Studies* have reported that morbidity/mortality and rehabilitation outcomes are positively affected by special stroke units (vs. general medical or neurologic units).[16,19] *A Very Early Rehabilitation Trial* (AVERT), a phase II randomized controlled trial (RCT), reported that earlier and more intensive mobilization after stroke is both feasible and improves walking and functional recovery.[20] A follow-up RCT by the AVERT group, however, reported that a high-dose very early mobilization protocol was associated with reduced odds of a favorable outcome at 3 months (where favorable outcome was defined as MRS <3).[21]

REFERENCES

The full complete reference list for this chapter appears in the digital version of the chapter, available at http://connect.springerpub.com/content/book/978-0-8261-5628-0/part/part03/chapter/ch24

CHAPTER 25

MULTIPLE SCLEROSIS

Sarah M. Eickmeyer, Aimee Lambeth, and Khulan Sarmiento

EPIDEMIOLOGY

Multiple sclerosis (MS) is the most prevalent chronic inflammatory demyelinating disease. It is thought to be immune-mediated and is characterized by areas of central nervous system (CNS) demyelination which are disseminated in time and space. The prevalence is about 309 per 100,000, or 727,433 adults, in the United States. There is a female to male ratio of 2.8:1.[1] The onset of MS is typically between 20 and 40 years of age, with a mean onset of 30. The incidence and death rates are higher in the northern latitudes, although this differential appears to be decreasing. Factors that increase the risk of developing MS include genetic and epigenetic factors, geographic latitude, socioeconomic status, tobacco exposure, obesity, and exposure to Epstein–Barr virus. The strongest genetic predictor is HLA-DRB1*1501, which has a twofold to fourfold increased risk.[2]

DIAGNOSIS AND CLINICAL FEATURES

The initial episode of MS is typically referred to as "clinically isolated syndrome" (CIS). This is generally synonymous to an attack or exacerbation when discussing MS. CIS is defined as subjective symptoms and/or objective findings that reflect focal or multifocal inflammatory demyelinating events in the CNS, lasting at least 24 hours, in the absence of fever or infection. Signs and symptoms vary depending on the location of the lesion. Common presenting symptoms include unilateral optic neuritis (with vision changes, such as blindness or scotoma), focal supratentorial syndromes (with focal weakness and sensory changes), focal brainstem or cerebellar syndromes, or transverse myelitis (also often presenting with focal weakness or sensory changes). Clinical features can also include fatigue, cognitive changes, vertigo, spasticity, neuropathic pain, depression and mood changes, dysphagia, bladder dysfunction, and sexual dysfunction. Patients may exhibit the Uhthoff phenomenon, or a transient worsening of symptoms by heat, and the Lhermitte sign, or an electric shock-like pain with neck flexion. Diagnosis may be made clinically, but corroboration with objective tests (e.g., MRI and visual evoked potentials) is recommended.

MS is formally diagnosed using the McDonald criteria (see Table 25.1), which were revised in 2017. A diagnosis of MS requires demonstration of CNS demyelinating lesions disseminated in time and space and exclusion of other diagnoses. Dissemination in space (DIS) can be

TABLE 25.1 Summary of the 2017 Revised McDonald Criteria for Diagnosis of MS

Clinical Signs and Symptoms	Additional Requirements to Make Diagnosis
Two or more attacks Two or more lesions on MRI One MRI lesion with evidence of a prior attack	None
Two or more attacks One lesion on MRI	Demonstrate DIS with additional MS attack implicating a different CNS site, or by MRI
One attack Two or more lesions on MRI	Demonstrate DIT with additional clinical MS attack or MRI lesions, or with CSF-specific oligoclonal bands
One attack One MRI lesion	Demonstrate DIS with additional MS attack implicating a different CNS site, or by MRI *plus* Demonstrate DIT by additional clinical attack or MRI, or with CSF-specific oligoclonal bands

CNS, central nervous system; CSF, cerebrospinal fluid; DIS, dissemination in space; DIT, dissemination in time; MS, multiple sclerosis.

Source: Thompson AJ, Banwell BL, Barkhof F, et al. Diagnosis of MS: 2017 revisions to the McDonald criteria. *Lancet Neurol.* 2018;17:162–173.

shown by T2 lesions in at least two MS-typical regions (juxtacortical or cortical, periventricular, infratentorial, and spinal cord). Dissemination in time (DIT) can be demonstrated by the presence of both gadolinium-enhancing and nonenhancing lesions at any time seen on a single scan, or by new T2 hyperintense or enhancing lesions on follow-up MRI which were not seen previously. MRI lesions may be symptomatic or asymptomatic. In the 2017 revisions of the McDonald criteria, with CIS and MRI with evidence of DIS, the presence of cerebrospinal fluid (CSF) oligoclonal bands allows for the diagnosis of MS (Table 25.1).[3]

CLINICAL CATEGORIES AND TREATMENT

There are four major clinical categories of MS: CIS, relapsingremitting MS (RRMS), primary progressive MS (PPMS), and secondary progressive MS (SPMS). CIS refers to the initial attack which may be compatible with MS, in which full diagnostic criteria may not be met. Once the diagnosis has been made, it is estimated that 85% of patients will have RRMS, characterized by intermittent acute attacks with return to neurologic baseline or near baseline between episodes. Patients with PPMS have a gradual progression of symptoms from the onset of the disease, and patients with SPMS start with RRMS but later develop a progressive course. An older term, relapsing-progressive MS, is

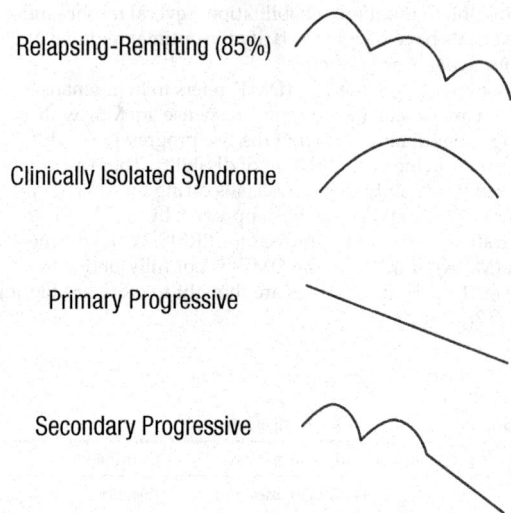

FIGURE 25.1 Schematic of the types of multiple sclerosis and their progression over time (left to right).
Source: Adapted from Thompson AI, Banwell BL, Barkhoff F, et al. Diagnosis of MS: 2017 Revisions to the McDonald Criteria. *Lancet Neurol*. 2018;17:162–173.

thought to be a combination of these types and is becoming less widely used. After 10 to 20 years, many patients with RRMS develop a progressive course (Figure 25.1).[2,4–6]

The pathophysiology of MS is thought to differ between clinical categories, although there is some overlap, and between different individuals with the disease. As discussed, geographic location and genetic factors play a role in the development of the disease. Generally, RRMS is thought to have a more prominent inflammatory component, and progressive types of MS are thought to have less active inflammation. Recent studies have looked into the possibility of a neurodegenerative process underlying progressive MS. T cells, both CD4+ and CD8+, have been found in both human studies and animal models of MS. B cells are thought to play a role as well, whether they are directly involved or indirectly involved as antigen-presenting cells. The CSF oligoclonal bands seen in MS represent antibodies which are produced by B cells. These mechanisms are important to consider when discussing medications used to treat MS.[2,6]

Acute exacerbations of MS are generally treated with corticosteroids, such as intravenous (IV) methylprednisolone. While at times this may be done in an outpatient setting, often patients are admitted to an acute care hospital to begin treatment. They may need to continue a course of IV corticosteroids during the first several days of their admission to inpatient rehabilitation. Several recent randomized controlled trials have sought to clarify the optimal regimen of corticosteroids for acute exacerbations.[7,8]

Disease-modifying therapy (DMT) refers to maintenance medications which modulate the immune response in MS, with goals of decreasing inflammation, slowing disease progression, reducing MRI lesions, and reducing accumulation of disability. These are likely to be encountered by rehabilitation physicians caring for MS patients. As of 2021, there are 23 DMTs for MS approved by the Food and Drug Administration, with most approved for RRMS. While the mechanism of action (MOA) of many of the DMTs is not fully understood, major mechanisms by which the drugs are thought to work are highlighted in Table 25.2.

TABLE 25.2 Examples of DMT for Multiple Sclerosis[5,9-12]

DMT	Mechanism of Action	Comments
Interferon-beta[a]	Effects on cytokines and cellular immunity	Injection; decreases brain atrophy, reduces MRI lesions, and slows progression of disease
Glatiramer acetate[a]	Expansion of regulatory T cells and production of neurotrophic factors	Injection; approved for treatment of CIS
Dimethyl fumarate[a]	Anti-inflammatory and cytoprotective mechanisms	Oral; 53% and 44% reductions in ARR
Teriflunomide[a]	Interferes with de novo pyrimidine synthesis	Oral; 36% and 31% reductions in ARR
Fingolimod[b]	Sphingosine-1-phosphatese receptor modulator	Oral; 54% decrease in ARR
Cladribine[b]	Inhibits DNA synthesis and promotes apoptosis in lymphocytes	Oral; 57.6% reduction in ARR
Natalizumab[b]	Monoclonal antibody against alpha-4 integrin and a selective adhesion molecule inhibitor	Monthly infusion; 68% reduction in ARR, risk of progressive multifocal leukoencephalopathy
Ocrelizumab[b]	Anti-CD20 monoclonal antibody	Biannual infusion; 40% reduction in ARR

[a]Moderately effective.

[b]Highly effective.

ARR, annual relapse rate; CIS, clinically isolated syndrome; DMT, disease-modifying therapy.

Traditionally patients are escalated from moderately effective to highly effective DMTs later in the course of the disease, but there is a trend toward using highly effective DMTs earlier in the course of the disease. Plasma exchange for treatment-resistant MS and stem cell therapies are being investigated, but are not yet commonly used. Vitamin D supplementation has been shown to be associated with decreased lesions on MRI in several studies; this should be considered for MS patients as well.[5,9,12]

REHABILITATION

Rehabilitation of MS patients varies considerably based on each patient's individual needs. However, areas that frequently deserve attention include cognitive impairment, chronic fatigue, spasticity management, mobility and assistive devices, vision impairment and its impact on function, and bladder dysfunction. Cognitive impairment is common in MS; brain atrophy is a hallmark of the disease. Brain atrophy may be seen prior to clinical symptoms and tends to worsen with disease progression. Cognitive rehabilitation is an essential component in helping MS patients function in work, social, and home environments.

Chronic fatigue is also very common in MS, reported in greater than 80% of patients, and can be very debilitating. Treatment of chronic fatigue includes working with therapists to develop energy-conserving strategies, minimizing sedating medications as able, and possibly prescribing stimulant medications such as amantadine, methylphenidate, or modafinil. A recent meta-analysis looked at studies of drugs for MS-related fatigue and concluded that amantadine has good evidence to support its use for this.

Spasticity management, similar to other neurologic disorders, should include stretching and positioning considerations. It may also involve oral medications such as baclofen, tizanidine, and others, botulinum toxin injections, and intrathecal baclofen pumps, which may be considered in patients with severe lower extremity spasticity.

MS patients frequently have gait impairment, and assessment for need of any assistive devices (canes, walkers, or wheelchairs) is essential to ensure they stay as safe and as active as possible in their daily lives. A regular exercise regimen, as allowed by the patient's mobility, is also important to maintain mobility and physical health. A newer medication, dalfampridine, has been approved for MS patients specifically to improve walking speed; multiple studies have demonstrated improvements in standardized measurements such as the 25-foot walk test. Patients are considered dalfampridine "responders" if they demonstrate at least 20% improvement in walking speed. This medication has also been investigated to see if it can improve other aspects of MS; a recent randomized controlled trial looked at its impact on cognition but found no significant impact outside on cognition.[2,9,13,16,17]

PROGNOSIS

Classically, some factors are reported to have favorable prognosis at diagnosis, including presentation with optic neuritis, female gender, and younger age at onset.[13] Unfavorable factors include spinal cord lesions, presence of CSF-specific oligoclonal bands, male gender, and older age at onset.[13,14] In addition, the increase in lesion volume during the first 5 years of the disease is associated with greater disability 20 years later.[13]

Tools including the Kurtzke Disability Scale, Expanded Disability Status Scale (EDSS), or Patient-Determined Disease Steps (PDDS) may be used clinically as measures of disability affecting persons with MS.[14] In RRMS, patients who experience three or more relapses in the first 2 years reached a higher level of disability on the EDSS 7.6 years earlier compared with those who only had one attack during this time.[15]

Receiving a disease-modifying treatment before the second attack is associated with lower risk of disability in relapsingremitting disease.[14] For RRMS patients, continuing disease-modifying treatments may reduce the risk of transitioning to SPMS to only 11.3% over 10 years.[14] Vitamin D deficiency, smoking, and some comorbidities have been associated with higher rates of relapse and disability progression.[15] Fertility is not affected by MS. There are fewer MS exacerbations during pregnancy, but the risk of exacerbation is increased early postpartum.

Overall, a relapsingremitting course generally has a better prognosis than a primary progressive or secondary progressive course. PPMS and SPMS are considered analogous because both have similar age of onset and rates of disability accumulation.[15] Spinal cord lesions and male sex are predictive of PPMS.[13] In primary progressive disease, imaging and clinical measures can help with early prediction of worsening disability.[13]

Future advances in disease biomarkers may include brain atrophy or volume seen on advanced imaging or laboratory markers such as serum or CSF neurofilaments, but these are still in development.[14,15]

REFERENCES

The full complete reference list for this chapter appears in the digital version of the chapter, available at http://connect.springerpub.com/content/book/978-0-8261-5628-0/part/part03/chapter/ch25

CHAPTER 26

MOVEMENT DISORDERS

Priya V. Mhatre

INTRODUCTION

Movement disorders are a group of central nervous system (CNS) degenerative diseases associated with involuntary movements or abnormalities of skeletal muscle tone and posture. They can be broadly classified as hypokinetic (too little) or hyperkinetic (too much) movement disorders.

HYPOKINETIC MOVEMENT DISORDERS (PARKINSON DISEASE)

Pathophysiology of Parkinson Disease

Key pathologic findings in Parkinson disease (PD) include loss of dopamine-producing neurons in the substantia nigra and abnormal alpha-synuclein protein aggregates (individually known as a "Lewy body").[1] This results in degeneration of the nigrostriatal pathway and thereby causes decreased dopamine in the corpus striatum, ultimately resulting in loss of inhibitory input to the cholinergic system, allowing excessive excitatory output. The pathologic features of PD also include pathology in other brain regions and other neurotransmitters, including serotonin, acetylcholine, and norepinephrine.[1,2]

Epidemiology

The incidence and prevalence of PD increase with age, with peak prevalence occurring between the ages of 85 and 89.[1,2] The prevalence of PD is expected to increase as the global population ages.[2] PD is more common in men than in women. Although most cases of PD are idiopathic, there have been associations with genetic and environmental factors (pesticide, herbicide, and heavy metal exposure).[1,2] Smoking and caffeine are associated with a decreased risk of PD.[1]

Clinical Presentation

PD is associated with both motor and nonmotor symptoms. Nonmotor symptoms may be present for years prior to PD diagnosis and onset of motor symptoms, although may not be recognized by patients or discussed with healthcare providers. Motor symptoms affect movement and physical tasks, whereas nonmotor symptoms are associated with other organ systems (Table 26.1).[1,3] The Hoehn and Yahr scale can be used to assess the clinical severity of disease (Table 26.2).[4] Independent of the severity of disease, motor, and nonmotor symptoms can cause various disabilities in individuals with Parkinson Disease (Table 26.3).

TABLE 26.1 Motor and Nonmotor Symptoms Seen in Parkinson Disease

Motor Symptoms	Nonmotor Symptoms
Bradykinesia Rigidity Resting tremor: typically pill-rolling quality in the hands, 4–6 Hz Postural instability	Decreased or absent sense of smell (anosmia) Sleep dysfunction Constipation Urinary urgency and frequency Orthostatic hypotension and blood pressure variability Psychiatric abnormalities (depression, anxiety, apathy, psychosis) Cognitive impairment ranging from mild to dementia Fatigue Hypophonia Dysphagia, speech impairment, and drooling

TABLE 26.2 Assessment of Clinical Disease Severity in Parkinson Disease

Stage 1: unilateral involvement only, minimal or no functional disability
Stage 2: bilateral or midline involvement, no impairment of balance
Stage 3: bilateral involvement, mild to moderate disability, impaired postural reflexes
Stage 4: unable to walk or stand unassisted, severe disability
Stage 5: confined to bed or wheelchair unless assisted

TABLE 26.3 Causes of Disability in Parkinson Disease

Social isolation
Decreased manual dexterity and coordination (inability to perform activities of daily living, such as dressing, cutting food, and writing)
Gait impairments: stooped posture, reduced gait speed, and retropulsion/propulsion, resulting in loss of balance and increased risk of falls
Speech impairments: difficulty communicating, dysphagia, and drooling
Psychiatric dysfunction and mood disorders

Treatment

Pharmacologic Treatment for Motor Symptoms[1]

1. *L-dopa:* precursor of dopamine; given with carbidopa (a dopa decarboxylase inhibitor), which prevents systemic metabolism of L-dopa (e.g., Sinemet)
2. *Dopaminergic agonists:* pramipexole (Mirapex), ropinirole (Requip), and rotigotine (Neupro patch), a once-daily transdermal (skin) patch that is changed every 24 hours
   a Ergot derivatives: bromocriptine (stimulates D2 receptors) and pergolide (stimulates D1 and D2 receptors)Nonergot derivatives

(possible neuroprotective): ropinirole (Requip) and pramipexole (Mirapex)
3. *Amantadine:* an antiviral that potentiates release of endogenous dopamine and has mild anticholinergic activity
4. *Anticholinergics:* effective in relieving tremor; include trihexyphenidyl (Artane), benztropine (Cogentin), procyclidine, and orphenadrine
5. *Inhibitors of dopamine metabolism:* inhibit monoamine oxidase (MAO)-B that is predominant in the striatum
   a *Selegiline and rasagiline:* decrease oxidative damage in the substantia nigra and slow disease progression
   b Tolcapone: catechol-O-methyltransferase inhibitor, inhibits metabolism of dopamine in the liver, gastrointestinal (GI) tract, and other organs

Pharmacologic Treatment for Nonmotor Symptoms

1. *Rivastigmine:* cholinesterase inhibitor, utilized for PD dementia
2. *Selective serotonin reuptake inhibitors (SSRIs), selective serotonin norepinephrine reuptake inhibitors (SNRIs), and tricyclic antidepressants (TCAs):* for treatment of depression in PD, with mechanism of action that varies on the subtype of the neurotransmitter affected
3. *Pimavanserin:* selective inverse serotonin 5-hydroxy-tryptamine 2A (5-HT2A) receptor agonist, approved for PD psychosis, although requires delivery via a specialty pharmacy
4. *Clozapine:* serotonin 5-HT2A receptor antagonist and dopamine D1 to D4 receptor antagonist, improves PD psychosis, with use that requires registration into the Risk Evaluation and Mitigation Strategy (REMS) program and with regular monitoring for neutropenia
5. *Quetiapine:* strong serotonin 5-HT2A receptor antagonist and weak dopamine D2 receptor antagonist, widely used for PD psychosis given the relative convenience of prescription compared with pimavanserin and clozapine
6. *Melatonin:* endogenous hormone secreted by the pineal gland for circadian rhythms, used for treatment of rapid eye movement sleep behavior disorder
7. *Fludrocortisone and midodrine:* mineralocorticoid analog and alpha-1 adrenergic agonist for treatment of orthostatic hypotension
8. Docusate, senna, and polyethylene glycol: prokinetic motility agents and laxatives for treatment of constipation

Nonpharmacologic Treatment for Motor and Nonmotor Symptoms[1,5]

1. *Cognitive behavioral therapy:* for treatment of depression in PD
2. Repetitive transcranial magnetic stimulation: may be useful for treatment of depression in PD, although definitive evidence is insufficient at this time

Surgical Treatment

Surgical treatment is indicated in patients with advanced disease in whom medical treatment is ineffective or poorly tolerated. It is mostly effective in the relief of tremor. Complications include brain hemorrhage, infection, and device failure.

1. *Destructive surgery*: thalamotomy or pallidotomy
2. *Deep brain stimulator*: electrode placed into the subthalamic nucleus or the ventral intermediate nucleus of the thalamus
3. Rehabilitation interventions with physical, occupational, and speech therapy (Table 26.4)

HYPERKINETIC MOVEMENT DISORDERS

Hyperkinetic movement disorders are classified by the form of movement, with a description based on characteristics such as rhythm, location (focal vs. generalized, unilateral vs. bilateral), duration (repetitive vs. nonrepetitive), and amplitude.[6] Subtypes include tremors, tics, Tourette syndrome, dystonia (generalized and focal), dyskinesia, chorea, hemiballismus, myoclonus, and asterixis.

Tremor: This is characterized by an involuntary, rhythmic oscillation of a body part which can occur at rest or with action, most commonly essential tremor. Whereas resting tremor occurs commonly with PD, a postural and action tremor is seen frequently with essential tremor. Essential tremor increases in prevalence with age and may be familial or progressive.[6] Treatment of essential tremor includes propranolol, primidone, benzodiazepines (BZDs), anticonvulsants (gabapentin and topiramate), and botulinum toxin injections.

Tics: These are sustained nonrhythmic muscle contractions that are rapid and stereotyped and often occurring in the same extremity or body part during stress. Movements can be suppressed temporarily with concentration. These are seen more often in children than adults.[6]

Tourette syndrome: The syndrome is characterized by multifocal tics and compulsive behavior, and may include involuntary use of obscenities (coprolalia) and obscene gestures (copropraxia). Onset occurs in childhood and is more common in boys.[6] It is treated using neuroleptics (pimozide and haloperidol).

Dystonia: This is characterized by sustained contractions of the muscles, which frequently cause twisting movements or abnormal postures. Movements tend to be patterned, occurring in recurrent locations, rather than random.[6] Subtypes include the following:

- Idiopathic
- Focal (torticollis, blepharospasm, oromandibular dystonia, and writer's cramp)

TABLE 26.4 Rehabilitation Strategies in Parkinson Disease

Physical therapy

- Posture training (hip extension, pelvic tilt, and standing)
- Postural reflexes
- Range of motion (passive/active and relaxation techniques)
- Progressive resistance training
- Ambulation: use of appropriate assistive device, including cane for early symptoms, wheeled walker, or weighted walker (to prevent retropulsion) for more advanced symptoms
- Conditioning (quadriceps and hip extensor strengthening)
- Wobble board or balance feedback trainers to improve body alignment and postural reflexes
- Fall prevention: home assessment, modification of environment

Occupational therapy

- Adaptive equipment such as plate guards, cups/utensils with large handles, and swivel forks and spoons
- Replace buttons on clothing with Velcro/zipper closures
- Management and compensatory strategies for micrographia
- Visuospatial evaluation
- Functional cognition strategies

Speech therapy

- Swallow evaluation and dysphagia management strategies
- Diaphragmatic breathing exercises to improve dysarthria
- Amplitude-based vocal exercises to improve dysarthria
- Cognitive evaluation and strategies to address executive function, attention, and memory

Other strategies

- General aerobic exercise
- Strength training
- Dance- and music-based exercise approach
- Tai chi and yoga

- Generalized (Wilson disease and lipid storage disorders)
- Neurodegenerative diseases such as PD and Huntington disease
- Acquired with perinatal brain injury, carbon monoxide poisoning, and encephalitis

Treatment includes anticholinergics, baclofen, carbamazepine, clonazepam, and botulinum toxin for focal dystonias.

Tardive dyskinesia: This is characterized by involuntary choreiform movements of the face and tongue, such as chewing, sucking, licking, puckering, and smacking, due to hypersensitivity of dopamine receptors due to long-term-blockade. It is associated with long-term neuroleptic medication use (20%). There has been decreased incidence since the advent of atypical neuroleptics such as clozapine, risperidone, and olanzapine. Treatment includes BZDs.

Ataxia: This is usually associated with cerebellar disease. Causes include stroke, multiple sclerosis (MS), acute/chronic alcohol toxicity, and hereditary Friedreich ataxia.

Treatment includes compensatory techniques, gait training, and assistive devices.

Athetosis: This is characterized by slow, writhing, and repetitive movements that may affect the face, trunk, and extremities. Movements may lead to an appearance of constant motion, although can be precipitated by voluntary activity in another body part; movements are not present during sleep.[6]

Chorea: This is characterized by nonstereotyped, unpredictable, jerky movements that are variable in type and location across body parts. Movements are present at rest but can be increased by activity and stress.[6]

Hemiballismus: This is characterized by extremely violent flinging of unilateral arm and leg and is classically secondary to infarct or bleeding in the subthalamic nuclei, although can also be seen with nonketotic hyperglycemia. Movements are involuntary, involve the proximal portions of the extremities, and disappear with deep sleep.[6]

Myoclonus: This is characterized by sudden, jerky, irregular contractions of the muscle. Types of myoclonus include the following:

- Can be physiologic (sleep jerks and hiccups)
- Essential (increasing with activity)
- Epileptic
- Symptomatic (part of underlying encephalopathy or stroke)
- Spinal myoclonus (group of muscles innervated by spinal segments), occurs in spinal cord disorders such as tumor, trauma, or MS

Treatment includes clonazepam, valproate, and levetiracetam.

REFERENCES

The full complete reference list for this chapter appears in the digital version of the chapter, available at http://connect.springerpub.com/content/book/978-0-8261-5628-0/part/part03/chapter/ch26

CHAPTER 27

OTHER NEUROLOGIC DISORDERS

Haibi (Daniel) Cai and Nassim Rad

MOTOR NEURON DISEASES

Amyotrophic Lateral Sclerosis

Amyotrophic lateral sclerosis (ALS) is a progressive neurodegenerative disease affecting the motor neurons in the brain and spinal cord. The hallmark of the disease is a combination of upper and lower motor neuron signs and symptoms, although a spectrum exists with only lower motor neuron disease (progressive muscular atrophy) and only upper motor neuron disease (primary lateral sclerosis; Table 27.1). The clinical presentation is diverse and initial symptoms can be weakness in a limb muscle (spinal onset) or speech and swallowing difficulties (bulbar onset). Respiratory weakness is common as the disease progresses and requires close monitoring so that noninvasive ventilation can be initiated when appropriate. Optimal care is provided in a multidisciplinary setting and should address dysphagia, dysarthria, sialorrhea, weight loss, respiratory function, cognitive changes, weakness, and spasticity.[1] ALS has a rapidly progressive course, with an average life expectancy of 2 to 3 years after the onset of symptoms. There is currently no cure for ALS. Two medications approved by the Food and Drug Administration (FDA), riluzole and edaravone, have been shown to slow disease progression and improve survival by 2 to 3 months.[2,3] The majority of cases are considered sporadic. Of those with a familial form, repeat expansion in the C9orf72 gene is the most common mutation. The diagnosis is largely clinical, although workup should be completed to exclude diseases that may mimic ALS.

Electrodiagnostic Findings

Electrodiagnosis criteria to support a diagnosis of ALS include the El Escorial criteria-revised and the Awaji criteria.

Nerve conduction studies (NCS): normal-low compound muscle action potential (CMAP) amplitudes; normal conduction velocities; normal sensory nerve action potential (SNAP) amplitudes

Electromyography (EMG): fibrillation potentials, positive sharp waves, and fasciculation potentials; large-amplitude, long-duration, and polyphasic motor unit action potentials (MUAPs) with reduced recruitment; evidence of active denervation and chronic reinnervation potentials in multiple body regions (bulbar, cervical, thoracic, and lumbar)[4]

TABLE 27.1 Physical Examination Findings in Upper and Lower Motor Neuron Disease

Upper Motor Neuron	Lower Motor Neuron
Weakness	Weakness
Hyperactive reflexes	Hypoactive reflexes
Spasticity	Atrophy
Dystonia	Fasciculations

X-Linked Spinobulbar Muscular Atrophy (Kennedy Disease)

Kennedy disease is a rare hereditary motor neuron disease affecting the lower cranial nerve motor nuclei and the anterior horn cells of the spinal cord. Affected males typically present with symptoms in their 30s to 50s. Symptoms include proximal muscle weakness (difficulty going upstairs, getting out of a chair, or with sustained overhead activities), dysarthria, and dysphagia. On examination, there is symmetric weakness in the proximal muscles (hips, shoulders, and neck) and bulbar muscles (cheek puff, lips, and tongue).[5] Fasciculations in the mouth and lips are pathognomonic of Kennedy disease. Life expectancy is near normal. Creatine kinase is moderately elevated. Kennedy disease is caused by CAG repeats on an androgen gene located on the X chromosome.[6] As a result, patients can also have gynecomastia, infertility, or endocrine dysfunction. A concomitant and asymptomatic sensory neuropathy is often diagnosed on electrodiagnostic testing.

Electrodiagnostic Findings

NCS: usually normal CMAP amplitudes (as the proximal muscles are more affected); often have decreased or absent SNAP amplitudes

EMG: fibrillation potentials, positive sharp waves, fasciculation potentials with large-amplitude, long-duration, and polyphasic MUAPs with reduced recruitment in the proximal and facial muscles

Spinal Muscular Atrophy

Spinal muscular atrophy (SMA) is a progressive neuromuscular disorder that results in the degeneration of the anterior horn cells of the spinal cord. The most common form of SMA results from mutations in the spinal motor neuron (SMN) gene, also known as 5qSMA, and presents with proximal symmetric weakness often accompanied by varying degrees of respiratory failure from weakness of the muscles of respiration. SMA is classified into four types based on onset of symptoms and maximum achieved motor milestone: type I: onset of symptoms less than 6 months, never achieve independent sitting; type II: onset of symptoms 6 to 18 months, achieve independent sitting but not independent standing; type III: onset of symptoms after 18 months, achieve independent ambulation; and type IV: adult onset of symptoms.[7]

Genetic testing has largely replaced electrodiagnostic studies in the diagnosis of SMA. In recent years, novel treatments such as nusinersen, risdiplam, and onasemnogene abeparvovec-xioi have drastically improved survival rates and slowed the progression of muscle weakness.

DEMYELINATING POLYNEUROPATHIES

Acute Inflammatory Demyelinating Polyneuropathy

Acute inflammatory demyelinating polyneuropathy (AIDP), also known as Guillain–Barre syndrome, is an acquired autoimmune disease characterized by ascending paresthesias, sensory loss, and weakness that can progress to total body paralysis, autonomic disturbances, and respiratory failure.[8] A mild flu-like illness often precedes the onset of symptoms by 1 to 4 weeks. *Campylobacter jejuni*, Epstein–Barr virus, and cytomegalovirus are frequently associated with AIDP. Extraocular muscles and sphincter function are typically spared. On examination, there are progressive symmetric sensory and motor deficits with hypoactive or absent reflexes. Cerebrospinal fluid (CSF) shows cytoalbuminologic dissociation (elevated protein, <10 mononuclear cells/mm^3). Patients require frequent pulmonary function testing to assess for impending respiratory dysfunction. Transfer to ICU and intubation should be considered for forced vital capacity less than 20 mL/kg, maximal inspiratory pressure above −30 cm H_2O, or maximal expiratory pressure below 40 cm H_2O (the 20/30/40 rule).[9] Later on in the course, autonomic symptoms such as tachycardia, urinary retention, hypertension, hypotension, orthostatic hypotension, arrhythmias, ileus, and bradycardia can occur. Clinical nadir occurs at about 4 weeks, with gradual recovery afterward. Most patients recover completely or nearly completely, although recovery time can be weeks to months, or up to 6 to 18 months if axonal damage has occurred. Of the patients, 10% have pronounced residual disability. First-line treatments are intravenous immunoglobulin (IVIG) and plasma exchange (PLEX).[10]

Electrodiagnostic Findings

NCS: absent or prolonged F-wave minimal latency as the earliest sign, with motor studies showing slowed conduction velocities and conduction blocks and sensory studies often showing low or absent SNAP responses

EMG: can show fibrillation potentials and positive sharp waves due to secondary axon loss; normal morphology MUAPs with reduced recruitment

Chronic Inflammatory Demyelinating Polyneuropathy

Chronic inflammatory demyelinating polyneuropathy (CIPD) is pathologically similar to AIDP but tends to have a more subacute onset of at least 2 months. CIDP can have a relapsing and remitting course, with periods of spontaneous improvement and worsening of symptoms.[11] Weakness is symmetric with both distal and proximal involvement. Differentiation between AIDP and CIDP is based primarily on temporal presentation. Whereas AIDP is an acute monophasic event, CIDP is a subacute event with relapses requiring sustained treatment. First-line treatment is immunomodulatory therapy with either high-dose corticosteroids or IVIG. Following strict electrodiagnostic criteria such as the European Federation of Neurological Societies/Peripheral Nerve Society (EFNS/PNS) criteria for diagnosis of CIDP is important to avoid misdiagnosis.

NEUROMUSCULAR JUNCTION DISORDERS

Myasthenia Gravis

Myasthenia gravis (MG) is a neuromuscular junction disorder caused by an autoimmune-mediated attack on acetylcholine receptors on the postsynaptic membrane. Fluctuating muscle weakness and fatigue are characteristic of MG, and symptoms are usually better in the morning and then worsen throughout the day.[12] Symptoms can progress subacutely over a few days to months, with a nadir around 2 years.[13] Ocular, bulbar, and proximal muscles are the most severely affected. Asymmetric ptosis and extraocular muscle weakness are common. Patients typically complain of double or blurry vision, which corrects when closing one eye. Weakness in the proximal muscles causes difficulty going upstairs, getting up from chairs/toilets, and prolonged overhead activities. Patients often also develop dysarthria and dysphagia. Respiratory dysfunction can occur in myasthenic crisis, necessitating intubation and aggressive immunotherapy. Muscle fatigability can be demonstrated on physical examination by (a) having the patient look up for greater than 2 minutes, (b) repeated strength testing of shoulder abduction or finger extension, or (c) having the patient count aloud and listening for slurring of speech. Acetylcholine receptor autoantibodies are found in the serum in 75% to 94% of generalized MG patients and 36% to 79% in ocular MG patients.[11] Muscle-specific kinase (MuSK) and lipoprotein-related protein 4 (LRP4) autoantibodies should be checked in patients who test negative for acetylcholine receptor antibodies. Pyridostigmine (acetylcholinesterase inhibitor) can be taken for symptomatic treatment. First-line immunomodulatory therapy is corticosteroids until the disease stabilizes and then transition to steroid-sparing agents such as azathioprine or mycophenolate mofetil. IVIG or PLEX can be used in myasthenic exacerbation or refractory disease. Thymectomy can be considered in patients less than 65 years with acetylcholine receptor-positive MG.[14]

Electrodiagnostic Findings

NCS: normal SNAP amplitudes; normal CMAP amplitudes but can be low in severe disease

EMG: no abnormal spontaneous activity; fibrillation potentials and positive sharp waves can be seen in severe disease; MUAPs show variability and blocking; MUAPs can be small amplitude with early recruitment in severe disease

Repetitive nerve stimulation (RNS): CMAP amplitude drop of greater than 10% from baseline on low-frequency RNS

Single-fiber EMG (SFEMG): increased jitter and blocking; SFEMG is the most sensitive test for MG (>90%), but is not specific; SFEMG can be abnormal in neuropathic or myopathic conditions

Lambert-Eaton Myasthenic Syndrome

Lambert-Eaton myasthenic syndrome (LEMS) is a neuromuscular junction disorder characterized by an immune-mediated attack on the presynaptic membrane's voltage-gated calcium channels (VGCC). Dysfunction of these calcium channels results in the inability to release acetylcholine from the presynaptic membrane. Patients present with proximal muscle weakness and can have mild dysphagia and dysarthria.[15] Patients may have autonomic symptoms such as dry mouth and orthostasis, distinguishing LEMS from other neuromuscular disorders. In LEMS, brief exercise or repeated deep tendon reflex testing can temporarily increase strength or tendon reflexes exhibiting postexercise facilitation. LEMS has a bimodal distribution, affecting young adults in their 20s (female predominance) and older adults in their 60s (male predominance). There is a strong correlation with small cell lung cancer in older adults, which initiates the autoimmune process. Autoantibodies to VGCC can be instrumental in making the diagnosis of LEMS.

Electrodiagnostic Findings

NCS: normal SNAP amplitudes; diffusely low CMAP amplitudes; brief isometric exercise (10 seconds) results in a marked increase (100%) of CMAP amplitude (postexercise facilitation)

EMG: no abnormal spontaneous activity; MUAPs can show variability and blocking; MUAPs can be small amplitude with early recruitment in severe disease

RNS: CMAP amplitude drop of greater than 10% on low-frequency RNS; high-frequency RNS results in postexercise facilitation and an increase in CMAP amplitude of greater than 100%

MYOPATHY

Polymyositis and Dermatomyositis

Polymyositis (PM) and dermatomyositis (DM) are classified as inflammatory myopathies. In both diseases, symmetric proximal muscles weakness develops and progresses subacutely over weeks to months, and in some cases of DM more acutely. Neck muscles can be significantly affected and head drop is common. Dysphagia and respiratory dysfunction can occur later on in the disease course.[16] Both PM and DM have a strong association with autoimmune disorders such as rheumatoid arthritis, lupus and Sjogren disease. The incidence of cancer is increased in adult DM, and if associated usually develops within 2 years of diagnosis. As such, a malignancy workup should be completed. In DM, patients also develop characteristic skin manifestations such as heliotrope rash in the upper eyelids, erythema over the cheeks and nasal bridge, a "shawl sign" of erythema over the posterior neck and shoulders, and Gottron papules which are erythematous or violaceous papules over the dorsal metacarpophalangeal (MCP) and interphalangeal (IP) joints. Creatine kinase is significantly elevated in PM and mildly to moderately elevated in DM. Muscle biopsy in PM shows inflammatory cells infiltrating nonnecrotic muscle fibers. Muscle biopsy in DM shows perifascicular distribution of atrophy and degenerating myofibers. Treatment requires immunomodulatory therapy with agents such as corticosteroids, IVIG, azathioprine, and methotrexate.[17]

Electrodiagnostic Findings

NCS: CMAP amplitudes usually normal (proximal muscles more affected); SNAP amplitudes normal

EMG: fibrillation potentials and positive sharp waves in the proximal muscles; small-amplitude, polyphasic MUAPs with early recruitment

Inclusion Body Myositis

Inclusion body myositis (IBM) is the most common inflammatory myopathy in older individuals. Unlike other inflammatory myopathies, IBM usually presents asymmetrically and has a more indolent course. Classically the long finger flexors, knee extensors, and ankle dorsiflexors are preferentially affected.[18] Dysphagia develops in up to 60% of patients and may be the presenting feature. Creatine kinase is normal to mildly elevated. Muscle biopsy characteristically shows inflammatory cells infiltrating myofibers and rimmed vacuoles. Despite classification as an inflammatory myopathy, IBM does not respond to immunomodulating therapy.

Electrodiagnostic Findings

NCS: can have mild sensorimotor polyneuropathy; low CMAP amplitudes; low SNAP amplitudes

EMG: fibrillation potentials and positive sharp waves; can have both small-amplitude, short-duration MUAPs and/or large-amplitude, long-duration MUAPs; early recruitment can help distinguish IBM from neuropathic conditions

Steroid Myopathy

Patients on chronic steroid therapy can develop proximal muscle weakness. Higher doses of steroids (>30 mg/d) and longer course of therapy exacerbate risk of developing steroid myopathy. Steroid myopathy preferentially causes atrophy of type II muscle fibers.[19] Creatine kinase is normal or decreased. Nerve conduction and EMG studies are normal in steroid myopathy.

REFERENCES

The full complete reference list for this chapter appears in the digital version of the chapter, available at http://connect.springerpub.com/content/book/978-0-8261-5628-0/part/part03/chapter/ch27

CHAPTER 28

COGNITION

Sony Issac, Natalia Del Mar Miranda-Cantellops, and Lauren T. Shapiro

INTRODUCTION

Cognition is defined as the "mental activity associated with obtaining, converting, and using knowledge."[1] Cognitive impairment may impede one's ability to learn and carry over new rehabilitation techniques, make appropriate decisions, safely live independently, and/or return to work, school, and/or driving. A change in cognition may be physiologic, as seen in normal aging, or pathologic, as a result of injury, disease, sleep deprivation, and/or exposure to or withdrawal from a substance. Such changes may come on acutely or insidiously, and may be temporary, permanent, or progressive.[2] The evaluation and treatment of cognitive impairment often require a comprehensive and multidisciplinary approach.

COGNITIVE DOMAINS AND PROCESSES

- *General intelligence* refers to the innate ability to problem-solve, adapt to surroundings, and learn from experiences.[1]
- *Learning* is the process by which changes in thought and/or behavior occur as a result of one's experiences.[1]
- *Memory* refers to the processes by which one remembers that which has been learned, and includes the encoding, storage, and retrieval of information.[1,2]
- *Spatial cognition* pertains to the acquisition and use of knowledge about one's environment. Impairments in this domain include difficulty navigating within one's home or community, and hemispatial neglect, in which one does not attend to the side contralateral to their brain lesion.[3]
- *Executive functioning* describes the group of skills required for planning, self-control, problem-solving, adaptation, and organization. Impairments may significantly impact the ability to perform daily tasks, including managing finances, driving, shopping, preparing meals, and work or school obligations.[1,3]
- *Social cognition* includes the social skills, personality traits, and psychological processes utilized to effectively engage with others. Impairments may impact one's relationships and worsen caregiver stress.[3]
- *Reaction time* refers to the ability to integrate and respond to stimuli with speed and accuracy.[3]
- *Attention* is the ability to focus on a sensory stimulus.[2]

- *Concentration* refers to sustained attention.[2]
- *Working memory* refers to the ability to retain information for its adaptive use.[2,3]
- *Self-awareness* refers to one's recognition of one's abilities and disabilities.[3]

DIFFERENTIAL DIAGNOSIS OF COGNITIVE IMPAIRMENT

Intellectual disability: This is characterized by deficits in mental abilities and adaptive functioning relative to one's peers. It may result from a genetic syndrome, hypoxic ischemic injury, infection, or head trauma during the developmental period. Such conditions usually result in lifelong impairment, but, with the exception of some genetic diseases, the intellectual disability is usually nonprogressive.[4]

Age-related changes: Older adults often have difficulty remembering recent experiences, as well as a slower rate of new learning. Older adults may also need additional time to complete cognitive tasks. Even so, one should not assume cognitive decline is secondary to normal aging. The American Academy of Neurology recommends assessment for cognitive impairment whenever a patient and/or a close contact expresses concern about their impaired memory or cognition.[5]

Dementia: Dementia, or major neurocognitive disorder, refers to a significant decline in one or more cognitive domains relative to premorbid performance that interferes with one's ability to independently perform activities of daily living (ADLs). It typically presents with insidious onset and progressively worsens over time. Alzheimer disease is the most common cause of dementia and is believed to affect 1 in 10 Americans over the age of 65. Dementia may also occur secondary to HIV infection, chronic traumatic encephalopathy, vasculopathy, Parkinson disease, and other neurodegenerative disorders.[2,5]

Mild cognitive impairment (MCI): MCI refers to a modest cognitive decline in one or more cognitive domains, without interference in one's independence with ADLs. An individual with MCI may still require more time and effort and/or the use of compensatory strategies in order to complete their ADLs. Patients with MCI have an increased risk of developing dementia.[2,5]

Pseudodementia: Depression and other psychiatric diseases may mimic dementia, especially in older adults. Its onset and course may be variable. Affected individuals often present with apathy and/or anhedonia (the loss of pleasure in usually enjoyable activities) and may exhibit hypersomnia.[2,5]

Acquired brain injury (ABI): Traumatic brain injury, anoxic brain injury, stroke, brain tumors, demyelinating diseases, and encephalitis may impair cognitive function.[2]

Delirium: Delirium is typically of acute onset, over hours to days, and affected individuals usually demonstrate fluctuating levels of arousal and confusion. They may have periods during which they are lucid and they may have hallucinations. It usually results from a reversible cause, such as infection, intoxication, or metabolic disturbance. Hyponatremia, hypernatremia, and hypercalcemia may result in delirium. Withdrawal from alcohol may result in delirium tremens, starting 3 to 5 days from cessation.[2,5]

Medication/substance use: Medications that commonly cause or contribute to cognitive impairment include benzodiazepines, barbiturates, opioids, tricyclic antidepressants, antihistamines, and antineoplastic drugs. The use of steroids may cause changes in memory and/or behavior. Cannabis use results in acute impairments in learning, memory, and attention, and habitual users perform worse than nonusers on neuropsychological tests.[2,5,6]

Systemic diseases: Individuals with hypothyroidism and survivors of COVID-19 may both experience impaired memory and attention. Persons with syphilis may exhibit signs of dementia and/or psychosis. Advanced liver disease and vitamin deficiencies may both impair cognition.[2,7]

EVALUATION OF THE COGNITIVELY IMPAIRED PERSON

History: Determine the onset and progression of symptoms, making note of any potential triggers, such as trauma, infection, or new medication. Inquire about any waxing or waning of symptoms, particularly worsening of confusion in the late afternoon or early evening (sundowning). Ask how the change in cognition has impacted the individual's function and safety. Review the medical and family history, with a focus on neurologic and psychiatric conditions, as well as systemic diseases that increase one's risk of cognitive impairment, such as liver and thyroid disease. Obtain birth history and information concerning school performance in those with impaired cognition due to developmental or early-onset disabilities. Inquire about their diet as well as their use of alcohol. Review all medications, herbal or nutritional supplements, and any recreational drugs the individual has been taking. Perform a thorough review of systems to identify potential clues as to the underlying cause.[2,5]

Physical examination: The examination should include vital signs, an assessment of one's general appearance, and a comprehensive neurologic examination, including speech, muscle strength and coordination, sensation, reflexes, balance, and gait. One should evaluate for any signs of physical trauma, as well as an assessment of one's mood, affect, and behavior.

Cognitive examination: Table 28.1 highlights an initial cognitive evaluation that may be conducted in an examination room or at a patient's

TABLE 28.1 Cognitive Examination

Cognitive Function	Means of Assessment on Examination
Level of consciousness	Assess if the patient is awake or easily awakened and if they respond appropriately to commands, questions, and/or cues.
Orientation	Ask the patient to identify their name, location, date, and situation.
Attention/concentration	Ask the patient to repeat digits (5–7 is normal), count backwards from 100 by 7s, and/or spell WORLD backwards.
Abstraction ability	Ask the patient to interpret a culturally relevant proverb, such as "People in glass houses shouldn't throw stones."
Judgment	Ask the patient what they would do if they found a stamped and addressed envelope on the street near a postal collection box.
Recall	Ask the patient to repeat three words immediately and again 3–5 minutes later.
Remote memory	Ask the patient about a verifiable personal experience or a major historic event.
Fund of knowledge	Ask the patient to name the current president.

bedside. Modifications may be necessary in case of hearing or communication impairments. It should be conducted in the patient's preferred language.[2,8]

Screening tools that are commonly used to identify cognitive impairment include the following:

- *Brief Interview for Mental Status (BIMS):* BIMS tests immediate and delayed recall of three items (blue, bed, and sock) and determines orientation to the year, month, and day. It is currently included on the Patient Assessment Instrument for patients admitted to inpatient rehabilitation facilities.[9]
- *Mini-Mental State Examination (MMSE):* MMSE is a set of 30 questions used to assess cognition by analyzing orientation, language, attention, memory, and visuospatial skills.[5]
- *Montreal Cognitive Assessment (MoCA):* The MoCA is a rapid screening tool for MCI that assesses executive function, memory, concentration, language, calculation, orientation, and visuospatial skills.[2]

Laboratory: To identify reversible causes of cognitive impairment, one should order serum thyroid-stimulating hormone (TSH), liver function tests, metabolic panel, and vitamin B_{12} level. Testing for HIV and syphilis is also indicated. In the event of cognitive decline with acute onset, one should also assess for possible underlying infection with a complete blood chemistry (CBC) and urinalysis/culture. Lumbar puncture with evaluation of the cerebrospinal fluid may also be necessary.[2,5]

Imaging: CT scan of the brain may identify traumatic injuries, hemorrhagic stroke, nonacute ischemic stroke, hydrocephalus, and/or brain tumors. MRI is used to identify acute ischemic stroke and multiple sclerosis plaques, and may be useful in helping to differentiate between Alzheimer, frontotemporal, and vascular dementias.[2,5]

Neuropsychological test: This includes a battery of tests to assess neurocognitive and psychological functioning. It may be used to identify the impaired cognitive domains, as well as areas of relative strength, enabling more targeted treatment planning. It may also aid in the differential diagnosis of cognitive impairment and help identify comorbid conditions, including mental health disorders, which may affect cognitive function and/or one's perception thereof.[10]

TREATMENT OF COGNITIVE IMPAIRMENT

Reversible causes of cognitive impairment, when identified, should be treated. One should re-evaluate the need for any medication that may be contributing to the impairment and avoid polypharmacy. Stimulants, such as amantadine and methylphenidate, may be used to enhance alertness and attention.[11] Donepezil (anticholinesterase inhibitor) and memantine (N-methyl-D-aspartate [NMDA] receptor antagonist) are used in the treatment of Alzheimer disease.[2]

Cognitive rehabilitation refers to interventions aimed at improving cognitive function in individuals with brain injury and other neurocognitive disorders. It is most often provided by speech and language pathologists, occupational therapists, and psychologists; however, other members of the rehabilitation team often assist in identifying relevant functional goals and reinforcing the use of strategies to aid memory and ensure safety. Goals of cognitive rehabilitation include maximizing the remaining function, improving lost functions, learning adaptive techniques, family training, and addressing safety and independence. *Restorative interventions* are aimed at the impairment itself, whereas *compensatory strategies* enable one to use their current abilities to circumvent the impairment. Such strategies may be external to the patient (e.g., using a memory notebook or setting reminder alerts on a phone) or internal, as in the use of a self-generated cue like a mnemonic device.[12]

Safety Interventions

While in the hospital and/or a postacute care setting, persons with cognitive impairment may demonstrate disorientation, agitation, and/or nonadherence to safety precautions. They may benefit from frequent reorientation to time, place, and situation and avoidance of overstimulation. Restraints should be avoided when possible, but may be needed to prevent injury and/or protect a medically necessary line, tube, or device. Decision-making capacity should be assessed, and when necessary a healthcare proxy may be designated to make medical decisions on their behalf.

Persons with impaired cognition may need assistance with management of their medications and finances. The use of a pillbox or pill packs may promote compliance and reduce risk of medication errors.

Those with impaired cognition may be unable to safely operate household appliances, firearms, and/or motor vehicles. Supervision may be necessary while preparing meals. Safe storage of firearms should be discussed with the patient and/or their caregiver(s). Driving requires both cognitive and physical skills, as well as an awareness of one's surroundings. A formal driving evaluation may be indicated when it is unclear if an individual is safe to continue or resume driving.

REFERENCES

The full complete reference list for this chapter appears in the digital version of the chapter, available at http://connect.springerpub.com/content/book/978-0-8261-5628-0/part/part03/chapter/ch28

CHAPTER 29

SPASTICITY

Gary Vargas and Amy Mathews

DEFINITION

Spasticity is a disorder of impaired muscle tone regulation that leads to a velocity-dependent hypertonicity in response to passive range of motion (ROM). It also involves impaired sensorimotor control presenting as intermittent or sustained involuntary activation of muscles.[1] Spasticity is part of the upper motor neuron (UMN) syndrome, which includes positive symptoms of hyperreflexia and clonus and negative symptoms such as weakness and impaired dexterity. Untreated spasticity can lead to a number of sequelae, including pain, limb contracture, skin breakdown, joint deformity, and loss of function.[2]

ASSESSMENT

Assessment of spasticity should include an evaluation of the impact of the patient's spasticity on their function. Some patients may experience activity limitations or increased caregiver burden due to their spasticity; however, in other cases, it may be desirable for a patient to have increased tone to facilitate activities of daily living (ADLs)/mobility.[2] For example, patients may "use" their leg extensor spasticity for transfers or their finger flexor spasticity to assist with grasp.

Scales commonly used in the assessment of spasticity include the Modified Ashworth Scale (MAS) and the Tardieu Scale (Table 29.1).[3,4] The Tardieu Scale demonstrates higher interrater reliability and reproducibility than the MAS in patients with traumatic brain injury (TBI), yet requires practitioners to precisely measure ROM, which may pose practical limitations to regular clinical practice.[5]

TREATMENT

Discussing meaningful and realistic treatment goals is an important step in spasticity management. Goals of treatment may be directed at improving mobility/function, relieving pain, reducing caregiver burden, improving hygiene, improving cosmesis, or preventing need for surgery.[6] Another important initial step in the treatment of spasticity is addressing any noxious stimuli that could be exacerbating spasticity, including urinary tract infections (UTIs), constipation, pressure injuries, ingrown toenails, fractures, and pain. Treatment for spasticity is multimodal and may include positioning, stretching, bracing/splinting, physical modalities such as heat/cold, pharmacologic management, chemodenervation, and neurolysis.[7] Figure 29.1 outlines a treatment paradigm. Starting early after the neurologic injury and continuing through all stages of treatment, correct positioning is essential

TABLE 29.1 Scales for Assessing Spasticity

Modified Ashworth Scale	
0	No increase in tone with passive stretch
1	Slight increase in tone manifested by a catch, followed by release at the end of ROM
1+	Slight increase in tone, followed by minimal resistance throughout the remainder (<50%) of ROM
2	Increase in tone affecting >50% of ROM, with joints being easily moved
3	Considerable increase in muscle tone affecting >50% of ROM, passive movement is difficult
4	Limb fixed in position, unable to range
Tardieu Scale	
Quality of muscle reaction	
0	No increase in tone
1	Slight resistance with no clear catch
2	Catch followed by release at precise angle
3	Fatigable clonus at precise angle (<10 sec)
4	Nonfatigable clonus at precise angle (>10 sec)
5	Limb fixed in position
Velocity of stretch	
V1	Limb ranged as slow as possible, less than that of gravity
V2	Limb ranged at speed of gravity
V3	Limb ranged as fast as possible
Spasticity angle	
R1	Angle of catch when stretching at fast velocity of V3
R2	Angle of catch when stretching at slow velocity of V1

ROM, range of motion.

Source: Adapted with permission from Bohannon RW, Smith MB. Interrater reliability of a modified Ashworth scale of muscle spasticity. *Phys Ther*. 1987;67(2):206–207; Boyd RN, Graham HK. Objective measurement of clinical findings in the use of botulinum toxin type A for the management of children with cerebral palsy. *Eur J Neurol*. 1999;6:s23–s35.

in controlling spasticity and preserving ROM. Early and frequent mobilization of patients with repositioning in bed, sitting out of bed, and standing can help provide prolonged stretching of spastic muscles. Splints and other orthotics can also be used to provide sustained stretch. Commonly used orthoses include elbow extension splints, resting hand splints, and rigid anklefoot orthoses.[8] For significant contracture, serial casting with progressively increased ROM every few

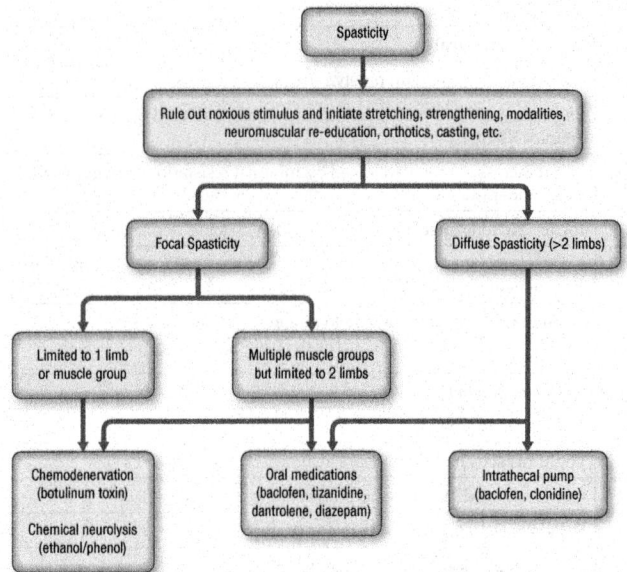

FIGURE 29.1 Spasticity treatment paradigm.
Source: Adapted with permission from Francisco G, Li S, Cifu DX, et al. Chapter 23: Spasticity. In: *Braddom's Physical Medicine and Rehabilitation*, 6th ed. Elsevier; 2021:447–468.

days may improve available ROM. Regular active ROM (AROM) and passive ROM (PROM) are essential in controlling tone. Heat modalities work to relax muscles and can be applied to spastic muscles via fluidotherapy, ultrasound, or direct application. Cold directly inhibits the stretch reflex inhibiting tone, although transiently. While massage has been shown to significantly improve MAS scores in patients with cerebral palsy, the evidence for acupuncture remains inconclusive.[9,10] Functional electrostimulation, concurrent physical therapy, casting, and dynamic splinting have been shown to enhance the effect of botulinum toxin (level 1a evidence for electrical stimulation).[11,12] Commonly used medications for diffuse spasticity are listed in Table 29.2.[13]

Focal spasticity is commonly managed with chemodenervation and/or neurolysis. In the United States, Food and Drug Administration (FDA)-approved toxins include botulinum toxin-A (BoNT-A) formulations (onabotulinumtoxinA, incobotulinumtoxinA, abobotulinumtoxinA) and botulinum toxin-B (BoNT-B) formulation (rimabotulinumtoxinB). BoNT-A and BoNT-B block the presynaptic release of acetylcholine (ACh), thus inhibiting neuromuscular junction (NMJ) transmission. BoNT-A acts at the sensory nerve action potentials (SNAP)-25 protein and BoNT-B acts at the synaptobrevin protein. Onset of effect is 3 to 5 days post injection, with peak effect around 3 to 6 weeks. The average duration of clinical

TABLE 29.2 Common Medications for Spasticity

Name	Mechanism of Action	Common Dosage	Common Side Effects	Laboratory Monitoring
Baclofen	GABA-B agonist within the spinal cord	Starting dose: 10 mg BID, max dose: 80120 mg/d	Sedation, urinary retention, nephrotoxicity, decreases seizure threshold, withdrawal risk	Cr
Dantrolene	Binds ryanodine receptor 1 in skeletal muscle	Starting dose: 25 mg BID, max dose: 400 mg/d	Hepatotoxicity, nausea, diarrhea	LFTs
Tizanidine	Alpha-2 adrenergic agonist (ceruleospinal tract)	Starting dose: 2 mg QHS, max dose: 36 mg/d	Hepatotoxicity, sedating, hypotension, bradycardia	LFTs
Diazepam	GABA-A agonist	Starting dose: 2 mg QHS, max dose: 60 mg/d	Sedation, decreased REM, impaired memory	

Cr, Creatinine; GABA A/B, Gamma-Aminobutyric Acid A/B; LFTs, Liver Function Tests; REM, Rapid Eye Movement sleep.

Source: Adapted with permission from Elovic E, Baerga E, Escalidi SV, et al. Associated topics in physical medicine and rehabilitation. In: Cucurullo SJ. ed. *Physical Medicine and Rehabilitation Board Review*. 3rd ed. Demos Medical Publishing; 2015:861–963.

effect is 3 months.[14] Tables 29.3[15,16] and 29.4[17] list the current FDA-approved indications for botulinum toxin and dosing for selected muscles, respectively. Botulinum toxin should be administered in intervals of at least 3 months to minimize antibody formation, which could decrease the efficacy of chemodenervation. Contraindications to treatment with BoNT-A formulations include pregnancy, NMJ disease, infection at the site of injection, concomitant aminoglycoside use, or hypersensitivity to toxin preparation or any components in the formulation.

Chemical neurolysis with 5% to 7% phenol (carboxylic acid) or 50% to 100% alcohol induces Wallerian degeneration of peripheral nerves, resulting in relaxation of musculature. Onset of effect is typically within 1 hour and lasts 6 to 12 months, at which time axons regenerate. Neurolysis is typically performed using ultrasound or electrical stimulation guidance to ensure sufficient proximity to the nerve.[18] Compared with botulinum toxins, phenol is more cost-effective, with a longer therapeutic effect. Potential adverse effects

TABLE 29.3 FDA-Approved Indications for Botulinum Toxin

Toxin	Indications
Onabotulinumtoxin A	Upper and lower limb spasticity in adults Upper and lower limb spasticity in children >2 years Cervical dystonia in adults Strabismus and blepharospasm Primary axillary hyperhidrosis Chronic migraine Bladder dysfunction
Incobotulinumtoxin A	Upper limb spasticity in adults Upper limb spasticity in children (excluding spasticity due to cerebral palsy) Cervical dystonia in adults Blepharospasm Sialorrhea in adults and children >2 years
Abobotulinumtoxin A	Upper and lower limb spasticity in adults and children Cervical dystonia in adults
Rimabotulinumtoxin B	Cervical dystonia in adults Sialorrhea in adults

FDA, Food and Drug Administration.

Source: Adapted from BOTOX® (onabotulinumtoxinA) for Medical Professionals. Evidence-based Dosing for Adult Upper Limb Spasticity. Upper Limb Spasticity Dosing and Administration; n.d.; BOTOX® (onabotulinumtoxinA) for Medical Professionals. Evidence-based Dosing for Adult Lower Limb Spasticity. Lower Limb Spasticity Dosing and Administration; n.d.; ipsen.com. Highlights of Prescribing Information; n.d.; myobloc.com. Highlights of Prescribing Information; n.d.

include excessive weakness and, if treating mixed motor/sensory nerves (e.g., main tibial nerve, median nerve), painful paresthesias. A reversible, diagnostic block using a local anesthetic such as lidocaine or marcaine may be utilized to predict treatment response and potential adverse effects. Chemical neurolysis may be done as an adjunctive treatment to chemodenervation, with neurolysis used to target severe diffuse spasticity and botulinum toxin used in the remaining muscles.

Intrathecal baclofen (ITB) therapy may be indicated in the treatment of diffuse and severe spasticity. ITB is an implantable infusion system that allows delivery of baclofen directly into the intrathecal space, often causing less central side effects than oral agents. Prior to pump implantation, patients are administered a test dose of 50 to 75 mcg baclofen via epidural injection and assessed for changes in tone and function. If the ITB trial yields favorable results, the patient undergoes a scheduled surgery where a reservoir pump is placed in the left or right lower quadrant of the abdomen with the catheter extending intrathecally.[19] After placement, ITB dosing is titrated under clinical supervision and may include basal, bolus, and flexible dosing schemes.

TABLE 29.4 Onabotulinumtoxin A Dosing in Selected Muscles

Clinical Presentation	Muscles Involved	Dose Range (Units)	Number of Injection Sites
Internally rotated/adducted shoulder and arm	Pectoralis major	75–100	3–4
	Latissimus dorsi	75–150	3–4
	Subscapularis	25–75	1
Flexed elbow	Brachialis	75–100	2
	Brachioradialis	75–100	1
	Biceps	100–200	4
Pronated forearm	Pronator teres	50–75	1
	Pronator quadratus	25–50	1
Flexed wrist	Flexor carpi radialis	25–50	1
	Flexor carpi ulnaris	25–50	1
Clenched fist	Flexor digitorum superficialis	50	1
	Flexor digitorum profundus	50	1
Flexed hip	Iliopsoas	50–150	2
	Rectus femoris	75–150	2
Adducted thigh	Adductor brevis	50–100	2
	Adductor longus	50–100	2
	Adductor magnus	50–100	2
Flexed knee	Semimembranosus	100–150	3
	Semitendinosus	100–150	3
	Biceps femoris	100–150	3
Extended knee	Quadriceps femoris	100–200	3–4
Equinovarus foot	Gastrocnemius	75–150	3 (for each head)
	Soleus	75–100	3
	Tibialis posterior	50–150	1–2
	Tibialis anterior	50–150	1–2
Cervical dystonia	Sternocleidomastoid	15–100	3–5
	Scalene	15–50	1
	Splenius capitis	15–100	1
	Levator scapula	20–100	1
	Trapezius	20–100	3

Source: Adapted with permission from Brin MF. Dosing, administration, and a treatment algorithm for use of BTX-A for adult-onset spasticity. *Muscle Nerve.* 1997;6(suppl):S214.

Pumps require refills every 1 to 6 months and surgical replacement approximately every 5 to 7 years. Providers should preemptively counsel patients and caregivers about the frequency of follow-up appointments and pump maintenance. Regular clinical care is required to minimize adverse medication effects, such as baclofen withdrawal, and to monitor for device malfunctions such as catheter malfunction or hardware infection.[20]

Tendon lengthening and selective dorsal rhizotomy (SDR) are surgical interventions that address contracture and diffuse spasticity. Tenotomies along the length of contracted tendons can stretch tendons and address joint deformities such as equinovarus contractures.[21] In SDR, a laminectomy exposes the dorsal roots of the lumbar spine. Using electromyography (EMG) guidance, abnormal dorsal roots are selectively severed. This has been shown to be effective in reducing pain, ROM, and improving gait in studies of children with cerebral palsy (CP).[22] The benefits of SDR are permanent but must be followed by intense inpatient and outpatient physical therapy, requiring good family support.[23]

Experimental treatments for spasticity include neuromodulation with repetitive transcranial magnetic stimulation (rTMS) and cannabinoids. rTMS has been shown to improve MAS scores, Penn Spasm Frequency Scale scores, and overall quality of life when it was repeated over 2 weeks in patients with multiple sclerosis (MS).[24] Similar findings have been reproduced in the stroke population as well. Use of smoked cannabis has been shown to significantly reduce MAS scores and Visual Analog Scale (VAS) scores compared with placebo in patients with MS, although evidence for its use is limited.[25]

REFERENCES

The full complete reference list for this chapter appears in the digital version of the chapter, available at http://connect.springerpub.com/content/book/978-0-8261-5628-0/part/part03/chapter/ch29

CHAPTER 30

NEUROGENIC BLADDER AND BOWEL

Stephanie Hendrick and Ishaan Hublikar

NEUROGENIC BLADDER

Neuroanatomy and Physiology

The urinary system is composed of the upper urinary tracts (kidneys and ureters) as well as the lower urinary tracts (bladder and urethra). The bladder consists of the detrusor and the trigone. The urethra is considered to have both internal and external sphincters. The internal sphincter is not a true anatomic sphincter but rather a functional sphincter composed of smooth muscle fibers and connective tissue under autonomic control. The external sphincter is composed of striated skeletal muscle fibers under voluntary control.

Bladder filling and emptying relies on the coordinated interplay between the peripheral nervous system (parasympathetic, sympathetic, and somatic) and the central nervous system (Figure 30.1).[1] *Sympathetic efferents* (arising from T10L2 via the hypogastric nerve) promote bladder storage by stimulating *beta-3 adrenergic* receptors in the body and dome (relaxation) and *alpha-adrenergic receptors* near the base of the bladder and prostatic urethra (contraction) via norepinephrine. *Parasympathetic efferents* (arising from S2–S4 via the pelvic nerve) promote bladder emptying by stimulating muscarinic (M2 and M3) receptors in the bladder (contraction) via acetylcholine. A helpful mnemonic is sympathetic for *s*torage and *p*arasympathetic for *p*eeing. Voluntary control of the external urethral sphincter (continence) is mediated via *somatic efferents* (Onuf's nucleus at S2–S4 via the pudendal nerve). The *afferent* system includes small myelinated *A-delta* and unmyelinated *C fibers*.

Bladder distention activates A-delta receptors, which provide feedback to the *sacral micturition center* at spinal segments S2 to S4 via the afferent nerves. An intact cerebral cortex, however, inhibits the sacral micturition center and reflex bladder contraction until a threshold is met. Bladder filling is initially sensed at ~100 mL and a feeling of fullness with urge to void is typically sensed at ~300 to 400 mL. During physiologic voiding, the sacral micturition center stimulates detrusor contraction via the *parasympathetic fibers*. The *pontine micturition center* (PMC) coordinates a synergic interaction between the contracting detrusor and a relaxing urethral sphincter, allowing urine to be excreted (Figure 30.2).[2]

Neurogenic bladder results from the disruption of nervous system input, leading to bladder dysfunction. Classification of neurogenic

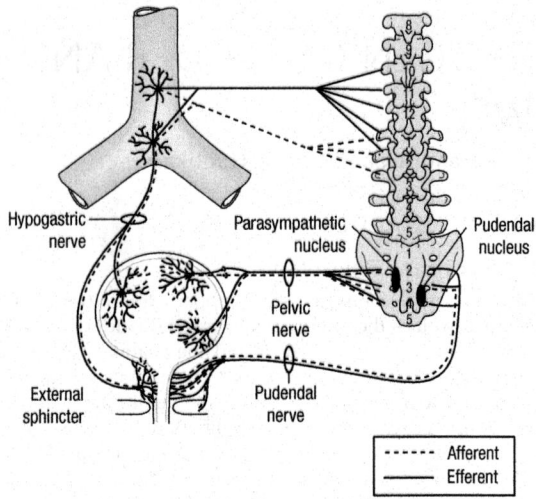

FIGURE 30.1 Bladder innervation.
Source: From Blaivas JG. Management of bladder dysfunction in multiple sclerosis. *Neurology.* 1980;30:12–18. doi:10.1212/WNL.30.7_Part_2.12.[1]

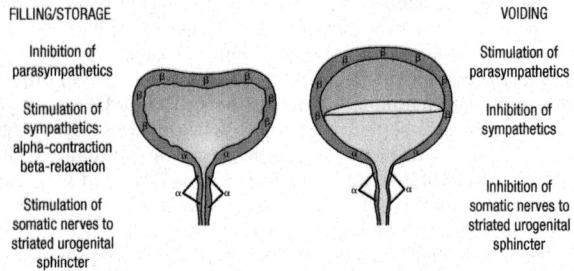

FIGURE 30.2 Bladder physiology.

bladder can be approached by anatomic lesion or by function with failure to store and failure to empty (Table 30.1). A *suprapontine* lesion (e.g., traumatic brain injury or stroke) results in detrusor hyperreflexia or overactivity due to a lack of cerebral inhibition of the sacral micturition reflex. Neurogenic bladder from a suprapontine lesion clinically manifests as failure to store with urinary frequency and/or urinary incontinence. *Detrusor sphincter dyssynergia* (DSD) is not seen with these lesions because the PMC's synergic control of the detrusor and sphincter remains intact. A *suprasacral* lesion (e.g., spinal cord injury) results in disruption of the cerebral input inhibiting the micturition

TABLE 30.1 Functional Classification of Neurogenic Bladder

Type of Failure	Bladder Factors	Outlet Factors
Failure to store	Hyperactivity	
	Decreased compliance	Denervated pelvic floor
		Bladder neck descent
		Intrinsic bladder neck sphincter failure
Failure to empty	Areflexia	
	Hypocontractility	Detrusor sphincter dyssynergia (striated sphincter and bladder neck)
		Nonrelaxing voluntary sphincter
		Mechanical obstruction (benign prostatic hypertrophy or stricture)

Source: From Goetz L, Klausner A. Chapter 20: Neurogenic lower urinary tract dysfunction. In: Cifu DX, Eapen BC, Johns JS, et al., eds. *Braddom's Physical Medicine and Rehabilitation*, 6th Ed. Elsevier; 2021. Table 20.2, p. 392.

reflex as well as disruption of the PMC's synergic control of the detrusor and sphincter. This can lead to DSD from detrusor contraction with simultaneous failure of the sphincter to relax. Consequences of DSD include urinary retention, high bladder pressures, bladder diverticula, vesicoureteral reflux, hydronephrosis, urinary tract infections, and autonomic dysreflexia. Chronic detrusor hyperactivity can lead to diminished bladder capacity over time. Of note, during the initial spinal shock period, neurogenic bladder from a suprasacral lesion clinically manifests as detrusor areflexia with urinary retention or overflow incontinence. A *sacral* or *infrasacral* lesion (e.g., conus medullaris syndrome, cauda equina syndrome, or peripheral nerve injury) results in detrusor areflexia or hypocontractility with high bladder volumes. Neurogenic bladder from a sacral or infrasacral lesion classically presents as a failure to empty with urinary retention with or without overflow incontinence.[2,3]

Management of Neurogenic Bladder

The overall treatment goals for neurogenic bladder are to maintain urinary continence and optimize quality of life while preserving renal function and preventing upper and lower urinary tract complications. Management is largely driven by addressing the underlying dysfunction (i.e., failure to store or failure to empty). Approach to management should be determined on an individual basis with consideration of anatomy, medical comorbidities, history of complications, cognition, functional assessment, lifestyle, and social support.

Suprapontine

Treatment for neurogenic bladder from suprapontine lesions is directed toward addressing neurogenic detrusor overactivity. Behavioral management includes instituting a timed voiding program (e.g., toileting every 2 hours) while monitoring and adjusting fluid intake. This can be combined with the use of anticholinergic medications (e.g., oxybutynin, tolterodine, and solifenacin) to suppress detrusor overactivity and increase bladder capacity. The use of alpha-adrenergic antagonist medications (e.g., tamsulosin) may be beneficial in addressing sphincter resistance. Urinary collective devices such as external catheters may be considered, but caution must be taken to monitor for skin breakdown.

Suprasacral

Treatment for neurogenic bladder from suprasacral lesions is directed toward addressing detrusor hyperreflexia and sphincter dyssynergia. Treatment options include intermittent catheterization (IC), indwelling catheterization, reflex voiding, surgical interventions, and pharmacologic management. IC is often performed four to six times a day with the goal to keep volumes less than 500 mL. Alternatives to IC should be considered when the individual does not have sufficient hand function or a willing caregiver to perform IC, as well as in the setting of urethral anatomic abnormalities, bladder capacity less than 200 mL, poor cognition, or a tendency for autonomic dysreflexia. Indwelling catheterization includes both urethral and suprapubic catheters. Indwelling catheterization is considered when less invasive methods have been unsuccessful or in the setting of elevated detrusor pressures, high fluid intake, and urologic complications. The primary disadvantages of an indwelling catheter over properly performed IC include increased risk of infection, autonomic dysreflexia, urolithiasis, and bladder neoplasm. Indwelling urethral catheters increase the risk of urethral strictures, hypospadias, prostatitis, and epididymitis. Suprapubic catheterization involves surgical placement of the catheter through the lower abdomen directly into the bladder. Indwelling suprapubic catheters should be considered with urethral abnormalities, difficulty with urethral catheterization, recurrent urethral catheter obstruction, psychological considerations (e.g., body image or personal preference), or to improve sexual function. In general, indwelling catheters should be changed every 4 weeks or more frequently in the setting of catheter encrustation or stones. Reflex voiding relies on spontaneous involuntary bladder contractions and is often paired with the use of an external catheter in males. This may require an endourethral stent, transurethral surgical sphincterotomy, or pharmacologic interventions (e.g., botulinum toxin injections to the urethra or alpha-adrenergic medications) to reduce the risk of DSD. Other options to enhance bladder storage include oral anticholinergic medication, intravesical botulinum toxin injections, and bladder augmentation surgery. Options to enhance bladder emptying include oral alpha-adrenergic antagonist medication, urinary diversions, or neurostimulation with implanted sacral nerve modulators. An example of a continent urinary diversion is the *Mitrofanoff appendicovesicostomy*, in which the appendix is used to create a conduit from the bladder to the abdominal skin with a catheterizable stoma.

Sacral and Infrasacral

Treatment for neurogenic bladder from sacral or infrasacral lesions is directed toward implementing techniques to facilitate bladder emptying. Treatment options include the use of IC, indwelling catheterization, as well as the Valsalva and Credé maneuvers. The Valsalva maneuver involves bearing down to increase intra-abdominal pressure, whereas the Credé maneuver involves application of suprapubic pressure to express urine from the bladder. The use of cholinergic agonists (e.g., bethanechol) can be considered in select patient populations, but clinical evidence for routine use is lacking.

Surveillance of neurogenic bladder is driven by the severity of dysfunction (risk stratification) and the presence of urinary symptoms. Surveillance monitoring can include renal function assessment, upper tract imaging, urodynamic study, cystoscopy, and voiding cystourethrogram.[3,4]

NEUROGENIC BOWEL

Neuroanatomy and Physiology

The gastrointestinal tract has its own unique innervation with the *intrinsic (enteric) nervous system* that can function independently with a network of sensory neurons, interneurons, and motor neurons. The intrinsic nervous system is composed of the *submucosal (Meissner's) plexus* and the *myenteric (Auerbach's) plexus*. The submucosal plexus is located in the submucosal layer of the intestinal wall and serves to regulate secretion and absorption. The myenteric plexus is located in the muscularis propria, layered between the circular and longitudinal muscles. This plexus coordinates motor function which facilitates propulsion and excretion of stool. Despite the intrinsic nervous system's ability to function independently, the optimal function of the gastrointestinal system relies on communication with the *extrinsic nervous system* (parasympathetic, sympathetic, and somatic).

Parasympathetic innervation through the vagus nerve (originating at the level of the medulla) innervates the proximal gastrointestinal

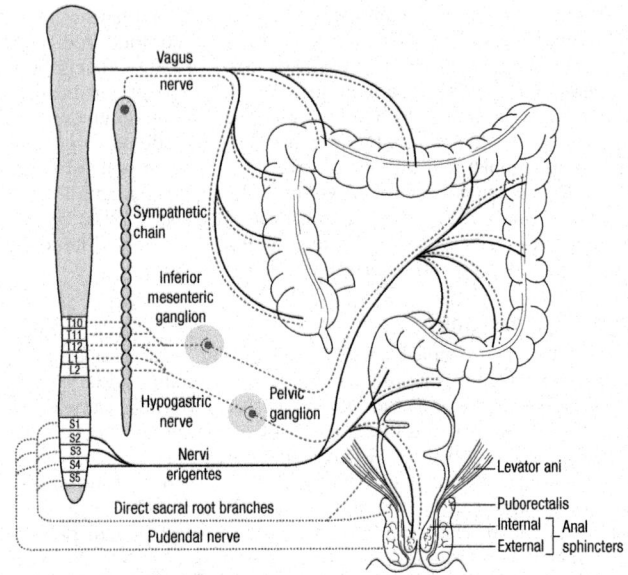

FIGURE 30.3 Bowel innervation.

Source: From Rodriguez G, Stiens S. Chapter 21: Neurogenic bowel: Dysfunction and rehabilitation. In: Cifu DX, Eapen BC, Johns JS, et al., eds. *Braddom's Physical Medicine and Rehabilitation*, 6th ed. Elsevier; 2021; Fig. 21.2, p. 409.

tract from the esophagus to the midtransverse colon, while the pelvic splanchnic nerve (arising from S2–S4) innervates the distal transverse colon to the anorectal region. Stimulation of the parasympathetic system promotes defecation through increasing peristalsis, stimulating secretions, and relaxing sphincters. *Sympathetic* innervation through the preganglionic fibers (arising from T5–L2) as well as the postganglionic fibers (arising from T10–L2 via the hypogastric nerve) promotes storage of stool by decreasing peristalsis, inhibiting secretions and absorption, and contracting sphincters. *Somatic* innervation through the pudendal nerve (arising from S2–S4) innervates the external anal sphincter and pelvic floor musculature (Figure 30.3).[5,6]

Neurogenic bowel results from an impairment in the neuroregulatory control of the gastrointestinal tract, leading to failure to evacuate stool and/or failure to store stool. Neurogenic bowel is typically classified as either an *upper motor neuron (UMN) bowel* or a *lower motor neuron (LMN) bowel*. The UMN bowel is known as the reflexic bowel as

TABLE 30.2 Classification of Neurogenic Bowel

	Upper Motor Neuron Bowel	**Lower Motor Neuron Bowel**
Localization of lesion	At or above the conus	Below the conus
Causes	Spinal cord injury, brain injury, stroke, multiple sclerosis, etc.	Conus medullaris syndrome, cauda equina syndrome, polyneuropathy, pelvic trauma, etc.
Presentation	Intact sacral reflexes	Absent sacral reflexes
	Normal or spastic anal sphincter	Flaccid or hypotonic anal sphincter
Bowel dysfunction	Slowed colonic transit	Slowed colonic transit
	Constipation	Constipation
	Fecal impaction	Fecal incontinence

reflex defecation remains intact, whereas the LMN bowel is known as the areflexic bowel as reflex defecation is absent (Table 30.2).

Management of Neurogenic Bowel

The goals of neurogenic bowel management are to facilitate bowel emptying in a timely and predictable manner, minimize bowel incontinence, and prevent gastrointestinal complications. Similar to the approach for neurogenic bladder management, treatment should be determined on an individual basis with consideration of premorbid bowel function, medical comorbidities, history of complications, functional assessment, lifestyle, and social support. An effective bowel program begins with establishing a consistent schedule (every day or every other day) and ideally is completed within 1 hour. Components to consider include dietary and fluid intake, stool consistency, physical activity, medications, positioning (side-lying or upright), and presence of reflexes. Collaboration with the interdisciplinary team, patient and caregiver education, as well as frequent reassessment of the bowel regimen are all key to optimizing the success of the bowel program.

Several reflexes are utilized during a bowel program to facilitate defecation. The *gastrocolic reflex* is a cholinergic-mediated reflex that results in increased colonic motility after consuming a meal. The *colocolonic reflex* is mediated by the myenteric plexus and results in forward propulsion of stool by constricting the muscles proximal to colonic distention and relaxing the muscles distal to colonic distention. The *rectocolic reflex* is mediated by the pelvic nerve and results in colonic peristalsis after mechanical or chemical stimulation of the anorectal region.

Upper Motor Neuron Bowel

Management is largely driven by utilization of intact sacral reflexes to trigger defecation. This can be achieved by use of chemical, mechanical, and electrical stimulation. Traditional approaches will pair the use of a suppository followed by digital stimulation. Digital stimulation is performed by inserting a lubricated, gloved finger into the rectum and gently moving the finger in a circular fashion along the rectal wall in 20-second intervals. This can be repeated every 5 to 10 minutes until the rectal vault is empty or if there are no results following two consecutive stimulations. Complications of mechanical rectal stimulation include irritation of hemorrhoids and autonomic dysreflexia. The goal stool consistency is soft and formed (Bristol Stool Scale score 4) to allow easy evacuation with the above methods of stimulation.

Lower Motor Neuron Bowel

In the absence of sacral reflexes, chemical and mechanical stimulation with use of suppositories and digital stimulation is ineffective in the management of LMN bowel. Manual removal or disimpaction is most effective for bowel emptying. In the setting of weak pelvic floor muscles and a flaccid sphincter, these individuals are prone to bowel incontinence. Thus, fiber and fluid intake must be adjusted to ensure the stool is formed and bulky (Bristol Stool Scale score 3) to allow the stool to be retained in the rectum between bowel programs. Individuals may need to perform manual removal multiple times a day.

Bowel programs can be further augmented by the use of various medications. Oral stimulants (e.g., senna) promote peristalsis by stimulating the *myenteric (Auerbach's) plexus*. Contact irritant agents (e.g., bisacodyl) promote peristalsis by direct irritation of the colonic mucosa. Saline and osmotic laxatives (e.g., polyethylene glycol, lactulose, and magnesium citrate) promote colonic motility and water retention in the colon. Stool softeners (e.g., docusate sodium) emulsify fat and reduce water retention in the colon. Bulk-forming agents (e.g., psyllium and calcium polycarbophil) promote stool bulk by absorbing water into the stool. Changes to the bowel program, including titration of medications, should allow three to five bowel programs to assess the efficacy of each change. If an effective bowel program cannot be achieved with the above interventions, alternatives include the use of a retrograde enema continence catheter, transanal irrigation systems, and surgical interventions (antegrade continence enema or colostomy).[6,7]

REFERENCES

The full complete reference list for this chapter appears in the digital version of the chapter, available at http://connect.springerpub.com/content/book/978-0-8261-5628-0/part/part03/chapter/ch30

CHAPTER 31

LANGUAGE, SPEECH, AND SWALLOWING

Kathryn DeMarco and Kathleen Webler

APHASIA

Aphasia is an acquired neurogenic language disorder caused by brain damage that may affect:

- Spoken language expression and comprehension
- Written expression and reading comprehension

Stroke, including ischemic and hemorrhagic stroke, is the most common cause of aphasia. Other etiologies include, but are not limited to, traumatic brain injury (TBI), brain tumor, brain surgery, brain infections, and progressive neurologic diseases.[1] About 25% to 40% of stroke survivors acquire aphasia.

Aphasia can be classified as fluent or nonfluent (Table 31.1). Fluent aphasia is characterized by more connected speech but lacking in meaning. Comprehension may be intact or more impaired. In individuals with nonfluent aphasia, speech production is effortful, grammar is impaired, and sentences are lacking in content. It is important to remember that an individual's symptoms may not fit into a single aphasia type. Additionally, aphasia symptoms can co-occur with speech impairments such as dysarthria and apraxia of speech (AOS).

Aphasia Prognosis and Treatment

Aphasia outcomes will vary and are generally influenced by the site of the lesion and the severity of brain injury; however, age, education level, and comorbidities will also factor into recovery.[1] Although most recoveries will tend to occur within the first year post injury, patients may continue to make gains for many years after. Consulting a speech language pathologist to assist in recovering linguistic ability and training family members on the use of communication strategies will maximize a person's quality of life and communication success.

Impairment-based therapy focuses more on restoring the language skills affected.

- *Constraint-induced language therapy (CILT):* treatment method focused on constraining compensatory strategies while providing mass practice communication targets
- *Oral reading for language in aphasia (ORLA):* oral reading of scripts in unison with melody and intonation to improve reading comprehension

- *Melodic intonation therapy (MIT):* utilizes the right hemisphere areas responsible for singing to increase expression, typically in nonfluent aphasia
- *Semantic feature analysis (SFA):* utilization of semantic features (what does it do, where do you find it) to increase word retrieval

Communication-based therapy focuses on compensatory strategies to increase functional communication.

- *Promoting aphasics' communication effectiveness (PACE):* focus on conversation skills through communicating a target message to a listener using a multimodal approach
- *Supported conversation:* focus on using a variety of communication strategies with emphasis on communication partner training to support conversation
- *Augmentativealternative communication (AAC):* intact communication skills supplemented with other communication modes, pictures, gestures, and more complex devices to aid in expression and comprehension

It is important to remember that aphasia is a disorder of language. Individuals with aphasia may have intact cognitive skills, such as memory and executive function; however, comorbid cognitive deficits may be present as a result of other co-occurring medical complexities.[1]

RIGHT HEMISPHERE DISORDER

Right hemisphere disorder (RHD) is the result of an acquired brain injury such as TBI, stroke, or tumor. RHD can impact cognitive domains such as attention, memory, and executive functioning, which can result in cognitive communication disorders. The characteristics of RHD include deficits in organization, reasoning, sequencing, problem-solving, attention, and pragmatic skills. Anosognosia (reduced deficit awareness) may occur in up to 40% of individuals with RHD,[2] and visual neglect is a common impairment that can directly impact verbal and written language. RHD deficits may only present during completion of more complex tasks, such as activities of daily living, conversation, and vocational tasks, and may have a significant impact on functional performance and safety.

Interventions for RHD can be either restorative (improving impaired skills) or compensatory (strategies for overcoming deficits) in nature. RHD can impact patient function and safety upon discharge. Recommendations for supervision are often dependent on the patient's cognitive communication status and self-awareness of deficit.[2]

TABLE 31.1 Types of Aphasia

	Type of Aphasia	Site of Lesion	Language Characteristics	Other Characteristics
Non-fluent	Broca aphasia	Broca area; left, frontal lobe or Brodmann area 44 in the posterior inferior frontal gyrus	*Impaired:* naming, writing, limited repetition *Intact:* auditory comprehension for simple material	Associated with right hemiparesis and oral apraxia
	Transcortical motor aphasia	Anterior cerebral artery and/or the anterior middle cerebral artery, supplementary motor area	*Impaired:* difficulty initiating speech and completing a thought, reading skills, writing skills *Intact:* naming skills relatively intact, repetition, auditory comprehension good for conversational interaction	Difficulty initiating speech and completing a thought, also echolalia
	Transcortical mixed aphasia	Anterior and posterior watershed area, multifocal cerebral emboli	*Impaired:* little to no spontaneous verbal speech, echolalia, and severely impaired auditory comprehension, reading comprehension, and writing skills *Intact:* relatively intact repetition	May have visual field deficits
	Global aphasia	Extensive damage to the language centers of the left hemisphere	*Impaired:* deficits across all modes of communication, naming, repetition, auditory comprehension severely impaired *Intact:* limited intact skills, severe aphasia	Right hemiparesis and right visual field deficits common
Fluent	Wernicke aphasia	Posterior superior temporal gyrus of the left hemisphere of the brain	*Impaired:* severe anomia with paraphasic errors and neologisms (made up words), significantly impaired repetition skills and auditory comprehension *Intact:* grammatically correct utterances, prosody and intonation[1]	Motor deficits not typically present, right visual field deficits may be present

Anomic aphasia	Basal temporal lobe, anterior inferior temporal lobe, temporo-parieto-occipital junction, inferior parietal lobe	*Impaired*: impaired naming skills *Intact*: normal utterance length, and auditory comprehension good for everyday conversation, oral reading and reading comprehension, repetition skills	Notable for circumlocutions
Conduction aphasia	Left hemisphere supramarginal gyrus and the arcuate fasciculus	*Impaired*: phonemic paraphasias and word-finding errors common, repetition skills, deficits in writing skills *Intact*: relatively intact auditory comprehension	Individuals typically aware of errors, but have significant difficulty self-correcting
Transcortical sensory aphasia	Temporal-occipital or parietal-occipital areas adjacent to the Wernicke area	*Impaired*: significantly impaired naming skills, reading comprehension *Intact*: repetition skills, intact oral reading	Paraphasic errors
Subcortical aphasias	Associated with damage to the basal ganglia, internal capsule, and left thalamus	*Impaired*: difficulty with complex information, deficits in articulation and word-finding *Intact*: repetition skills, auditory comprehension good for everyday conversation	

MOTOR SPEECH DISORDERS

Dysarthria

Dysarthria is a speech impairment resulting from weakness, discoordination, and abnormal tone.[3] Multiple attributes, including speed, accuracy of articulation, prosody, resonance, and coordination of respiration for phonation, affect speech intelligibility (Table 31.2).

Treatment options can focus on restorative or compensatory strategies or maintenance of skills. Restorative therapy targets the individual speech components of respiration, phonation, articulation, resonance, and prosody. Compensatory treatment focuses on teaching communication strategies to repair communication breakdowns, modifying the communication environment, or using AAC. Maintenance focuses on preservation of skills in the presence of a progressive disease process.[3]

Apraxia of Speech

AOS is an impairment in the ability to plan speech movements. AOS is unrelated to errors of articulation due to muscle weakness, as in dysarthria, and impairments in language, such as aphasia, but can co-occur with either. In AOS, the message is formulated correctly but the expression is inefficient, marked by a slower rate of speech and difficulty changing the rate, imprecise articulation, impaired prosody, decreased fluency, and speech production errors.[3] Oral apraxia, or nonspeech oral praxis, is an impairment in volitional nonspeech movements. The most common etiologies include vascular lesions to the dominant hemisphere where motor speech is programmed, typically the left hemisphere; other common etiologies include neurodegenerative diseases and toxic metabolic disorders. Evaluation of AOS includes assessment of the structures and functions of the body systems to produce speech, perceptual speech characteristics, and motor speech. Evaluation is heavily focused on the differential diagnosis of AOS from dysarthria and aphasia.[1,3]

Treatment of apraxia can be restorative with focus on facilitating efficiency and prosodic elements. Targets are selected on a hierarchy of complexity. Depending on the severity of symptoms, treatment can also have a compensatory focus of using multimodal communication, including verbal expression combined with gestures, written expression, or augmentative communication devices.[3]

Neurogenic Stuttering

Neurogenic stuttering (NS), which is a dysfluency characterized by syllable repetitions, prolongations, and hesitations, can be a result of a central nervous system disease. It can occur independently or co-occur with other motor speech disorders, or may occur as a psychological response to neurologic disease. NS has also been associated with various medications associated with anxiety, depressions, seizures, and

Parkinson disease. Tricyclic antidepressants, antipsychotics, benzodiazepine derivatives, and phenothiazine anticonvulsants are just a few drug groups that have been associated with NS. Effects typically resolve with withdrawal of medication.[3]

VOICE

A voice disorder occurs when vocal quality, intensity, and/or pitch are atypical as compared with age, geographic location, or cultural background. Symptoms may include rough or breathy vocal quality, hypophonia, or aphonia. Organic etiologies of voice impairment are the result of physiologic changes of the vocal structures, which can be either *structural* (changes in the structures that create voice) or *neurologic* (atypical central or peripheral nervous system innervation with the laryngeal mechanism). *Functional voice disorders* are the result of atypical vocal behaviors in the presence of normal physical vocal structures.[4]

Voice rehabilitation includes direct and indirect approaches. Direct approaches rehabilitate the mechanisms that produce voice in order to improve vocal behaviors and vocal quality. Indirect approaches include patient education to improve vocal behaviors and to adapt environmental factors that impact voice.[5]

DYSPHAGIA

Dysphagia involves impairment in the oral, pharyngeal, and/or esophageal stages of swallowing.

- Oral phase dysphagia symptoms can include pocketing of food/liquid material in the oral cavity, reduced mastication, or reduced management of oral secretions.
- Pharyngeal phase dysphagia symptoms can include reduced management of pharyngeal secretions, a wet vocal quality, a delayed or absent swallow reflex, immediate or delayed coughing or clearing of the throat before or after the swallow, and changes in respiration and/or respiratory rate.
- Esophageal phase dysphagia symptoms can include globus sensation, laryngeal pharyngeal reflux, and difficulty swallowing.

Penetration describes when food or liquid enters the laryngeal vestibule but does not pass below the vocal folds.

Aspiration occurs when food or liquid passes below the level of the vocal folds and falls into the trachea. Silent aspiration occurs when the patient is not sensate to the aspirated material and no reflexive response in the form of cough or throat clearing occurs.

Etiologies can be due to adverse neurologic events, degenerative disease, infectious processes, impaired cognition, metabolic disorders, and myopathic conditions. Structural etiologies such as cricopharyngeal bar, Zenker diverticulum, oropharyngeal tumor, or skeletal abnor-

TABLE 31.2 Categories of Dysarthria

Type of Dysarthria	Site of Lesion	Speech Characteristics	Neuromuscular Deficits	Common Etiologies
Spastic dysarthria	Upper motor neuron	Strained and harsh vocal quality, hypernasality, slow and monotonous speech	Bilateral facial weakness may be present, hypertonia, weakness, reduced range and speed of movement	Parkinson disease
Hypokinetic dysarthria	Basal ganglia	Reduced loudness, monotone voice, rapid rate of speech, imprecise articulation	Rigidity and reduced range and speed of movement	
Ataxic dysarthria	Cerebellum	Excess and equal stress, monotone pitch, monoloudness, reduced rate of speech, irregular articulatory breakdowns	Hypotonia, slow and inaccurate movements of the oral musculature	Inflammatory degenerative diseases, stroke, tumor, alcohol abuse
Flaccid dysarthria	Lower motor neuron	Weak and breathy voice, reduced rate of speech, hypernasality	Weakness, hypotonia, fasciculation	Often damage to the brainstem but could be peripheral nerve damage, myasthenia gravis, bulbar palsy
Hyperkinetic dysarthria	Basal ganglia	Varying impairments in voice quality, interruptions in speech flow, involuntary vocal output	Abnormal rhythmic or irregular and unpredictable, rapid or slow involuntary movements[3]	Huntington disease, athetosis, spasmodic dysphonia, tremor, myoclonus
Mixed dysarthria	Variable; upper and lower motor neurons; cerebellar, damage from more than one neurologic event	Harsh vocal quality, monopitch, hypernasality, slow rate of speech		Toxic metabolic conditions, infectious processes, tumors of the brainstem, closed head injuries, neurodegenerative diseases, multiple cerebral infarcts

TABLE 31.3 Cranial Nerve Functions in Swallowing[7]

Number	Cranial Nerve	Major Function
V	Trigeminal	Sensory: facial sensation Motor: open/close mouth, mastication
VII	Facial	Sensory: facial sensation, taste Motor: facial expression
IX	Glossopharyngeal	Sensory: taste, sensation from the tonsil and pharynx Motor: elevates the pharynx and larynx
X	Vagus	Sensory: sensation from the pharynx, larynx, and trachea Motor: velopharyngeal closure, pharyngeal constriction, and airway closure
XII	Hypoglossal	No sensory component Motor: lingual movement

mality are often associated with dysphagia. Trauma to the larynx related to intubation can cause difficulty swallowing. Table 31.3 outlines the cranial nerves involved in swallow function.

Dysphagia as a Side Effect of Medications

Medications that affect the smooth and striated muscles of the esophagus (anticholinergic or antimuscarinic effects) may cause symptoms of dysphagia. Medications can cause injury to the esophagus due to irritation. When an inadequate amount of fluid is taken with the medication and it remains in the esophagus too long, damage can occur. Chemotherapeutic (anticancer) preparations may cause muscle wasting or damage to the esophagus.[6] ACE inhibitors, diuretics, and antipsychotic or neuroleptic medications may affect swallowing as they can cause xerostomia.[6] Medications that depress the central nervous system may reduce awareness and voluntary control, causing dysphagia.

Clinical Swallow Evaluation

A speech language pathologist will complete a clinical evaluation of swallowing, which consists of obtaining a comprehensive medical and surgical history, current medications, symptoms and risk factors for dysphagia, and a physical examination. Based on presentation, the patient may be presented with varying consistencies of food and liquid, which aid in establishing the presence of dysphagia. An instrumental swallow evaluation is required to determine the presence of aspiration and severity of dysphagia, and to create a plan of care for the patient, including diet modifications and/or interventions needed. An individual's cognitive status, such as alertness level and awareness of and orientation to feeding, should be assessed.[7]

Instrumental Assessment of the Swallow Mechanism

A videofluoroscopic swallow study (VFSS; also known as VFSS, modified barium, cookie swallow) is an examination that allows for visualization of the bolus movement through the oral, pharyngeal, and upper esophageal areas in real time by having the patient ingest barium with foods and liquids under fluoroscopy guidance. A variety of bolus volumes, consistencies, and compensatory strategies can be trialed.[8]

Fiberoptic endoscopic evaluation of swallowing (FEES) is an examination in which a flexible fiberoptic endoscope is passed transnasally, giving a direct visualization of the laryngeal and pharyngeal structures of the swallow. Varying consistencies of foods and liquids are administered to assess structure and function of the swallow mechanism. FEES provides visualization of secretions, degree of residue, and vocal fold pathology that cannot be detected during VFSS.

When there is a concern for esophageal dysphagia, other studies such as a barium swallow or an esophogram can better assess the esophagus.[7]

Management and Treatment of Dysphagia

A speech language pathologist can make recommendations based on the instrumental swallow assessment, including compensatory strategies or diet modifications to support safe oral intake and reduce patients' risk for aspiration. Diet modifications can include changes in bolus volume or texture by changing the viscosity of liquids or by softening, chopping, or pureeing foods. The International Dysphagia Diet Standardization Initiative provides a standardized vocabulary around diet modifications for interdisciplinary use (Figure 31.1).[9]

Food preferences, patient and family wishes regarding oral versus nonoral means of nutrition, and cultural background should be taken into account when developing a treatment plan for dysphagia.

Treatment of Dysphagia

- Compensatory
  - Diet modifications
  - Postural techniques (redirect the movement of the bolus or improve physiologic function)
  - Swallow behaviors or maneuvers (strategies to improve the timing or coordination of the swallow)
- Rehabilitative
  - Enhance motor learning by use of resistance—changing the load, volume, or number of repetitions; and specificity
  - Dysphagia exercises that target oral and pharyngeal strength and coordination[8]

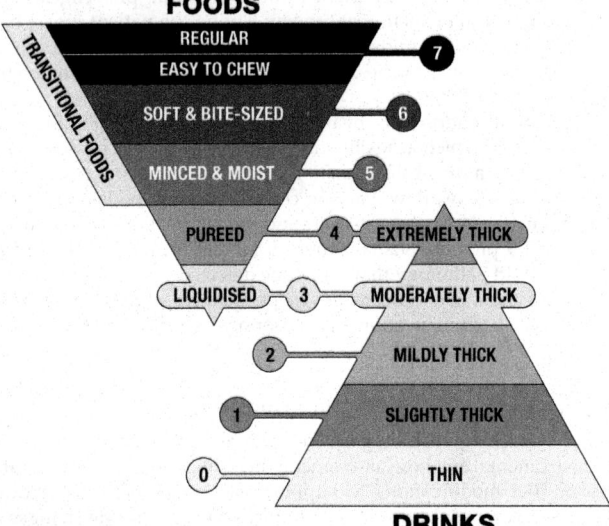

FIGURE 31.1 International Dysphagia Diet Standardization Initiative (IDDSI) framework.

Source: From the International Dysphagia Diet Standardization Initiative 2019. https://iddsi.org/framework.

- Medical intervention
  - Antireflux medication
  - Prokinetic agents
  - Salivary management
- Surgical interventions
  - Surgery includes medialization of the vocal folds, stents, laryngotracheal separation, laryngectomy, and tracheostomy tubes. Intervention in PES opening can be done through dilation, myotomy, and botulinum toxin injections.
  - Alternative means of nutrition include nasogastric tube, gastrostomy tube, or jejunostomy tube when swallow is severely impaired and the patient cannot safely tolerate hydration or nutrition per oral.[7]

Once the treatment plan for dysphagia has been established, families and caregivers should be educated and trained to carry over the specific airway protection strategies and/or changes in diet to reinforce safe swallowing at home.

REFERENCES

The full complete reference list for this chapter appears in the digital version of the chapter, available at http://connect.springerpub.com/content/book/978-0-8261-5628-0/part/part03/chapter/ch31

PART IV

MUSCULOSKELETAL REHABILITATION

CHAPTER 32

ELECTRODIAGNOSTIC TESTING

Danielle Powell and Aleks Borresen

DEFINITION

Electrodiagnostic testing (EDx) is used to assess the health of peripheral nerves and muscles. There are two components of EDx testing: nerve conduction studies (NCS) and electromyography (EMG). EMG and NCS can be used to diagnose the following conditions: mononeuropathy, plexopathy, radiculopathy, polyneuropathy, neuromuscular junction (NMJ) disorder, myopathy, and motor neuron disease. EDx testing can aid in diagnosis, guide treatment (surgical vs. nonsurgical) and prognosis, monitor disease progression and response to treatment, and can assess chronicity, localization, symmetry, and severity.

RELATIVE CONTRAINDICATIONS/PRECAUTIONS[1]

- *Pacemaker/defibrillator:* There is no evidence of safety hazard in EMG/NCS testing.
- *Deep brain stimulators:* Get clearance from neurology before testing and weigh the risks and benefits.
- *Wounds/soft tissue infection:* Avoid EMG due to risk of infection.
- *Lymphedema:* Limit EMG due to infection risk/worsening lymphedema.
- *Pregnancy:* There is no evidence of safety hazard in EMG/NCS testing.
- *Neuropathic/insensate skin:* Caution with EMG testing and use of heating pads.
- *Anticoagulation use:* Perform EMG with caution and watch for bleeding.

PATIENT CONSIDERATIONS FOR TESTING

- *Informed consent:* Discuss the risks, benefits, and reasonable alternatives to EMG/NCS and inform the patient that they are in control and can stop the test at any point in time.
- *NCS:* This portion of the test can be uncomfortable but does cause any permanent damage.
- *EMG:* EMG may be painful and comes with risk of bleeding/bruising, damage to underlying tissues or structures (pneumothorax if needling the trapezius, chest, or thorax), infection, and pain.

Tips for patient comfort:
- Remind the patient that they are in control and the test can be stopped at any time.
- Insert the needle quickly after a quick verbal warning.

- When able, use isometric contraction to evaluate motor unit action potential (MUAPs) to prevent painful bending of the needle in the muscle.
- Plan out and minimize the number of nerves and muscles tested.
- Keep the patient updated on the status of the test.
- Make the patient comfortable with pillows/positioning.

ELECTRODIAGNOSTIC TESTING HISTORY AND PHYSICAL EXAMINATION

- *History:* family history of neurologic conditions, occupation, comorbid medical conditions, medications (including prior chemo or radiation), prior surgeries or trauma, thyroid disorder, diabetes, and general medical conditions
- *Physical examination:* atrophy, tone, sensory testing, manual muscle testing, muscle stretch reflexes, surgical scars, bony deformities, and presence of any skin changes over the limbs to be tested
    Limb factors affecting NCS: lotion, sweat, or oils on the skin, edema, obesity, thick skin/scleroderma, and obstructive jewelry

NERVE CONDUCTION STUDY

NCS consists of motor and sensory studies. Which nerves are tested depends on the question being asked and the clinical presentation, and can be dynamically changed based on incoming NCS data.

During NCS, an electric stimulus is applied to the nerve; this impulse propagates through the nerve to an electrode which records the motor or sensory response, producing a waveform known as the compound motor action potential (CMAP) or the sensory nerve action potential (SNAP). The SNAP waveform is recorded over a patch of skin innervated by the sensory nerve and represents the cutaneous response of all stimulated sensory nerve fibers (Figure 32.1). The CMAP waveform is recorded over the muscle belly innervated by the motor nerve and represents muscle contraction. Waveforms are characterized by their latency, amplitude, duration, and temporal dispersion.

Terminology

- *Latency* is the delay between the initial stimulus and the onset of the SNAP or CMAP waveform and requires the distance between the stimulation site and the recording site to be calculated. Onset latency is the time from the stimulus to the first deflection from baseline and represents the fastest nerve fiber transmission time. Peak latency is the time from the stimulus to the waveform peak and is only ever used for sensory NCS and even then only in some EDx labs.
- *Conduction velocity (CV):* Sensory nerve CV (speed) is calculated by dividing the distance traveled by the latency. Motor nerve CV calculation requires distal segment latency and another more proximal

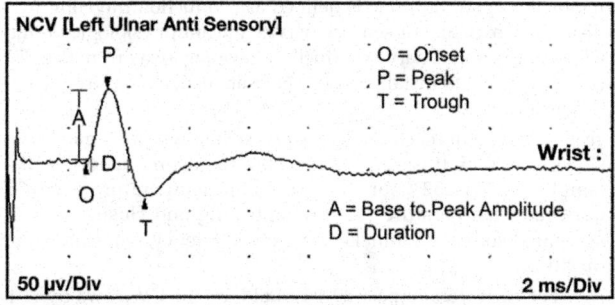

FIGURE 32.1 Outline of a typical sensory nerve conduction response showing component parameters. The x-axis shows the time in milliseconds/division, while the y-axis shows voltage/division (μV/div for sensory, mV/div for motor). By convention the downward direction is positive.

NCV, nerve conduction velocity.

Source: From Chu SK, Jayabalan P, Visco CJ. *McLean EMG Guide*, 2nd ed. Springer Publishing Company; 2019.

segment latency to eliminate NMJ/muscle contraction time. *Demyelination prolongs (increases) latency.*

- *Amplitude* is the height of the waveform. Motor amplitudes are typically measured from baseline to peak, while sensory amplitudes are measured peak to peak. The amplitude of motor waveforms compound muscle action potential scheme (CMAPs) is 5 to 15 mV (100 × larger compared with sensory amplitude, which is 10–20 μV) Axon loss leads to decreased amplitude. The presence of a drop in CMAP when measuring across a known focal entrapment site may represent a conduction block if the decrease in proximal CMAP is greater than 20% compared to the CMAP at the distal stimulation site.

- *Duration* is the time from onset of potential to the first baseline crossing and can be prolonged by demyelinating lesions, leading to dispersion of the waveform on the x-axis or to temporal dispersion.

  It is possible for distal motor latency to be significantly prolonged yet for the median nerve conduction velocity (MNCV) to remain in the normal range if a demyelinating lesion occurs near the muscle being tested.

- *Orthodromic* refers to nerve conduction and recording occurring in the physiologic direction of the nerve being tested. Thus, for motor nerves which transmit efferent signals, orthodromic is defined as conduction traveling from proximal to distal along the motor nerve. For sensory nerves, which transmit afferent signals, orthodromic is defined as conduction traveling toward the central nervous system (CNS). Motor NCS are usually performed orthodromically.

- *Antidromic* refers to nerve conduction and recording occurring in the antiphysiologic direction from the nerve being tested. Thus, for motor nerves, antidromic is defined as conduction traveling from distal to proximal. For sensory nerves, the antiphysiologic or antidromic direction is nerve conduction traveling away from the CNS (from proximal to distal). Sensory NCS are usually performed antidromically.

- *Temperature:* For each degree Celsius below 34°C, motor CV slows 1 m/sec^2. It is standard practice to ensure the upper limb temperature is ≥32°C or the lower limb temperature is ≥30°C. Cool limb temperature → slower opening and closing of voltage-gated sodium channels → increased latency, amplitude, and duration.
- *Age:* For each decade past 20 years old, motor CV slows by .4 to 1.7 m/sec and sensory conduction slows by 2 to 4 m/s^2.
- *High-frequency filter (low pass):* This filters out frequencies above a certain threshold and allows frequencies below the threshold to pass unaffected "low pass." Adjusting a filter's threshold has a predictable impact on NCS waveforms. Decreasing the high-frequency filter threshold (e.g., 10 → 1 kHz) causes ↑ peak/onset latency and ↓ amplitude.
- *Low-frequency filter (high pass):* This filters out frequencies below a certain threshold and allows frequencies above the said frequency to pass unaffected "high pass." NCS waveforms change predictably if the low-frequency filter is elevated. For example, increasing the low-frequency filter (e.g., 20 → 200 Hz) causes ↓ peak latency, unchanged onset latency, and ↓ amplitude.
- *Differential amplifier:* This is used to reduce noise artifacts from the surrounding electromagnetic radiation, such as fluorescent lights, Wi-Fi, nearby power sources, electronics, or even NCS electrode wiring.

Nerve Conduction Study Setup

- Typical sensory NCS settings (in microvolts, µV): sweep 1 to 2 msec/division, gain 20 µV/division (i.e., .02 mV/division), low-frequency filter 2 to 10 Hz, and high-frequency filter 2 kHz (Figure 32.2).
- *Active (recording) electrode = A (usually black in color; "blacktive" electrode):* For motor studies, place over the bulk of the muscle being studied; for sensory studies, place over the nerve being studied (preferably where it runs as superficial as possible).
- *Reference electrode = R (usually red in color; "redference" electrode):* For sensory studies, the reference electrode is placed ~3 cm downstream from the active electrode over a patch of skin innervated by the nerve being studied. For motor study reference electrode placement, place over an electrically neutral site, such as the tendon or the bone, further downstream from the active electrode (ideally 5 cm or more).

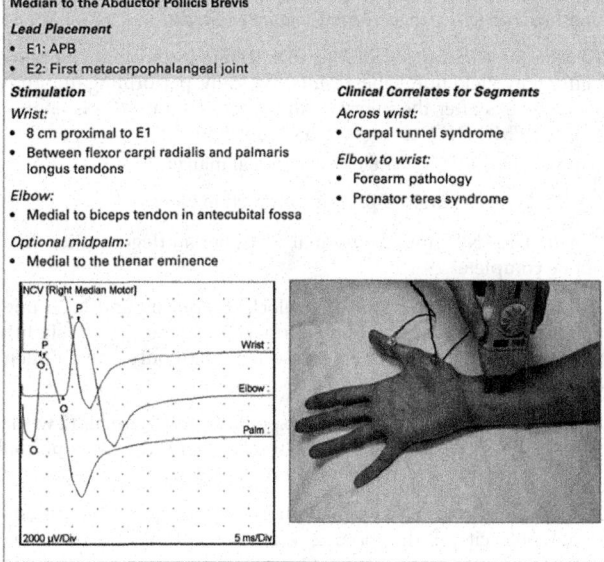

FIGURE 32.2 Median motor study nerve conduction study setup.

NCV, nerve conduction velocity.

Source: From Chu SK., Jayabalan P, Visco CJ. *McLean EMG Guide*, 2nd ed. Springer Publishing Company; 2019.

- *Ground electrode = G (usually green in color; green for ground):* It is a known zero-voltage comparison point usually placed in between but outside the direct path of the impulse between the stimulator cathode terminal and the active (recording) electrode (e.g., dorsum of the hand for upper limb studies).

    In radiculopathy, nerve impingement occurs at the level of the sensory nerve root *prior to the sensory nerve ganglion*, which houses the sensory nerve cell body. During sensory NCS, only the postganglionic sensory nerve fibers are tested (which are intact in the setting of a radiculopathy), and thus sensory NCS will be normal in radiculopathies (a rare exception is for lateral L5 radiculopathy, which may impinge at the ganglion). The brachial plexus is entirely postganglionic. The "roots" of the brachial plexus are actually ventral rami which contain motor and postganglionic sensory fibers. Thus, an injury to the brachial plexus "root" (e.g., rami) *will* affect sensory NCS (in contrast to the preganglionic sensory nerve root lesions found in radiculopathy).

- *Abnormal findings:* In general, more than 50% asymmetry between sides (amplitude, CV) is significant (relative rule). There also exist specific cutoffs which can vary by age and limb temperature. For normal latency, CV, amplitude values, refer to the EDx software or Buschbacher's *Manual of Nerve Conduction Studies*.[2]

- *Timeline for obtaining NCS/EMG:* EDx testing too soon after a nerve injury may yield unreliable results. Typically, performing the study 4 to 6 weeks after the injury or the onset of symptoms is enough time for EMG/NCS changes to have developed.
- Time course of EDX changes after axonal injury:
- *Less than 3 days:* can find pseudo-conduction block
- *3 to 10 days:* NCS may be normal as Wallerian degeneration may not be complete
- *2 to 6 weeks:* pseudo-conduction block disappears and NCS now abnormal with ↓ amplitude and normal CV/latency (can be slightly prolonged if the fastest fibers transected), with only ↓ recruitment on EMG
- *2 weeks to 2 months:* EMG now with spontaneous potentials (2 weeks paraspinals, 6 weeks distal leg, 4 weeks thigh), can have normal MUAP with only ↓ recruitment as no reinnervation yet
- *Less than 2 months:* EMG now with MUAP changes: ↑ amplitude, ↑ polyphasicity, ↑ duration, ± ↓ recruitment, and spontaneous potentials (Note: months to years after lesions [if no ongoing active lesion], spontaneous potentials will disappear and NCS CMAP greater than SNAP amplitudes may improve or normalize due to reinnervation.)
- *F-waves:* This is not a true reflex. These can be obtained from any muscle by applying a supramax retrograde motor impulse toward the anterior horn cell. A small subset of anterior horn cells will fire in response to this and send motor impulses down the nerve to the recording electrode. The waveform produced is of variable latency and configuration. Obtain 10 or more waves and find the earliest latency. F-waves have limited specificity as they assess the entire motor nerve pathway to the anterior horn cell.
- *H-reflex:* This is a true reflex. It is present in adults only. The H reflex is obtained by applying submaximal stimulus to the tibial nerve in the popliteal fossa with the cathode pointing proximal to the anode. The active electrode is placed over the soleus muscle. Similar to F-waves, H-reflex has limited specificity as it can be abnormal with injury anywhere along the pathway from the sensory nerve, spinal cord interneuron, anterior horn cell, motor nerve, NMJ, or muscle, but can be sensitive in S1 radiculopathy and Guillain–Barré syndrome (GBS). The waveform produced is typically of fixed latency and stable reproducible configuration. It is important to compare with contralateral H-reflex as side to side difference of less than 1.5 msec is considered significant. Normal

values can also be looked up in nomograms based on height and age. It can be "physiologically" absent in the older adults. H-reflexes may be seen in nonsoleus muscles when upper motor neuron (UMN) lesions are present or in infants.

Anomalous Innervations

- *Martin Gruber anastomosis:* Ulnar nerve fibers destined for the ulnar-innervated hand muscles form an anastomosis with the median nerve near the elbow. May be seen when testing abductor pollicis brevis (APB) motor NCS by stimulating the "median nerve" at the antecubital fossa, which also stimulates the martin gruber anastomosis. The adductor pollicis motor response arrives prior to the APB motor response, leading to a waveform with initial positive (downward) deflection, a larger amplitude, and decreased latency. Recognizing this pattern is important as stimulating the median APB at the wrist will lead to a latency and amplitude difference which when compared against the "median" APB antecubital fossa values may lead to an erroneous diagnosis of carpal tunnel syndrome (CTS).
- *Riche–Cannieu anastomosis:* This is rare and presents as an all-ulnar-innervated hand as ulnar motor fibers cross to innervate (normally median-innervated) the thenar muscles (APB, etc.). This may lead to a misdiagnosis of "severe CTS" and unnecessary surgery due to an absent median APB CMAP when stimulated over the median nerve at the wrist. However, in RicheCannieu, stimulating the ulnar nerve while recording over the APB will show a normal APB CMAP response. It should be suspected in the presence of median CMAP greater than SNAP amplitude loss, and one should measure the median APB CMAP while stimulating over the ulnar nerve at the wrist to rule out Riche–Cannieu anastomosis in this scenario. It can also present as an APB without EMG changes despite axonal injury of the median nerve at the carpal tunnel.
- *Accessory peroneal nerve:* This is a branch of the superficial peroneal nerve which comes off prior to the ankle and runs posterior to the lateral malleolus to innervate the lateral extensor digitorum brevis (EDB). The anomaly is revealed when the CMAP response below the fibular neck and popliteal fossa is higher than distal stimulation at the ankle. Stimulation posterior to the lateral malleolus will produce a CMAP response that if added to the CMAP response of the ankle will produce a larger response than the two proximal sites.

Nerve Conduction Study Troubleshooting[3]

- *Poor/absent NCS waveform:* Verify the following: (a) good adhesion of active, ground, and reference electrodes; (b) adequate electrolyte gel used on stimulator prongs; (c) cathode is pointing in the direction of the active (recording) electrode to avoid anodal conduction block; (d) electrode wires have not inadvertently been unplugged and are connected to the active amplifier channel; and (e) obtain the waveform in the contralateral limb (if present, its absence on the affected limb is more suspicious for pathology > technical error).

Unstable NCS baseline:
- Attempt to clean any sweat or lotion off the skin.
- Ensure electrode wires are plugged into the active amplifier channel and are not tangled.
- Rotate the simulator anode position medially and laterally while stimulating to change the polarity of the baseline until it is neutral.
- Limit electromagnetic interference (Wi-Fi or other electronics in adjacent rooms/floors can impact).

ELECTROMYOGRAPHY

Monopolar EMG needles require an *external reference* and ground electrode and a sample in 360° from a broader area of tissue. Due to broader sampling, MUAPs have larger amplitudes and up to 25% polyphasicity may be considered normal. Monopolar needles are typically smaller and Teflon-coated, which can make insertion less painful.

Concentric EMG needles only require an external ground electrode as the reference electrode is built into the needle. They only sample from a 180° field and thus MUAP amplitudes are smaller and only up to 15% polyphasicity may be considered normal.

- *Insertional activity:* Set gain to 50 to 100 μV. The needle is advanced into the muscle belly with the muscle at rest. Advance the needle slightly to depolarize the muscle membrane and stop; with normal insertional activity, a brief crisp popping noise will coincide with needle movements. Continue to repeat this process advancing 1 to 2 mm in several different quadrants of the area being tested to check for any aberrant waveforms/sounds. This is graded as normal, reduced, or increased (prolonged >.3 seconds) insertional activity.

- *Spontaneous activity:* Set gain to 50 to 100 μV. After initially inserting the needle and in between advances of the needle, briefly pause (few seconds) and observe for any spontaneous noises/waveforms that occur.

- *MUAP analysis:* Set gain to 200 μV and have the patient begin to gently engage the tested muscle while the needle is still in place. If the MUAP is distant (dull sound with prolonged rise time), gently move the needle until the sound becomes more crisp. With only a few motor units on screen, analyze the motor unit: (a) amplitude, (b) duration/rise time, (c) number of phases/turns, and (d) stability.

- *Recruitment (muscle firing characteristics) and activation:* The patient is asked to produce a gentle isometric force (against the examiner's resistance) and to gradually increase the magnitude of muscle contraction. During this time, the examiner is analyzing the rate at which individual motor units fire and the rate at which additional motor units are recruited to aid in increasing force generation. Recruitment can be normal, early (increased), reduced (decreased), or absent.

Interference pattern refers to how tightly MUAPs are grouped during maximal contraction and are usually graded 0%, 25%, 50%, 75%, and 100% (full). Less than 100% interference pattern can be seen in neuropathic conditions, submaximal effort (often due to pain), or CNS weakness (poor activation).

- In a healthy muscle, contraction force is increased via two mechanisms: (a) increased firing frequency of the current motor unit and/or (b) recruitment of additional larger motor units. For example, a motor unit already firing at 5 Hz will increase its frequency to 10 Hz and an additional (larger) motor unit will begin to fire at 5 Hz.
- Reduced recruitment is usually the result of a neuropathic process with axon loss or severe demyelination with conduction block. EMG will show only a few MUAPs that fire with increased frequency (>15–20 Hz) as the contraction force is increased and failure to recruit additional motor units to aid force creation.
- Early or increased recruitment is usually the result of a myopathic process. In a myopathic process, EMG will show rapid firing of many small-amplitude MUAPs when the examiner asks for a small force to be generated. This is because muscle fiber loss leads to ineffective motor units which generate only a fraction of their prior power when asked to contract. The patient compensates by ramping up the amount and frequency of motor nerves firing, leading to early recruitment (Box 32.1).

Motor Unit Action Potential Features

- *MUAP amplitude* is measured from positive peak to negative peak. For monopolar needles, it is around 1 to 7 mV and for concentric needles it is typically .5 to 5 mV. The needle EMG recording area is such that only 10 or less muscle fibers contribute to the MUAP amplitude. The number and size (diameter) of muscle fibers near

---

BOX 32.1 Difference Between Myopathic and Neuropathic EMG Pattern

A myopathic electromyography (EMG) pattern is differentiated from neuropathic EMG pattern as myopathic EMG demonstrates short-duration, short-amplitude (SDSA) waveforms with an early recruitment pattern, whereas neuropathic EMG demonstrates long-duration, large-amplitude (LDLA) waveforms with a late (decreased) recruitment pattern.

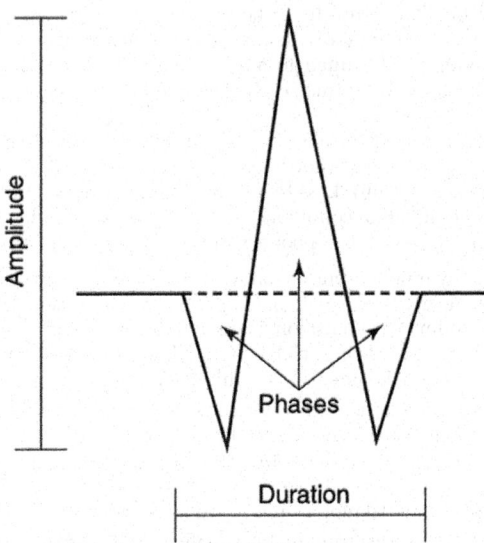

FIGURE 32.3 Normal motor unit action potential (MUAP). Phases are equal to the number of baseline crossings + 1. In this MUAP, there are two baseline crossings + 1 = 3 phases. The amplitude measures the entire vertical dimension of the MUAP. MUAP duration is measured from the onset of initial baseline deflection to the final return to baseline (the normal is generally <15 msec).

Source: From Chu SK, Jayabalan P, Visco CJ. *McLean EMG Guide*, 2nd ed. Springer Publishing Company; 2019. Figure 16.3.

the needle tip and how synchronously they are contracted determine the MUAP amplitude. Asynchronous firing (variable myelination) may lead to increased duration, polyphasicity, or turns.

- *MUAP duration* is directly proportional to the number of fibers making up a motor unit and inversely proportional how synchronously they fire. It is measured from the initial deflection from the baseline to the eventual return to baseline (after all phases) and is typically 5 to 15 msec.
- *Rise time* is a subset of duration and is measured from the initial positive (downward) deflection from baseline to the first negative peak. Rise time correlates with how close the needle is to the MUAP being measured and ≤.5 msec is ideal.
- *Phases* are the number of times that the MUAP *crosses the baseline* and are determined by counting the number of baseline crossings and adding one (Figure 32.3). Polyphasia is present when four or more baseline crossings (e.g., five phases) are present. For concentric needles, up to 10% polyphasia can be physiologic, and for monopolar needles up to 25% polyphasia can be physiologic. If a

greater percent of waves are polyphasic, the muscle is said to have polyphasia or polyphasic potentials. Polyphasia produces a clicking sound.
- *Serrations (or turns)* are changes in the direction of the MUAP waveform which do not cross the baseline (small peaks or valleys). They typically arise during an immature reinnervation process. Note: Serrations may resolve into discrete phases with slight needle movement.
- *Satellite potentials* are small delayed motor unit potentials time-locked with the main motor unit waveform firing pattern. They occur after denervation and represent collateral sprouting from neighboring motor units that have reinnervated muscle fibers (but are delayed due to poor myelination).

Stability refers to the reproducibility of MUAP waveform. Unstable waveform morphology is seen in NMJ disorders (amplitude change), but can also be seen with reinnervation due to immature NMJs.

Electromyography Waveforms[4]

Electromyography Waveform Sounds

The pitch of the sound correlates to quickly it rises (slope). The volume of the wave is proportional to the peak amplitude. The frequency or how closely spaced the waveforms are determines the tempo or "beat" of the sounds.

- *Spontaneous potentials generated by the muscle:* fasciculation potentials, positive sharp waves (PSW), fibrillation potentials, complex repetitive discharges (CRD), and myotonic discharges
- *PSW (sharps):* initiated by needle movement stimulating a single muscle fiber action potential which fires in a regular pattern and produces a recurring (low-pitch) "dull thuds"; appears as a biphasic wave with initial positive deflection; a grouping of PSWs is referred to as a "run" or "train" of PSWs (Figure 32.4)
- *Fibrillation potentials (fibs):* represent the contraction of a single muscle fiber firing spontaneously (fibrillating) or in response to needle electrode movement, producing a (usually) regular high-pitched sound like "rain on a tin roof," biphasic or triphasic spikes (<5 msec duration), and less than 1 mV peak to peak amplitude; initial deflection positive (downward) needle electrode is in the muscle fiber (Figure 32.4)
- *CRD:* may sound similar to myotonic discharge if it is not so complex CRD but will *not* have significant amplitude change; frequency is 20 to 150 Hz; abrupt onset with waning frequency and amplitude and abrupt offset; may begin spontaneously or after needle movement; can result from both myopathic and neurogenic processes; evidence of a chronic process of denervationreinnervationdenervation process, leading to ephaptic transmission where muscle fibers fire depolarizing neighboring fibers in a cyclic pattern; produces complex repetitive sound; previously termed bizarre repetitive discharge or pseudomyotonic discharge

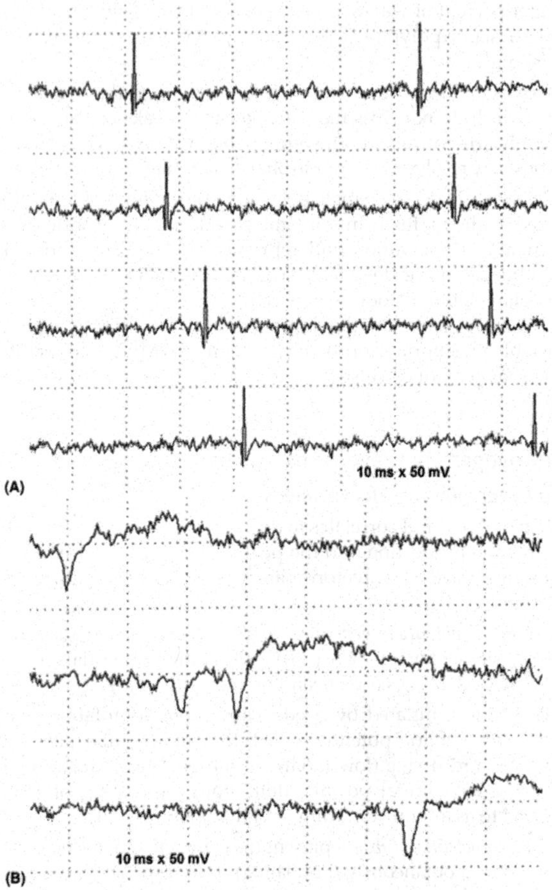

FIGURE 32.4 Fibrillation and positive sharp wave potentials.
Source: From Ferrante MA, Tsao B. *EMG Lesion Localization and Characterization*. Springer Publishing Company; 2019. Figure 5.1.

- *Myotonia/myotonic discharge:* repetitive discharges of single muscle fibers, fire at a rate of 20 to 80 Hz, dive bomber sound, waning and waxing frequency and amplitude, with abrupt onset and offset; may occur after needle insertion or muscle contraction/percussion; conditions with severe active denervation may cause myotonic discharges (polymyositis, chronic radiculopathy, and peripheral neuropathy), but diffuse myotonia with myopathic MUAPs and early recruitment is suggestive of myotonic muscle disorder (myotonic dystrophy, myotonia congenita, hyperkalemic periodic paralysis)

- *Spontaneous potentials generated by the nerves:* fasciculation potentials (fasics, myokymic discharges, cramp discharges, neuromyotonic discharges, tremors, doublets, triplets)
- *Fasciculation potentials:* involuntary (spontaneous) twitching of a group of muscle fibers that all belong to a single motor unit; look like normal MUAPs but fire irregularly and occur with patient at rest; in a large motor unit, fasciculations may yield grossly visible, writhing movement of the skin (or even joint movements); seen in normal individuals (benign fasciculation potentials), anterior horn cell disease, and radiculopathy
  - *Myokymia/myokymic discharges:* abrupt onset of tightly grouped repetitive bursts of nerve MUAPs firing semiregularly several times per second, often described as "soldiers marching in snow"; occur involuntarily and are subacute in onset; extremity myokymia *classically seen in radiation plexopathy* but can also occur in compression neuropathy; facial myokymia may occur in facial nerve lesions, brainstem lesions, polyradiculopathy, and multiple sclerosis
  - *Neuromyotonic discharges:* sporadic or recurrent bursts of MUAPs originating from rapidly firing (150–300 Hz) motor nerves, with abrupt onset and offset, usually with waning amplitude lasting a few seconds; may be triggered by needle advancement, voluntary contraction, percussion, or ischemia; note: may sound similar to CRD or myotonic discharge, but during neuromyotonia the bursts of MUAPs fire more rapidly (at a higher frequency), creating pulses of a fast buzzing or zipping sound (150–300 buzzes/sec); may be present in clinical neuromyotonia
  - *Miniature endplate potentials (MEPPs):* short-duration, tiny-amplitude (10–20 µV) monophasic negative waveforms which fire at a high frequency and sound like a seashell or low-volume TV static; quickly move the needle through or pull back as the needle is in the motor endplate, which can be painful

Nerve Injury Severity Grading (Seddon Classification)

- *Neuropraxia* (mildest injury) is the result of focal segmental demyelination interrupting nerve signal propagation leading to a conduction block. The underlying axon and neural connective tissue are intact and the axon can remyelinate. Prognosis for recovery is good and remyelination can occur on a timescale of weeks to months.
- *Axonotmesis* is the result of axonal disruption with Wallerian degeneration (nerve death) distal to the lesion. It is a more severe injury compared with neuropraxia. The neural connective tissue remains intact and the axon can regenerate with eventual reinnervation of its target tissue. Prognosis for recovery is fair but occurs on a timescale of months to years. Axon growth rate estimate is ~1 inch/mo or 1 mm/d.

  Neurotmesis (most severe injury) is the result of complete disruption of myelin, axon, and neural connective tissue scaffolding.

There is poor prognosis as regrowth of the axon is not anticipated due to loss of the neural connective tissue.

ELECTRODIAGNOSTIC TESTING PATHOLOGY PATTERNS

- *Entrapment neuropathies:* The nerve can be entrapped anywhere along its path. Classically this occurs at known anatomic entrapment sites, and areas with tight passages that may squeeze the nerve, leading to a mononeuropathy. An example is median mononeuropathy at the wrist, which can be assessed using the Combined Sensory Index.[5] Entrapment can also occur at nonclassic entrapment sites via many different compressive mechanisms. There my be trauma with hematoma or bony deformity (heterotopic ossification), muscular hypertrophy (pronator teres hypertrophy), presence of a mass (lipoma, synovial cyst, and tumor), anatomic variance (accessory cervical rib, piriformis syndrome), and external compression (crutches in axilla, fibular neck, and tight belt/obesity). Uncommon entrapment neuropathies include thoracic outlet syndrome/Pancoast tumor (lower trunk), piriformis syndrome (sciatic nerve), anterior tarsal tunnel (deep peroneal nerve), pronator syndrome (median nerve), superficial radial nerve, radial tunnel syndrome, and tarsal tunnel syndrome.
- *Peripheral neuropathies:* These may affect sensory fibers, motor fibers, or both; may cause axonal or demyelinating injuries or both; and may be segmental, uniform, focal, versus distal in location (see Table 32.1 for additonal EDx patterns of common conditions).

Distribution patterns

- Uniform demyelinating polyneuropathies show uniform slowing of CV (in a nonsegmental or length dependent manner). This is typically of congenital polyneuropathies, such as hereditary motor and sensory neuropathies or Charcot-Marie-Tooth.
- Segmental demyelinating polyneuropathies have CV slowing about a particular segment of the nerves (inflammatory polyneuropathies and some drug-induced).
- Distal polyneuropathies (diabetes, thyroid, renal disease, HIV, B_{12}/folate, ethyl alcohol, and heavy metals) are length-dependent axonal or demyelinating changes which progress from distal to proximal as disease worsens.
- Focal demyelinating/axonal pattern: If there is presence of axonal or demyelinating lesion about a common or known entrapment site (or uncommon site which may be caused by a tumor), this may be due to a focal conduction block. In these lesions, CMAP or SNAP amplitude, latency, and/or CV are abnormal when stimulating above a particular segment of the nerve and recording distally, but these amplitude/latency/CV abnormalities normalize when stimulating at a site distal to this particular segment of focal conduction block (for orthodromic

TABLE 32.1 EDx Patterns in Select Specific Conditions

AIDP/GBS/CIDP	Multifocal demyelinating motor > sensory neuropathy; prolonged F-waves and latencies
Critical illness neuropathy	Axonal sensorimotor polyneuropathy
Neuropathy associated with diabetes/chronic renal failure	Diffuse mixed axonal/demyelinating sensorimotor polyneuropathy distal and progressing proximal
Anterior horn cell disease/multifocal motor neuropathy	Normal sensory NCS with evidence of motor NCS and EMG findings consistent with axonal injury/denervation
Myopathy	Myopathic changes with small-duration, small-amplitude motor units with early recruitment pattern
Hereditary motor and sensory neuropathy	Diffuse demyelinating mixed sensorimotor polyneuropathy
Mononeuritis multiplex	Multiple focal axonal sensory and/or motor mononeuropathies

AIDP, acute inflammatory demyelinating polyneuropathy; EDx, electrodiagnostic testing; EMG, electromyography; GBS, Guillain–Barré syndrome; CIDP, chronic inflammatory demyelinating polyneuropathy; NCS, nerve conduction studies.

motor studies; e.g., ulnar neuropathy at the elbow testing abductor digiti minimi CMAP above-elbow vs. below-elbow stim).

ELECTRODIAGNOSTIC REPORT

- Include a brief history and physical examination including height/weight.
- Include documentation of patient consent to the procedure.
- Include EMG needle type.
- Include any complications.
- State and clearly answer the question from the referring physician.
- Note if findings are acute versus chronic or both, or demyelinating versus axonal, as well as the pattern (focal, generalized) and if the lesion occurs about a known entrapment site and the severity.
- Compare with prior study if available.
- Describe caveats upfront (if any) that is inability to tolerate EDx study, limitations due to edema, obesity, or previous surgery.

REFERENCES

The full complete reference list for this chapter appears in the digital version of the chapter, available at http://connect.springerpub.com/content/book/978-0-8261-5628-0/part/part04/chapter/ch32

/ CHAPTER 33

ULTRASOUND

Dayna M. Yorks, Matthew C. Sherrier, and Samuel K. Chu

INTRODUCTION

Ultrasound (US) is an invaluable tool for diagnosis and treatment of various musculoskeletal conditions and has become increasingly important in the field of physiatry. The advantages of US over other imaging modalities include its relative portability, low cost, high-quality spatial resolution of superficial soft tissue and neurovascular structures, no exposure to ionizing radiation, and capability for continuous needle visualization during interventions.

ULTRASOUND PRINCIPLES

Ultrasound Physics

The head of an US transducer contains piezoelectric crystals, which convert electric current into pulses of ultrasonic waves. These waves are conducted through the patient's skin with the use of a sonoconductive gel toward the target tissues, where they are reflected, absorbed, or penetrated through the tissue. An US image is produced when the US waves return to the transducer and are converted into electrical current. The US appearance of the tissue is based on tissue density. The term *hyperechoic* is used to describe bright-appearing structures that result from the reflection of greater amounts of US energy by denser tissues, such as the bone. *Hypoechoic* is used to describe dark-appearing structures that result from the reflection of lesser amounts of US energy by less dense tissues, such as the hyaline cartilage. *Anechoic* is used to describe black-appearing areas on US images that result from absorption of all US waves, such as simple fluid.

The amplitude and intensity of the US waves emitted from the US transducer decrease as they travel through the tissue. This will typically lead to deeper structures appearing more hypoechoic than superficial structures. This natural decrease in amplitude is referred to as *attenuation*. The amount of attenuation varies based on the density of the tissue. For example, denser structures, such as tendons, cause more attenuation than less dense structures, such as fluid or air.

Transducer Selection

Transducers vary by the range of US frequencies that they transmit. Frequencies are typically labeled on the body of the transducer in megahertz (MHz). Linear array transducers transmit higher frequency US waves that allow for greater detail and superior near-field resolution when imaging superficial structures. In contrast, curvilinear array transducers transmit lower frequency US waves that are less susceptible to attenuation as they penetrate to deeper tissues. Generally, a higher frequency linear array transducer will be preferable when imaging more superficial structures and a lower frequency curvilinear array transducer is preferable when imaging deeper structures. Appropriate US transducer selection is an important component of image optimization.

Image Optimization/Knobology

In addition to choosing the most appropriate transducer, there are many ways to optimize an US image. It is necessary for the sonographer to familiarize themselves with the layout of the functional knobs, switches, and touchscreen interfaces of each platform that they might utilize, as these will vary by US manufacturer and model. *Depth* refers to penetration of the sound beam into the tissue. Depth can be adjusted, typically by turning a dial or pushing a switch up or down, such that the target structure(s) is visible. Excessive depth leads to dead space on the image, which should be avoided. *Focal zones* can be selected to optimize resolution at a particular depth. The number and positioning of the focal zones should be chosen based on the size and depth of the target structure. *Gain* refers to the overall brightness of the US image. Increasing or decreasing the gain with a knob or switch adjusts the brightness of the entire image. *Time gain compensation (TGC)* allows for adjustment of gain at a specific depth and is typically set through a vertically oriented stack of sliding switches. Most US machines have *Doppler* features, which can be used to appreciate vascular flow. *Color Doppler* shows flow toward the transducer as red and flow away from the transducer as blue. *Power Doppler* is generally more sensitive than color Doppler and assigns a color to blood flow regardless of direction.

TRANSDUCER MOVEMENTS AND TERMINOLOGY

Orientation

Standard orientation on an US image includes superficial structures toward the top of the image and deeper structures toward the bottom of the image. The US transducer usually has an indicator (notch or dot) on one side, which typically corresponds to the left side of the image. Care should be taken when determining the orientation of the transducer on the patient and how that corresponds to the US image.

Transducer Movement

Moving the transducer results in real-time changes to the image that is produced.

- *Translating* or *sliding:* moving the entire transducer in the direction of the long axis of the transducer

- *Sweeping:* moving the entire transducer in the direction of the short axis of the transducer
- *Rock* and *heel-toe:* angling the transducer along its long axis by putting more pressure on one side of the transducer while maintaining the same location
- *Toggle* and *wag:* angling the transducer along its short axis while maintaining the same location
- *Rotate:* rotating the transducer around a center point/axis

Common Sonographic Artifacts

US imaging is fundamentally vulnerable to image artifacts as the appearance of a normal tissue can change based on the angle of US waves and the relative sonographic characteristics of the adjacent tissues. Knowledge and awareness of US artifacts are of vital importance to distinguish those artifacts from pathology and to avoid unnecessary interventions. Common sonographic artifacts are described in Table 33.1.

SONOGRAPHIC APPEARANCE OF NORMAL AND PATHOLOGIC STRUCTURES

Tendons, ligaments, muscles, bones, and peripheral nerves have characteristic sonographic appearances (Table 33.2 and Figure 33.1). Common pathologic findings are detailed in Table 33.2.

TABLE 33.1 Common Sonographic Artifacts

Artifact	Description
Anisotropy	When the US beam is perpendicular to the tissue, such as the tendons or ligaments, it appears hyperechoic. If the US beam is not perpendicular, the tissue can have varying echogenicity (referred to as anisotropy). This artifact can potentially be mistaken for pathology and should be considered when scanning tendons and ligaments in both short and long axes. Anisotropy can also be used to distinguish tendons from the surrounding structures, such as the median nerve in the carpal tunnel.
Reverberation	When the US beam hits a smooth, flat structure, such as a metal object or a needle, it reflects back and forth between the structure and the transducer, creating a series of linear echoes that extend beyond the structure.
Posterior acoustic shadowing	When the US beam is reflected, absorbed, or refracted from the surface of a structure, an anechoic area extends deep to the structure. This can be seen with bone or calcification.
Posterior acoustic enhancement	Tissues deep to the hypoechoic or anechoic structures (e.g., cysts) can appear relatively hyperechoic compared with adjacent soft tissue structures due to less beam attenuation or reflection.

US, ultrasound.

TABLE 33.2 Sonographic Appearance of Normal and Pathologic Musculoskeletal Structures

Structure	Normal Appearance on Ultrasound	Pathologic Features on Ultrasound
Tendon	*Long axis:* hyperechoic with fibrillar appearance *Short axis:* ovoid with homogeneously hyperechoic fibers, often referred to as a "broom-end"	*Tendinosis:* Ultrasound shows tendon thickening, loss of normal fibrillar echotexture, heterogeneity, and sometimes with hyperechoic calcification or neovascularization (Doppler). *Tendon tears:* Partial-thickness tears show focal hypoechoic regions, confirmed on both long- and short-axis images. Full-thickness tears show tendon gapping, typically occurring in the background of tendinosis-related changes. *Tenosynovitis:* Ultrasound shows peritendinous anechoic fluid.
Ligament	*Long axis:* homogenous, dense, and fibrillar hyperechoic structure *Short axis:* flattened structure, often referred to as a "broom-end" Can be distinguished from tendons by tracing the ligament to the bony structures to which it attaches	Similar to tendons, low-grade injuries manifest as ligament enlargement and hypoechogenicity. Partial- and full-thickness tears demonstrate fiber disruption.
Muscle	*Long axis:* hypoechoic tissue with hyperechoic fibroadipose septa epimysium and fascia, often referred to as "pennate" or "feather-like" *Short axis:* often referred to as a "starry night" appearance	Low-grade injuries show subtle hypoechoic regions accompanied by loss of normal pennate echotexture. High-grade injuries exhibit fiber disruption and may have heterogeneous fluid typical of a hematoma.

(continued)

TABLE 33.2 Sonographic Appearance of Normal and Pathologic Musculoskeletal Structures (continued)

Structure	Normal Appearance on Ultrasound	Pathologic Features on Ultrasound
Bone	Well-defined, linear, smooth, hyperechoic border	Cortical irregularities in the otherwise smooth surface of the bone may be indicative of overlying tendinosis, periostitis, or stress fracture and warrant further diagnostic evaluation.
Peripheral nerve	*Long axis*: fascicular appearance with hyperechoic epineurium surrounding hypoechoic fascicles *Short axis*: "honeycomb" appearance Can be differentiated from tendons due to relative lack of anisotropy	Ultrasound shows hypoechoic enlargement with loss of normal fascicular pattern. Sites of entrapment may demonstrate focal narrowing with proximal enlargement, known as "notch sign."
Fluid-filled structures	Anechoic *Vasculature*: anechoic tubular structures that exhibit blood flow on Doppler examination, with arteries less easily compressible and will remain pulsatile during compression, whereas veins are easily compressible and nonpulsatile	*Effusion*: Anechoic fluid is found in a joint. *Cyst*: Ultrasound shows anechoic, often circular structure emerging from a joint or tendon sheath. Knowledge of anatomy and use of Doppler can be used to differentiate between fluid-filled structures.

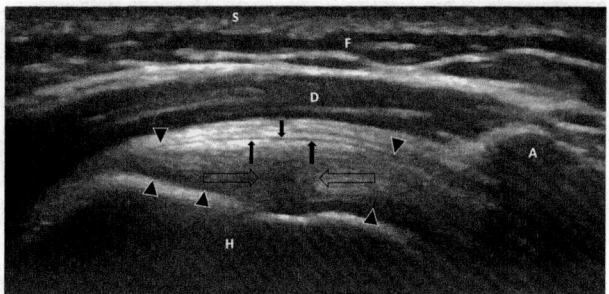

FIGURE 33.1 Supraspinatus tendon (arrowheads) in an anatomic transverse plane with anisotropy (open arrows) demonstrated visualized using a linear transducer. Trace anechoic fluid of the subacromial/subdeltoid bursa (closed arrows) can be seen superficial to the supraspinatus tendon. The overlying deltoid muscle (D) is seen in long axis demonstrating a characteristic "feather-like" echotexture. Hyperechoic, well-defined, and linear bony cortex of the humerus (H) and acromion (A) bones.
F, fat/subcutaneous tissue; S, skin.

Conventionally, when structures are imaged along their length, this is considered to be in *long axis* to the structure of interest. Conversely, if the structure is imaged on a plane transverse to its length, this is considered to be in *short axis*.

INTERVENTIONAL APPLICATIONS OF ULTRASOUND

Compared with palpation guidance, the use of US guidance for musculoskeletal interventions has the potential to improve accuracy, efficacy, and safety. The advantages of US procedural guidance over image guidance using CT and fluoroscopy include the lack of ionizing radiation, real-time visualization of neurovasculature, portability, and reduced cost. US guidance for procedures is indicated when there is close proximity to neurovascular structures, absence of surface landmarks due to body habitus, deeper target structures, as well as in cases where the diagnostic or therapeutic injection depends on precise injectate placement. As with all injections, US-guided procedures should not be performed in patients with known allergy to injectate or in the location of an active infection, rash, or skin breakdown. Although no absolute contraindications exist to the use of US guidance for procedures, a relative contraindication is the skill limitation of the user. It should be noted that proficiency in diagnostic US is the foundation of safe and effective US-guided interventions.

Important considerations prior to performing an US-guided intervention include informed consent, with discussion of risks and benefits, equipment preparation, ergonomics, and a thorough pre-scan of the intended area to identify the best approach, including identification of nearby neurovascular structures with use of Doppler and

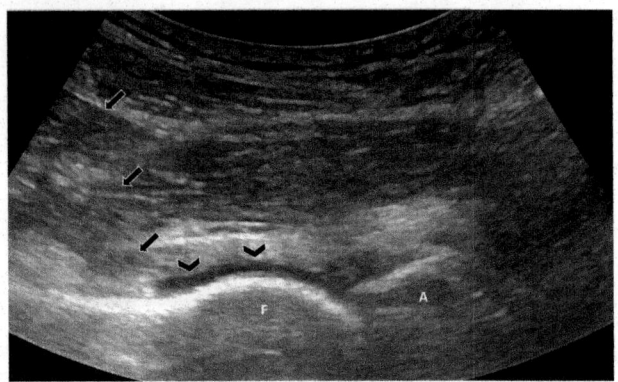

FIGURE 33.2 Hip joint injection using a curvilinear transducer. The needle (arrows) is visualized in-plane with the needle tip at the femoral head-neck junction and distension of the hip joint capsule with injectate (arrowheads).

A, acetabulum; F, femoral head.

documentation. With regard to needle visualization relative to the US transducer, the targeted structure can be approached in two ways—*in-plane* and *out-of-plane*. The in-plane approach involves orientation of the needle shaft parallel to the US transducer, allowing for visualization of the entire needle shaft (Figure 33.2). Generally, this is the preferred technique for most US-guided injections as it allows for continuous visualization of the needle and target during needle advancement and delivery of injectate. The out-of-plane approach involves orientation of the needle shaft perpendicular to the US transducer. In this technique, visualization of the needle shaft appears as a single hyperechoic dot and is generally used in the approach to superficial targets (e.g., acromioclavicular joint).

CHAPTER 34

PAIN MEDICINE

Ai Mukai and Edward Kim

TERMINOLOGY

Pain: a subjective unpleasant sensory or emotional experience due to actual or potential tissue damage[1]

Nociceptor: a receptor preferentially sensitive to a noxious stimulus or to a stimulus that would become noxious if prolonged

Allodynia: pain due to a stimulus that does not normally provoke pain

Dysesthesia: an unpleasant abnormal sensation, whether spontaneous or evoked

Hyperalgesia: an increased response to a stimulus that is normally painful

Hyperesthesia: increased sensitivity to stimulation

Hyperpathia: a painful syndrome characterized by an abnormally painful reaction to a stimulus, especially a repetitive stimulus, as well as an increased threshold

Hypoalgesia: diminished pain in response to a normally painful stimulus

Hypoesthesia: decreased sensitivity to stimulation, excluding the special senses

Neuralgia: pain in the distribution of a nerve or nerves

Neuropathic pain: pain initiated or caused by a primary lesion or dysfunction in the nervous system

Neuropathy: a disturbance of function or pathologic change in a nerve: in one nerve, mononeuropathy; in several nerves, mononeuropathy multiplex; if diffuse and bilateral, polyneuropathy

Paresthesia: an abnormal sensation, whether spontaneous or evoked

Somatic pain: superficial somatic pain is from nociceptive input from skin or subcutaneous tissues; may be characterized as localized, and sharp, throbbing, or burning; deep somatic pain arises from the joints, muscles, tendons, or bones, usually dull, aching, and less localized

Visceral pain: due to pathology involving an internal organ or parietal pleura, pericardium, or peritoneum; often described as dull and diffuse

Acute pain: pain occurring from tissue damage and resulting nociceptor activation; acute pain resolves once the tissue damage is repaired; often defined as pain lasting for less than 3 months

Chronic pain: pain lasting or recurring for more than 3 to 6 months, or lasting beyond the duration required for normal tissue healing; affects approximately 20% of all U.S. adults and is one of the most common reasons why patients seek care, according to estimates of a 2016 survey[2]

PATHOPHYSIOLOGY

The sensation of pain travels via three primary neuronal pathways that transmit noxious stimuli from the periphery to the brain. Primary afferent neurons contain cell bodies in the dorsal root ganglia, which are located in the vertebral foramina at each spinal cord level.

Each of these primary afferent neurons contains a single axon that bifurcates to the periphery and to the dorsal horn of the spinal cord.

In the dorsal horn, the primary afferent neuron synapses with a second-order neuron whose axon crosses the midline and ascends through the contralateral spinothalamic tract to the thalamus. These neurons then synapse in the thalamic nuclei with third-order neurons, which then transmit the signal to the internal capsule and corona radiata, and then to the postcentral gyrus of the brain cortex.

COMPLEX REGIONAL PAIN SYNDROME I/II

Complex regional pain syndrome (CRPS) is a chronic neuropathic pain condition that is poorly understood. CRPS I (previously known as reflex sympathetic dystrophy[RSD]) is in the setting of known injury or illness without specific nerve injury. CRPS II (previously known as causalgia) is in the setting of known injury to a nerve. Causes may include trauma, underlying neurologic pathology, musculoskeletal disorders, and malignancy.

Clinical Picture of Complex Regional Pain Syndrome

- Disproportionate extremity pain
- Swelling
- Autonomic (sympathetic) and motor symptoms

The condition can affect the upper or lower extremities, but is slightly more common in the upper extremities.

CRPS is subdivided into the following three phases:

- *Acute stage:* usually a warm phase of 2 to 3 months
- *Dystrophic phase:* vasomotor instability for several months
- *Atrophic phase:* usually cold extremity with atrophic changes

Diagnosis and Workup

- No single diagnostic test has proven sensitive and specific enough to diagnose CRPS.
- Radiographic findings
  - An x-ray imaging may show osteoporosis.
  - The *triple-phase bone scan* has also been useful in the diagnosis. In Kozin et al., scintigraphic abnormalities were reported in up

to 60% of CRPS patients and may be useful in arriving at the diagnosis of CRPS. The most suggestive and sensitive findings on bone scan included diffuse increased activity in the *delayed (third) phase*, including juxta-articular accentuation.[3]
- Skin thermography can reveal temperature disparities between the limbs.
- Quantitative sudomotor axon reflex testing (QSART)[4]
- Laser Doppler imaging

Budapest Criteria

Currently, the Budapest criteria is the most widely used diagnostic criteria for CRPS. In 1994, the International Association for the Study of Pain (IASP) published consensus-based diagnostic criteria for CRPS with the objective of becoming the internationally accepted standard. Ongoing research studies elucidated issues with validation and low specificity leading to potential overdiagnosis. This prompted an international task force to develop and validate CRPS diagnostic criteria with high sensitivity and improved specificity. In 2012, the Budapest criteria became the official IASP diagnostic criteria for CRPS.[5]

1. Continuing pain, which is disproportionate to any inciting event
2. Must report at least one symptom in *three of the four* following categories:
   - *Sensory:* reports of hyperesthesia and/or allodynia
   - *Vasomotor:* reports of temperature asymmetry and/or skin color changes and/or skin color asymmetry
   - *Sudomotor/edema:* reports of edema and/or sweating changes and/or sweating asymmetry
   - *Motor/trophic:* reports of decreased range of motion and/or motor dysfunction (weakness, tremor, and dystonia) and/or trophic changes (hair, nail, and skin)
3. Must display at least one sign at the time of evaluation in *two or more* of the following categories:
   - *Sensory:* evidence of hyperalgesia (to pinprick) and/or allodynia (to light touch and/or deep somatic pressure and/or joint movement)
   - *Vasomotor:* evidence of temperature asymmetry and/or skin color changes and/or asymmetry
   - *Sudomotor/edema:* evidence of edema and/or sweating changes and/or sweating asymmetry
   - *Motor/trophic:* evidence of decreased range of motion and/or motor dysfunction (weakness, tremor, and dystonia) and/or trophic changes (hair, nail, and skin)
4. No other diagnosis that better explains the signs and symptoms

Treatments/Medications

The mainstay of treatment for CRPS involves early restoration of function.

- *Physical therapy (PT)/occupational Therapy (OT):* Initiate PT/OT program with a focus on the affected limb. This may include desensitization techniques, mirror therapy, mobilization, and strengthening exercises.
- *High-dose vitamin C:* This has been shown to prevent the development of CRPS after wrist/ankle fracture.[6,7]
- *Oral steroids:* Oral steroids are beneficial in the early stages of CRPS.
- *Antidepressants:* Tricyclic antidepressants such as amitriptyline and nortriptyline have been widely used for CRPS. Selective serotonin reuptake inhibitors (SSRI)/serotonin and norepinephrine reuptake inhibitors (SNRI) have not demonstrated effectiveness.
- *Bone-targeting medications:* Intranasal calcitonin can be used to reduce pain associated with CRPS. Intravenous (IV) clodronate/alendronate can be used to reduce pain and swelling.[8]
- *Anticonvulsants:* Gabapentin, pregabalin, and carbamazepine may have mild benefit to pain and sensory symptoms.
- *Ketamine infusions:* There is weak evidence that these may provide reduction in pain.
- *Sympathetic blocks:* Sympathetic blocks are diagnostic and therapeutic.
  - Stellate ganglion blocks are good for upper extremity CRPS.
  - Lumbar sympathetic blocks are good for lower extremity CRPS.
- *Sympathectomy:* Sympathectomy can be performed interventionally (radiofrequency [RF] and cryoablation) or surgically.
- *Neurostimulation:* Dorsal column stimulation and dorsal root ganglion stimulation can be a tremendous help with upper extremity/lower extremity CRPS.
- *Intrathecal (IT) pumps:* IT ziconotide may be helpful in severe chronic pain. IT baclofen can be helpful in patients with dystonia associated with CRPS.[9]

NEUROMODULATION

Neuromodulation techniques represent an evolving interventional approach to treatment of chronic pain.

Spinal Cord Stimulation

Mechanism of action: Spinal cord stimulation (SCS) is a neuromodulation technique that involves placing electrodes into the posterior epidural space (either percutaneously or through an open incision), along with a generator unit that typically is implanted in the lower abdomen or the gluteal region. The mechanism of action for pain relief is complex and is dependent on the type of pain. Relief of neuropathic pain is likely mediated by inhibiting dorsal horn wide dynamic range (WDR) neurons that have become hyperexcitable after nerve injury. Relief of ischemic pain is likely mediated by reducing sympathetic outflow, which results in vasodilation and reduction in tissue ischemia.[10]

Indications/contraindications: Indications for SCS include failed back surgery syndrome (FBSS), chronic radicular pain, CRPS I/II, peripheral neuropathy, ischemic pain, and Raynaud syndrome. In addition to an indicated diagnosis, patients must meet the following criteria: (a) fail conservative therapy for at least 6 months, (b) undergo psychological screening and treatment of underlying mood disorders, and (c) no history of illicit drug use.[5] Preoperatively, it is important to set expectations and counsel patients to focus on functional improvement rather than pain relief. Contraindications include high bleeding risk (anticoagulant therapy, thrombocytopenia, etc.), uncontrolled psychiatric conditions, local/systemic infections.

Placement: Loss of resistance technique is used for percutaneous technique with fluoroscopic guidance. The stimulator leads are then placed through the Tuohy needle into the desired area. Intraoperative testing of the stimulator is often done to ensure good coverage of the painful area. An external control device is used for the duration of the trial.

Complications: Complication rates range from 28% to 42%, with the most common being lead migration/fracture (22%).[11] Other common complications include superficial wound infections, scar formation, dural puncture, and/or seroma formation. Serious/rare complications include deep infection, hematoma formation, paralysis, and death.

Other considerations

- *MRI compatibility:* 82% to 84% of patients with an SCS will require at least one MRI within 5 years of implantation.[12] MRI compatibility varies by manufacturer. The term *magnetic resonance (MR) conditionality* refers to items that have demonstrated to pose no known hazards in a specific MR environment. Most SCS are MR conditional for head/extremity scans, while newer devices are MR conditional for whole-body scans.
- *Newer developments:* Burst stimulation SCS (as opposed to tonic stimulation in conventional SCS) has been proposed as offering minimal paresthesias while providing superior pain relief. High-frequency SCS is another paresthesia-free modality that shows promising initial studies.

Peripheral Nerve Stimulation

Peripheral nerve stimulation (PNS) involves the percutaneous insertion of an electrode to a given peripheral nerve, using either fluoroscopy or ultrasound guidance. PNS is an emerging field that is currently used to treat neuropathic pain associated with peripheral mononeuropathy (including entrapment neuropathy), CRPS, occipital neuralgia, and phantom limb pain. The mechanism of action for PNS, similar to SCS, is complex and likely extends beyond the gate control theory of pain to include spinal/supraspinal descending modulation and neurotransmitter modulation. Similar to SCS, patients will typically undergo a PNS trial prior to permanent implantation. There are also PNS devices that are meant for 60 day use with some evidence indicating longer term relief after the trial. Common peripheral nerves that are targeted include the radial, ulnar, median, common peroneal, and posterior tibial nerves. The occipital nerve can also be targeted for chronic migraine. In addition to neuropathic pain, PNS has been used to target the hypoglossal nerve for sleep apnea, peroneal nerve for foot drop, and tibial nerve for overactive bladder and pelvic pain.[13–17] Complications include infection, lead migration/fracture, and hematoma formation. Long-term nerve damage is a serious but rare complication. The evidence for PNS is promising, and the hardware, systems, and techniques associated with PNS continue to evolve.

Dorsal Root Ganglion Stimulation

The dorsal root ganglion (DRG) is a group of bipolar cell bodies that are responsible for transmitting sensory information from the peripheral nervous system to the central nervous system (CNS). The DRG is located at the distal end of the dorsal root of the spinal nerves, in the intervertebral foramina. Neurostimulation of the DRG has been used as another minimally invasive option for treatment of CRPS, FBSS, painful peripheral neuropathy, and phantom pain.[18–20] It involves the use of fluoroscopic guidance to place leads into the intervertebral foramina near the DRG. These leads are connected to an external stimulator device during an initial trial. If the trial is successful, an implanted stimulator device is placed in the abdominal or gluteal region. The mechanism of action is similar to that of SCS. Compared with SCS, DRG stimulation offers the advantage of increased anatomic specificity and targeted coverage of painful areas (it is particularly useful when targeting specific dermatomes). DRG stimulation represents a promising modality; however, few randomized control trials or prospective studies have been published to date.

OTHER INTERVENTIONAL MODALITIES

Implanted Drug Delivery Systems/Pumps

Intrathecal pumps have a place in the management of chronic pain as well as spasticity. A catheter is inserted intrathecally and connected to a pump. Initially, during the trial, the pump is external. If a satisfactory result is achieved, a permanent catheter is placed intrathecally and is tunneled through the subcutaneous tissue to an internal pump that usually sits in a pocket in the anterior abdomen. The pump can then be adjusted to deliver different amounts of medication. IT infusion bypasses the blood–brain barrier and hence allows a more directed effect on brain and spinal neuroreceptors with less medication, thereby mitigating dose-dependent side effects. For example, IT morphine provides equal analgesia to oral morphine at 1/300th of the dose.

Complications associated with the implantation procedure include bleeding, local infection, meningitis, and postdural puncture headache. There are also risks intrinsic to the medication being delivered, ranging from adverse effects to medication withdrawal. Refill procedures of the pump can be done in the clinic setting but if the medication is injected outside of the pump, there is risk of both overdose from local soft tissue absorption and withdrawal from medication not being delivered via the pump.

Only four medications are Food and Drug Administration (FDA)-approved for IT use: morphine, baclofen, ziconotide, and clonidine.

Opioids: Opioids are the most commonly used IT medications for pain. The evidence for IT opioids in chronic pain is generally positive. In a 2002 study, 202 patients with refractory cancer pain were randomized to receive either IT analgesia or conventional medical management. At 4 weeks, significantly more patients treated with IT analgesia achieved at least a 20% reduction in the pain visual analog score compared with conventional medication management (85% vs. 71%).[21] Commonly used medications include morphine, hydromorphone, and fentanyl. Opioids are also commonly combined with other agents (such as bupivacaine, baclofen, clonidine, and ziconotide) to achieve synergistic effects and reduce the total dose of each individual medication. Adverse effects include constipation, urinary retention, and respiratory depression. IT morphine and hydromorphone are also associated with catheter-tip granuloma formation.

Baclofen: IT baclofen is primarily used for treatment of dystonia and spasticity. It is also established for treatment of pain associated with spasticity, dystonia, and muscle spasms. The evidence for its use in other chronic pain conditions is not well established. Adverse effects include weakness and sedation. Of note, withdrawal from baclofen is life-threatening and can occur in the setting of refill errors (pocket fills) or pump/catheter malfunction. Baclofen withdrawal presents with increased spasticity/rigidity, pruritus, hyperthermia, tachycardia, hypertension, and neuropsychiatric symptoms (hallucinations, altered mental status). In severe cases, patients can present with rhabdomyolysis, seizures, coma, multisystem organ failure, and even death. Patients typically require prompt evaluation in the ED, pump interrogation/evaluation, and administration of IT baclofen.

Ziconotide: Ziconotide is a calcium channel blocker that is used to treat neuropathic pain. Inhibition of voltage-gated calcium channels has been shown to reduce excitatory neurotransmitter release. As a result, calcium channel blockers can be effective in treating neuropathic pain. There is strong evidence to support the use of IT ziconotide for neuropathic pain. Adverse effects typically involve CNS effects such as dizziness, confusion, psychosis, and suicidal ideation. As a result, ziconotide is contraindicated in patients with a history of psychosis.

Clonidine: Clonidine is an alpha-2 adrenergic agonist that is commonly used in conjunction with other IT medications to treat neuropathic pain. Alpha-2 adrenergic receptor agonists work by decreasing presynaptic neurotransmitter release in the CNS. IT clonidine is rarely used as monotherapy; however, it has been shown to be highly effective when used in combination infusions. Adverse effects include hypotension, bradycardia, and sedation/drowsiness.

Bupivacaine: Bupivacaine is a sodium channel blocker that is commonly used in conjunction with other IT medications to treat chronic pain. The use of IT bupivacaine is not FDA-approved and therefore considered off-label. Sodium channel blockers work by inhibiting action potentials and therefore nerve transmission. It has been shown to be highly effective when used in combination infusions. In particular, it has an opioid-sparing effect. Compared with IT morphine monotherapy, IT morphine-bupivacaine infusions have been shown to reduce pain and total opioid doses. Bupivacaine, like clonidine, is rarely used as monotherapy. Adverse effects include bowel and bladder dysfunction.

PHARMACOLOGIC MODALITIES

Neuropathic Pain

- *Gabapentin:* calcium channel ligand that inhibits release of neurotransmitters; typical starting dose: 100 to 300 mg one to three times daily, max daily dose 3,600 mg; adverse effects: dizziness, sedation, respiratory depression, and weight gain
- *Pregabalin:* calcium channel ligand that inhibits release of neurotransmitters; typical starting dose: 50 mg BID, max daily dose: 300 mg; adverse effects: dizziness, sedation, respiratory depression, and weight gain
- *Amitriptyline:* tricyclic antidepressant that inhibits norepinephrine, 5 hydroxytryptophan reuptake; typical starting dose: 10 to 25 mg QHS, max daily dose: 300 mg; adverse effects: anticholinergic effects, cardiotoxicity, and CNS depression
- *Nortriptyline:* tricyclic antidepressant that inhibits NE/5HT reuptake; typical starting dose: 10 to 25 mg QHS, max daily dose: 300 mg; adverse effects: anticholinergic effects, cardiotoxicity, and CNS depression
- *Duloxetine:* serotonin/norepinephrine reuptake inhibitor; typical starting dose: 60 mg daily, max daily dose: 120 mg; adverse effects: drowsiness, nausea, vomiting, constipation, hepatotoxicity, sexual dysfunction, and activation of mania/hypomania
- *Venlafaxine:* serotonin/norepinephrine reuptake inhibitor; typical starting dose: 37.5 to 75 mg daily, max daily dose: 225 mg; adverse effects: hypertension, diaphoresis, drowsiness, nausea, vomiting, constipation, hepatotoxicity, sexual dysfunction, and activation of mania/hypomania

- *Tramadol:* weak mu opioid receptor agonist; typical starting dose: 25 to 50 mg daily, max daily dose: 400 mg; adverse effects: respiratory depression, drowsiness, gastrointestinal (GI) upset, constipation, and opioid-induced hyperalgesia; risk of dependence, addiction, and withdrawal
- *Topical lidocaine:* inhibits action potential propagation by inactivating voltage-gated sodium channels; typical starting dose: apply patch to intact, dry skin, apply for 12 hours, then remove for 12 hours before reapplying; adverse effects: local skin reaction, minimal systemic absorption
- *Topical capsaicin:* transient receptor potential cation channel subfamily V member 1 (TPRV1) receptor agonist which produces a burning/painful sensation; prolonged activation of TRPV1 is thought to desensitize nociceptors and thereby bring pain relief; available as cream or patch; adverse effects: skin irritation, erythema, and burning pain, minimal systemic absorption.

Nonopioid Analgesics

- *Nonselective nonsteroidal anti-inflammatory drugs (NSAIDs):* inhibit cyclooxygenase 1 (COX-1) and COX-2 enzymes, which inhibit the prostaglandin from arachidonic acid; meloxicam, etodolac, and diclofenac selectively inhibit COX-2 over COX-1; typical starting dose of meloxicam: 7.5 mg daily, max daily dose: 15 mg (meloxicam loses relative COX-2 selectivity at higher doses); adverse effects: increases risk of stroke and myocardial infarction increases risk of GI inflammation, ulceration, and bleeding, decreases platelet aggregation and adhesion; avoid in patients with renal disease
- *Celecoxib:* COX-2 selective NSAID with fewer GI side effects compared with nonselective NSAIDs; typical starting dose: 200 mg daily, max daily dose: 400 mg; adverse effects: similar to nonselective NSAIDs
- *Diclofenac gel, diclofenac patch, and diclofenac solution:* topical agents may limit systemic exposure and reduce risk of adverse effects; topical diclofenac has 3% to 5% of the systemic absorption of oral diclofenac; avoid concurrent use with systemic NSAIDs, unlikely to provide additional pain relief
- *Acetaminophen/paracetamol:* inhibits central prostaglandin synthesis; has antipyretic and analgesic effects but very limited anti-inflammatory effects; starting dose: 325 to 650 mg q4h to q6h, max daily dose: 4,000 mg; adverse effects: hepatotoxicity, GI upset, and skin reactions

Muscle Relaxants

- *Methocarbamol:* centrally acting medication with unclear mechanism of action; typical starting dose: 1.5 g TID, max daily dose: 8,000 g;

adverse effects: dizziness and drowsiness; avoid concurrent use with other sedatives; risk of hepatotoxicity; nephrotoxic only in IV form
- *Cyclobenzaprine:* centrally acting 5-HT2 receptor antagonist; typical starting dose: 5 mg TID, max daily dose: 30 mg; adverse effects: anticholinergic effects, dry mouth, headache, dizziness, drowsiness, constipation, and urinary retention; can cause serotonin syndrome and arrhythmias
- *Tizanidine:* alpha-2 adrenergic agonist, but unclear mechanism of action; typical starting dose: 2 to 4 mg q6h to q12h, max daily dose: 24 mg; adverse effects: dry mouth, dizziness, drowsiness, hepatotoxicity, and QT prolongation
- *Carisoprodol:* centrally acting medication with unclear mechanism of action; typical starting dose: 250 to 350 mg TID; adverse effects: headache, dizziness, somnolence, GI upset, and seizure; caution in patients with hepatic and renal dysfunction; significant risk of dependence, withdrawal, and addiction (Schedule IV controlled substance); carisoprodol metabolized to meprobamate, which is a highly addictive substance, and therefore should only be used for short periods of time (2–3 weeks)
- *Metaxalone:* centrally acting medication with unclear mechanism of action; typical starting dose: 800 mg TID, max daily dose: 3,200 mg; adverse effects: dizziness, drowsiness, and headache; relatively well tolerated compared with other muscle relaxants
- *Baclofen:* centrally acting gamma-aminobutyric acid B receptor agonist; typical starting dose: 5 mg TID, max daily dose: 80 mg; adverse effects: dizziness, drowsiness, somnolence, weakness, headache, urinary retention, and constipation; discontinuation may lead to withdrawal, needs to be tapered gradually
- *Chlorzoxazone:* centrally acting medication with unclear mechanism of action; typical starting dose: 250 mg TID, max daily dose: 3,000 mg; adverse effects: dizziness, drowsiness, nausea, vomiting, hepatotoxicity, and urine discoloration

Lidocaine/Ketamine Infusions

Intravenous infusion therapy is an emerging treatment option for patients with chronic pain who have failed conventional treatment. Lidocaine and ketamine infusions have been used to treat neuropathic pain, cancer pain, fibromyalgia, and CRPS.

Cannabinoids' Role in Pain

There is emerging evidence that cannabinoids may have a role in pain management, particularly in the setting of chronic neuropathic pain, spasticity, and cancer pain. There are many regulatory and legal issues associated with cannabinoid use that vary by state.

EQUIANALGESIC OPIOID CONVERSION

Step 1: Calculate the total daily dose of the starting opioid medication.
Step 2: Using Table 34.1, convert your starting opioid medication to oral morphine milligram equivalents (ORAL MME).
Step 3: Using Table 34.2, convert from ORAL MME to the desired opioid medication.
Step 4 (optional): When switching to a *new* opioid, the initial daily dose should be reduced by 25% to 50% (to adjust for incomplete mu receptor cross-tolerance). This step is not required when switching from IV/oral administration of the *same* opioid.

After completing the above steps, you now have the total daily dose of the desired opioid medication.

For example, to convert IV hydromorphone (scheduled at 1 mg every 6 hours) to oral oxycodone:

Step 1: Calculate total daily dose: 1 mg IV hydromorphone every 6 hours = 4 mg IV hydromorphone every 24 hours.

TABLE 34.1 Conversion of Starting Opioid Medication to ORAL MME

	Ratio	Calculation
Parenteral fentanyl to ORAL MME	1:300	Multiply your total daily dose by 300.
Parenteral oxymorphone to ORAL MME	1:30	Multiply your total daily dose by 30.
Parenteral hydromorphone to ORAL MME	1:20	Multiply your total daily dose by 20.
Oral hydromorphone to ORAL MME	1:4	Multiply your total daily dose by 4.
Oral oxymorphone to ORAL MME	1:3	Multiply your total daily dose by 3.
Parenteral morphine to ORAL MME	1:3	Multiply your total daily dose by 3.
Oral oxycodone to ORAL MME	1:1.5	Multiply your total daily dose by 1.5.
Oral hydrocodone to ORAL MME	1:1	Multiply your total daily dose by 1.
Oral tramadol to ORAL MME	1:.1	Multiply your total daily dose by .1.

ORAL MME, oral morphine milligram equivalents.

Source: National Center for Injury Prevention and Control. CDC Compilation of Benzodiazepines, Muscle Relaxants, Stimulants, Zolpidem, and Opioid Analgesics with Oral Morphine Milligram Equivalent Conversion Factors, 2018 Version. Centers for Disease Control and Prevention; 2018. Available at https://www.cdc.gov/drugoverdose/resources/data.html; Rosenquist R. Use of opioids in the management of chronic non-cancer pain. In: Post TW, ed. UpToDate. UpToDate; 2022.

TABLE 34.2 Conversion of ORAL MME to Desired Opioid Medication

	Ratio	Calculation
ORAL MME to parenteral fentanyl	300:1	Divide your ORAL MME by 300.
ORAL MME to parenteral oxymorphone	30:1	Divide your ORAL MME by 30.
ORAL MME to parenteral hydromorphone	20:1	Divide your ORAL MME by 20.
ORAL MME to oral hydromorphone	4:1	Divide your ORAL MME by 4.
ORAL MME to oral oxymorphone	3:1	Divide your ORAL MME by 3.
ORAL MME to parenteral morphine	3:1	Divide your ORAL MME by 3.
ORAL MME to oral oxycodone	1.5:1	Divide your ORAL MME by 1.5.
ORAL MME to oral hydrocodone	1:1	Divide your ORAL MME by 1.
ORAL MME to oral tramadol	.1:1	Divide your ORAL MME by .1.

ORAL MME, oral morphine milligram equivalents.

Source: Rosenquist R. Use of opioids in the management of chronic non-cancer pain. In: Post TW, ed. UpToDate. UpToDate; 2022; National Center for Injury Prevention and Control. CDC Compilation of Benzodiazepines, Muscle Relaxants, Stimulants, Zolpidem, and Opioid Analgesics with Oral Morphine Milligram Equivalent Conversion Factors, 2018 Version. Centers for Disease Control and Prevention; 2018. Available at https://www.cdc.gov/drug overdose/resources/data.html.

Step 2: Convert to ORAL MME: 4 mg × 20 = 80 ORAL MME.
Step 3: Convert to desired opioid: 80 ORAL MME/1.5 = 53.3 mg oral oxycodone.
Step 4: Reduce dose by 25% for incomplete cross-tolerance: 53.3 × .75 = 40 mg oral oxycodone (total daily dose).

REFERENCES

The full complete reference list for this chapter appears in the digital version of the chapter, available at http://connect.springerpub.com/content/book/978-0-8261-5628-0/part/part04/chapter/ch34

CHAPTER 35

SPINE

Jennifer G. Leet, Allen S. Chen, and David S. Cheng

AXIAL PAIN

Facet (Zygapophyseal) Joint Pain

Definition

Facet (zygapophyseal) joints are common and significant sources of axial pain in the aging population.[1] Facet joints are paired, diarthrodial joints that articulate with adjacent vertebral levels. Each joint is dually innervated by the medial branches of the dorsal rami. Pain is experienced with joint capsule distention, inflammation, or degeneration, which can lead to facet hypertrophy/arthropathy over time, and is commonly due to improper biomechanics, osteoarthritis, and trauma. Facet arthropathy typically affects the caudal levels of the lumbar spine, largely due to higher weight-bearing loads.[2] In the cervical spine, the most common level associated with whiplash is C5 and C6, followed by C2 and C3.[3]

Clinical Presentation

Facet joint pain can present as unilateral or bilateral paramedian axial pain, with characteristic referral patterns (Figure 35.1).

Pain is typically aggravated by activities that load the facet joints, such as prolonged standing or walking and spinal extension/twisting. Provocative maneuver such as the Kemp test places the patient in ipsilateral lumbar extension and rotation to reproduce typical symptoms; however, this test has poor accuracy, with a sensitivity of 50% to 70%[4] and a specificity of 67.3%.[5]

Diagnostic Workup

Although facet joints can be visualized on plain radiographs, CT, MRI, or single-photon emission CT (SPECT), the presence of degenerative changes on imaging does not predictably correlate with symptoms.[6] Plain radiographs can only detect late stages of facet arthropathy. Early signs of degeneration/inflammation can be detected on SPECT and some T2-weighted MRIs. History and physical examination can also be nonspecific. Medial branch blocks (MBBs) are considered the "gold standard" in the diagnosis of facet-mediated pain.[2] In the cervical spine, each facet joint is innervated by the medial branches of the levels comprising the joint (i.e., C4 and C5 facet joint is innervated by the medial branches of C4 and C5). In the thoracic and lumbar regions, each facet joint receives innervation from the medial branches of the cranial level involved in the joint and the level above it. For example, L3 and L4 facet joint is innervated by the medial branches of L2 and L3 (Figure 35.2).

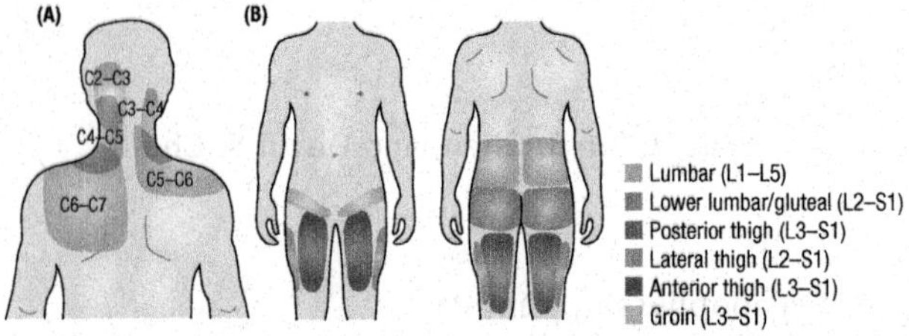

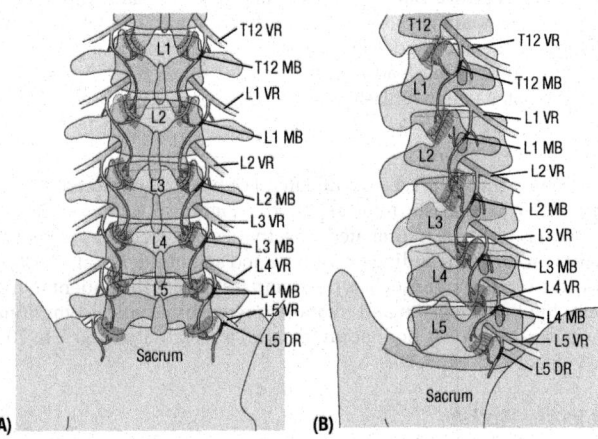

FIGURE 35.1 Referral pain pattern graphic. **(A)** Cervical facet joint referral pain pattern. **(B)** Lumbar facet joint referral pain pattern. The most common distribution is the lower lumbar/gluteal region.

Source: Reproduced with permission from Gellhorn AC, Katz JN, Suri P. Osteoarthritis of the spine: The facet joints. *Nat Rev Rheumatol.* 2013;9(4):216–224. doi:10.1038/nrrheum.2012.199.

FIGURE 35.2 Lumbar medial branch anatomy. **(A)** and **(B)** demonstrate the typical location and course of the medial branch nerves on AP (anteroposterior) and oblique views of the lumbosacral spine.

DR, dorsal ramus; MB, medial branch; VR, ventral ramus.
Source: Reproduced with permission from Furman MB, Berkwits L, Cohen I, et al. *Atlas of Image-Guided Spinal Procedures,* 2nd ed. Elsevier; 2017.

Treatment

Treatment includes trial of initial conservative treatment (see the Treatment section). Intra-articular facet injection and radiofrequency ablation (RFA) of the medial branches are widely used to treat facetogenic pain; however, evidence is lacking for intra-articular facet injections.[7] RFA candidates are chosen based off their responses to MBBs.

Sacroiliac Joint Dysfunction

Definition

The sacrum supports the axial spine and articulates with the iliac wings to form the left and right sacroiliac (SI) joints. Several ligamentous and muscle attachments contribute to the stability of this joint and can also be sources of pain. Imbalance or dysfunction in the SI joint can result from functional or anatomic leg length discrepancies, pelvic girdle imbalances, pregnancy, ankylosing spondylitis, connective tissue disorders, and history of lumbosacral fusion. Innervation of the SI joint is variable; however, the posterior SI joint complex is typically described as being innervated by the L5 dorsal ramus and S1 to S3 lateral branches.

Clinical Presentation

Clinical presentation of SI joint pain can vary widely; however, it is typically localized to the upper buttock below L5 and can refer to the thigh.[8] A variety of provocative maneuvers exist to evaluate for SI joint dysfunction, although their sensitivity and specificity vary across conflicting studies.[9,10] Laslett's cluster for SI joint pain reports increased diagnostic power if three or more examination maneuvers are positive (thigh thrust, SI distraction, SI compression, sacral thrust, and Gaenslen).[9]

Diagnostic Workup

There is no single diagnostic test for SI joint pain. Imaging findings of degenerative or erosive changes are late findings in the disease course and do not elucidate extra-articular causes of pain. As such, one must obtain appropriate history and physical examination and evaluate for systemic causes of sacroiliitis, such as ankylosing spondylitis.

Treatment

A trial of conservative measures including physical therapy (PT) to correct pelvic girdle mechanics and SI joint belt is a reasonable initial step in treatment. Intra-articular steroid injections are commonly used, although there is better evidence in cases of spondyloarthropathy.[11] Pain arising from extra-articular sources of the posterior SI joint can be effectively treated with L5 dorsal rami and sacral lateral branch RFA if there is adequate relief from blocks.[12]

Discogenic Pain

Definition

Intervertebral discs (IVDs) are composed of cartilaginous endplates with a central nucleus pulposus that is circumferentially contained by the annulus fibrosis. Degeneration of IVDs is not necessarily painful; it involves normal age-related desiccation, which is influenced by genetic and environmental factors and can be found in asymptomatic individuals as early as the second decade of life. Internal disc disruptions, such as annulus fibrosis fissures, can lead to disc bulge or herniation. Leaked contents of the nucleus pulposus through annular defects create a strong inflammatory reaction, which is responsible for the pain associated with acute disc herniations. Pain from chronic disc degeneration is less well understood; however, it is theorized to involve an ingrowth of innervation and vasculature mediated by growth factors and vascular granulation tissue.[13]

Clinical Presentation
Clinical presentation includes deep centralized axial pain, often poorly localized, worse with Valsalva-type maneuvers or sudden movements.

Diagnostic Workup
Discogenic pain is often a diagnosis of exclusion and is difficult to make given lack of a pathoanatomic gold standard. There are several imaging findings related to disc degeneration; however, it is important to remember that disc degeneration is frequently found in asymptomatic individuals. In T2-weighted sagittal MRIs, disc degeneration appears as decreased signal intensity, and high-intensity zones appear as a bright signal intensity contained within the annulus fibrosis. Modic changes refer to imaging findings of endplate marrow: type I appears as hyperintense on T2 MRI and hypointense on T1 MRI, representing infiltration of vascular granulation tissue and inflammation; type II appears as hyperintense on both T1 and T2 MRI, representing fatty infiltration. Provocation discography has been used to identify painful IVDs (typically for surgical planning); however, its use remains controversial given poor correlative fusion outcomes and concerns for accelerating degeneration.[14–16]

Treatment
There are no effective, well-established interventional treatments for discogenic back pain. Potential treatment options include intradiscal injections with regenerative techniques such as platelet-rich plasma (PRP), epidural steroid injections, RFA of the sinuvertebral nerves, disc biacuplasty, and discectomy and fusion.

RADICULAR PAIN

Radiculopathy

Definition
Radiculopathy refers to radicular pain with sensory and/or motor involvement in the setting of nerve root compression/inflammation and is commonly secondary to spondylotic changes such as disc herniation, facet hypertrophy, synovial cyst, and ligamentum flavum buckling.

Clinical Presentation
Radicular pain typically has neuropathic qualities (burning, shooting, and lancinating), follows a nerve root, or dermatomal, distribution,

and is typically more severe in the extremities. There can be associated neurologic deficits corresponding to the affected nerve root(s), such as loss of reflexes, dermatomal paresthesias or hypoesthesias, and myotomal weakness or atrophy.

Diagnostic Workup

Nerve root tension tests such as straight leg raise and seated slump tests are generally thought to be more sensitive than specific for lumbar radiculopathy; however, the evidence is variable.[17] Spurling's test is a provocative test for cervical radiculopathy that has reported high specificity with moderate sensitivity.[18] Advanced imaging (MRI, CT) is indicated in the presence of neurologic deficits and is useful in visualizing structural compression. MRI is usually preferred due to its superior ability to evaluate soft tissues. Electromyography (EMG) can detect active denervation and chronic neurogenic changes, localize a lesion, and define if a lesion is pre- or post-ganglionic.

Treatment

Treatment includes PT after acute pain subsides, medications (anti-inflammatory, neuropathic), and epidural steroid injections. An effective physical medicine and rehabilitation (PM&R) or spine physician will be able to assess if a patient is a candidate for surgical evaluation.

Spinal Stenosis

Definition

Spinal stenosis is an acquired or congenital narrowing of the spinal canal often resulting from disc herniation/bulges coupled with spondylitic changes such as facet joint and ligamentous hypertrophy. There are no universally accepted radiographic criteria for spinal stenosis; however, an anteroposterior diameter of the central canal of less than 10 mm is frequently used.[19] Symptoms result from mechanical compression and/or ischemic insult of nerve roots brought on by an upright or extended posture, which physically narrows the spinal canal and increases intrathecal pressure, and in turn causes venous congestion and reduced arterial flow. Symptoms may also be exacerbated by walking, referred to as *neurogenic claudication*, which is caused by increased metabolic demands and the combination explained above. Symptoms should improve with sitting, lying, or spinal flexion (a key differentiator from *vascular claudication*, which presents with leg pain worsened or brought on by walking and which improves with rest regardless of position).

Clinical Presentation

Pain typically has an insidious onset and variable pattern. Patients may complain of vague axial pain and more commonly bilateral leg symptoms, including diffuse pain, paresthesias, and weakness, worse with upright or extended postures and improves with flexion or sitting (shopping cart sign). Symptoms may have a dermatomal distribution but are typically more diffuse.

Diagnostic Workup

History and physical examination are often nonspecific. MRI is frequently used and can define the extent of narrowing.

Treatment

Treatment options include PT, medications, epidural steroid injections, and interspinous process spacers. An effective PM&R or spine physician will be able to assess if a patient is a candidate for surgical evaluation.

TREATMENT

Conservative Care

Physical Therapy

If pain is acute, a short period of rest is appropriate before initiation of PT. In general, PT should focus on restoring proper biomechanics by stretching/relaxing hypertonic shortened muscles, strengthening weakened muscles, reestablishing beneficial neuromuscular firing patterns and proprioception, and breaking kinesiophobic habits.

Pharmacologics

Consider initiation of nonsteroidal anti-inflammatory drugs (NSAIDs) and acetaminophen. If appropriate, a short course of muscle relaxants and/or neuropathic agents such as gabapentin can be considered. Various topical formulations exist, such as diclofenac, lidocaine, capsaicin, methyl salicylate-menthol, camphor, and so forth. A short course of oral steroids is commonly prescribed, but evidence supporting this practice is limited and prescribers should be aware of potential systemic adverse effects with regular use.[20] Opioid use is controversial and under increased scrutiny in light of the opioid epidemic. A short course of opioids might be considered for severe, debilitating pain after failing other measures.

Alternative Treatments

Alternative treatments include acupuncture, massage therapy, transcutaneous electrical nerve stimulation unit, ice/heat, myofascial release, and mindfulness/meditation.

SPINE INTERVENTIONS

Epidural Injections

Epidural injections involve the introduction of local anesthetics and/or steroids into the epidural space and are used in the management of radicular symptoms from radiculopathy or spinal stenosis. Steroids are used to provide short- to medium-term relief by reducing inflammation and are particularly useful in disc herniations.[21] Adverse neuroendocrine effects of cumulative steroid exposure must be considered.[22] Some studies show that multiple spinal conditions receive just as much benefit from injection of local anesthetic alone compared with local anesthetic plus steroid.[21] Complications include, but are not limited to, spinal cord or cerebral infarct, hemodynamic compromise from inadvertent intravascular or intrathecal injection, spinal cord or nerve root damage (needle placement, epidural hematoma, etc.), and infection.

Approaches include interlaminar, transforaminal, and caudal.

Radiofrequency Nerve Ablation

Radiofrequency nerve ablation (RFA) involves using a needle (electrode) to deliver an electric current to a nearby nerve supplying a painful structure for intermediate- to long-term pain relief. Only after a diagnostic nerve block (specific to a painful etiology) has provided significant relief should RFA be pursued. Traditional (or thermal) RFA causes neurolysis by heating the tissues surrounding the electrode tip to 80°C. Similarly, cooled RFA utilizes heat for neurolysis; however, water circulating in an inner cannula prevents tissue charring and in turn creates a larger lesion. Complications include, but are not limited to, local postprocedure soreness, post-RFA neuritis, vascular trauma, pneumothorax (thoracic), or direct disc, cord, and nerve root trauma. Interventionalists should discuss with all patients that an expected result of medial branch RFA is temporary denervation of the deep dorsal spinal musculature (multifidus in the lumbar region); however, the effects on spinal health and function remain unknown.

Vertebroplasty/Kyphoplasty

This procedure is aimed at treating pain and instability from acute or subacute vertebral compression fractures from the age of 2 weeks to 6 months. Although most compression fractures heal and pain from compression fractures generally improves with time, vertebroplasty can be considered in patients with refractory pain or vertebral body instability (tumor, osteoporosis). Absolute contraindications include discitis, sepsis, and osteomyelitis. Relative contraindications include significant spinal canal compromise secondary to bone fragments, fractures older than 2 years, less than 75% collapse of the vertebral body, fractures above T5, and traumatic compression fractures or disruption of the posterior vertebral body wall. While both vertebroplasty and kyphoplasty can treat pain from a compression fracture, kyphoplasty focuses on restoring stability and vertebral height. Vertebroplasty involves tunneling a large-gauge needle into the vertebral body and injecting 3 to 5 mL of methyl methacrylate cement into the vertebral body. In kyphoplasty, a balloon is introduced via a catheter into the vertebral body, restores height, and allows for filling with the cement.

REFERENCES

The full complete reference list for this chapter appears in the digital version of the chapter, available at http://connect.springerpub.com/content/book/978-0-8261-5628-0/part/part04/chapter/ch35

CHAPTER 36

MUSCULOSKELETAL—UPPER LIMB

Michael Catapano and Ashwin Babu

OSTEOARTHRITIS

Osteoarthritis (OA) is the most common musculoskeletal issue, especially older adults, and can present in any joint of the body. OA of the upper extremity is most common in the glenohumeral joint, acromioclavicular (AC) joint, and fingers. There is an increased rate of post traumatic OA in the upper extremity compared with the lower extremity, and prior intra-articular fractures resulting in posttraumatic OA must be considered. Common presenting symptoms include stiffness, pain, and loss of range of motion (ROM). Plain radiographs are the best diagnostic modality for arthritis, which will present as loss of joint space, sclerosis, subchondral cysts, and osteophytes.[1] Treatments range from therapeutic exercises to improve strength and neuromuscular control to support the joint, topical or oral nonsteroidal anti-inflammatory drugs (NSAIDs), analgesics, corticosteroid injection(s), and ultimately joint replacements or fusions. Additional options including viscosupplementation and platelet-rich plasma (PRP) injections can be considered.[2]

SHOULDER

Acromioclavicular Joint Separation

AC joint injuries are typically a result of impact on the lateral aspect of an adducted shoulder. AC joint injuries are classified on the Rockwood Scale (Table 36.1).[3] Treatment for type I and II injuries include nonoperative treatment consisting of symptomatic pain management with an arm sling, ice, analgesics, and progressive ROM. Type III lesions may be treated either nonoperatively or operatively depending on patient goals.[4] Nonoperative treatment of type III injuries consists of 2 to 4 weeks of supportive bracing with an arm sling, followed by a gradual return to activity. Type IV to VI lesions require operative consultation for potential open reduction and internal fixation (ORIF).

Rotatory Cuff Pathology

Rotator cuff conditions consist of a spectrum of disease that begins with subacromial impingement of the rotator cuff tendons between the humeral head and the acromion with associated subacromial bursitis, partial-thickness tears, full-thickness tears, and/or massive irreparable rotator cuff tears. The most common tendons affected are the supraspinatus and infraspinatus; however, the subscapularis tendon

TABLE 36.1 Types and Associated Causes and Findings of AC Separation

Type	AC Ligament	CC Ligament	Radiographs	Treatment
Type I	Sprain	Normal	Normal	Nonoperative
Type II	Torn	Sprain	Increased CC distance of <25%	Nonoperative
Type III	Torn	Torn	Increased CC distance of 25%–100%	Controversial
Type IV	Torn	Torn	Lateral clavicle displaced posterior through the trapezius on axillary lateral radiographs	Operative
Type V	Torn	Torn	Increased CC distance <100%	Operative
Type VI	Torn	Torn	Inferior displacement of the lateral clavicle into the subacromial or subcoracoid space	Operative

AC, acromioclavicular; CC, coracoclavicular.

can be involved as well. Most patients present with nighttime pain and pain with overhead activities.[5] In addition to pain and/or weakness with isolated activation of the affected tendon, specific examination maneuvers include the empty can, drop-arm, Hawkins–Kennedy, Neers, belly press, and lift-off tests.

Irrespective of grade of injury, those with rotator cuff pathology are suggested to undergo a rehabilitation program focusing on posture, flexibility, neuromuscular control, and strengthening.[6] Analgesics or subacromial-subdeltoid bursal injection with corticosteroids can be trialed to aid in symptomatic management or supplement rehabilitation. PRP may be considered in select cases; however, evidence is currently conflicting regarding its efficacy.[7] The exception to this is traumatic full-thickness, full-width tears of the supraspinatus, or any full-thickness, full-width tears of the subscapularis, which are suggested to have operative repair. In addition, surgery is an option for those who fail conservative treatment. Surgical options include, but are not limited to, primary repair, augmented repair, superior capsular reconstruction, latissimus dorsi or trapezius transfer, or reverse total shoulder replacement.[8]

Anterior Shoulder Instability and Labral Injuries

Anterior dislocations are the most common dislocations of the shoulder, and even after relocation may have long-term complications. These include axillary nerve injury, chronic anterior instability, bony or soft tissue Bankart lesions, Hill-Sachs lesions, and labral tears. Bankart lesions are described as avulsions of the anterior labrum from the anterior glenoid; a piece of bone may also be avulsed, described as a bony Bankart lesion. A Hill-Sachs lesion is a compression fracture of the humeral head when the posterolateral aspect of the humeral head compresses against the anterior glenoid while the humeral head is dislocated anterior to the glenoid.[9]

Anterior instability is typically described as recurrent dislocations of the shoulder or a feeling of imminent dislocation with glenohumeral stress. These pathologies may also present as pain during overhead or cross-body activities which engage the superior or anterior labrum. Although 1 to 3 weeks of sling immobilization followed by rehabilitation focused on neuromuscular control of the shoulder to improve stability is suggested after a single anterior dislocation, those with recurrent instability or pain may require surgical fixation.[10] Surgical options include Bankart and labral repair, capsulorrhaphy, and the Latarjet and Remplissage procedures.[11]

Alternatively, labral tears may occur independent from dislocation events. Although tears may happen at any point within the labrum, the most common are superior labral anterior to posterior (SLAP) tears. SLAP tears present with pain with overhead activities with associated clicking. Patients may also present with symptoms consistent with bicipital tendinitis due to the insertion on the long head of the biceps on the superior labrum. Initial management consisting of neuromuscular rehabilitation and strengthening. Those failing conservative therapy may benefit from arthroscopic labral repair.[12]

Adhesive Capsulitis (Frozen Shoulder)

Adhesive capsulitis is characterized by insidious and idiopathic inflammation and subsequent contracture of the glenohumeral capsule, resulting in a three-stage disease process.[13] Patients progress predominately from pain with subsequent loss of ROM in the initial 6 to 12 months and culminate with resolution of pain and a return of ROM over the subsequent 12-month to 18-month period. It most commonly occurs in patients in their 40s to 60s and is more frequent in women or those with diabetes or hypothyroidism. Suggested treatment is intra-articular corticosteroids, which have been supplemented with hydrodilatation or suprascapular nerve blocks by some practitioners. Surgical intervention, including arthroscopic capsular release, is an option in those who do not respond to conservative therapy, including multiple intra-articular steroid injections.[14]

(Long-Head) Bicipital Tendinitis

This syndrome is typically secondary to overuse or a result of another interarticular pathology.[15] As such, clinicians should be astute to other potential causes of glenohumeral swelling, including shoulder impingement syndrome, rotator cuff tears, or labral pathology (SLAP

TABLE 36.2 Causes and Associated Findings of Scapular Winging

Muscle	Direction of Winging	Physical Examination
Serratus anterior	Medially with superior migration and medial rotation of the inferior angle of the scapula	Push-up against the wall
Rhomboids	Lateral winging with lateral winging of the inferior angle of the scapula	Hands at the hip, resisted shoulder retraction
Trapezius	Lateral winging of the entire medial scapular border	Resisted abduction at 90°

lesions). Examination often reveals tenderness through the long head of the biceps within the bicipital groove, with some patients demonstrating subluxation with internal and external rotation of the humeral head. Treatments include NSAIDs, rest, activity modification, and soft tissue massage, with a progressive strengthening program. An ultrasound-guided injection of corticosteroids into the biceps sheath may be utilized to improve symptoms and enable rehabilitation.

Scapular Dyskinesis

Scapular dyskinesis refers to the incoordination of the scapula with glenohumeral motion and encompasses multiple conditions including those that result in scapular winging. Scapular dyskinesis is most notable when examining the patient from the posterior while they slowly and repeatedly abduct their shoulders. Side-to-side as well as interpersonal comparisons should be made of the quality and smoothness of scapular motion.[16] Treatments include guided rehabilitation focusing on neuromuscular control. Additional nonoperative and operative interventions are tailored to individual patients.

Historically, scapular winging may be caused by serratus anterior, rhomboids, or trapezius dysfunction. Weakness in these structures may be due to underlying muscular dystrophy, peripheral nerve injury, or acquired weakness. The location of winging and the associated physical examination maneuvers are demonstrated in Table 36.2.[17]

ELBOW

Medial Epicondylitis and Lateral Epicondylitis

Medial and lateral epicondylitis are considered tendinopathies of the flexor and extensor masses, respectively. As with most tendinopathies, a spectrum of disease is possible, ranging from thickening and loss of parallel fibrillar tendon pattern, to partial-thickness tears and rarely full-thickness tears. Patients present with focal tenderness surrounding the epicondyle and pain and/or weakness with upper extremity activities. Muscles that attach most proximally to the epicondyle, including the extensor carpi radialis brevis (ERCB) and the supinator laterally, and the flexor carpi radialis (FCR) and the pronator teres medially, tend to be the most painful with activation and passive stretch. Either MRI and ultrasound can be utilized for diagnosis depending on local availability of imaging techniques and experts.[18] Initial treatment with rest, ice, compression, and elevation (RICE) and NSAIDs is appropriate. Most patients require further treatments which can include local nitroglycerin patch, topical NSAIDs, bracing, therapy, injection, and/or surgery. An eccentric strengthening protocol is suggested for most patients both as initial treatment and to ensure reduction in disease recurrence. An elbow counterforce brace can be considered during symptomatic periods. A one-time injection of corticosteroids can be considered in symptomatic patients. However, treatment with PRP has been shown to be more effective than corticosteroids in patients who have failed conservative treatment and is suggested to those with access and partial tears.[19] Surgical fasciotomy, repair, or release of the tendinous attachment can be considered if all conservative and interventional measures fail.

WRIST AND HAND

de Quervain Tenosynovitis

The first extensor compartment consists of the abductor pollicis longus (APL) and the extensor pollicis brevis (EPB). Due to repetitive wrist extension and radial deviation, inflammation and irritation of this compartment can develop. Symptoms include focal swelling and pain over the dorsal radial wrist and pain and weakness with activities that necessitate radial deviation, including opening jars and picking up objects or young children. Ultrasound evaluation may demonstrate increased swelling in these tendon sheaths with or without focal tendinopathy of either tendon.[20] Treatment includes activity modification and thumb spica splint wrist in neutral position with the first metacarpophalangeal (MCP) immobilized (interphalangeal [IP] joint is free), which is helpful in resting the tendons. Local corticosteroid injection under ultrasound can be utilized to reduce acute inflammation while reducing the risk of intratendinous injection. Surgical decompression and synovectomy can be considered in severe, refractory cases.

Scaphoid Fractures

Those with pain to palpation in the anatomic snuff box or on the proximal pole of the scaphoid after trauma, including a fall on an outstretched hand, should be evaluated for a potential scaphoid fracture. Those with displaced fractures may require operative fixation as, due to retrograde blood flow, a high nonunion rate is associated.[21] However, initial radiographs may be negative in nondisplaced fractures. CT or MRI can be considered to diagnose those with initial negative radiographs.[20] Alternatively, most practitioners suggest conservative treatment in a short-arm cast or splint with a thumb spica for 2 weeks with repeat radiographs. Those with resolution of symptoms and no radiographic scaphoid fracture at 2 weeks can return to activities. Those demonstrating a nondisplaced fracture at 2-week radiographs should be treated with a short-arm cast for no less than 8 weeks and until radiographic healing is demonstrated. Unfortunately, despite treatment, a high rate of avascular necrosis (AVN) is common with waist and proximal pole fractures due to retrograde blood supply. Those who progress to AVN may require surgical fixation or excision.

Digital Stenosing Tenosynovitis (Trigger Finger)

Tendons and/or tendon sheaths of the flexor digitorum superficialis (FDS) and the flexor digitorum profundus (FDP) tendons may thicken or become inflamed, resulting in increased cross-sectional area of the tendon sheath complex.[22] This results in a reduction in the smooth pull-through of the tendon complex under the A1 pulley at the MCP head. In these cases, patients get 'stuck' fingers that need forced extension and/or flexion to get movement of the tendons. Local corticosteroid injection, either under ultrasound or landmark approach, may result in improved glide of these tendons. In those with recurrent triggering, ultrasound-guided or surgical release of the A1 pulley will improve tendon glide in the long term with a minimal to no recurrence rate.

Mallet Finger (Distal Extensor Tendon Rupture)

Forced flexion of a fully extended finger can result in disruption of the terminal extensor tendon distal to the distal interphalangeal joint (DIP). Patients present with a loss of terminal extensor of the DIP with a resting flexion deformity of the finger. The x-rays may demonstrate an avulsion fracture of the dorsal distal phalanx.[21] Those with bony avulsion fractures are suggested to be in a full-time extension splint for 6 to 8 weeks, while those with no bony avulsion a minimum of 8 weeks. Surgical repair is not routinely needed.

Jersey Finger (Flexor Digitorum Profundus Rupture)

Forced extension of a flexed finger can result in rupture of the FDP tendon from the distal phalanx with intact FDS. Patients lack active DIP flexion, but will maintain MCP and proximal interphalangeal joint (PIP) flexion. All ruptures require operative fixation due to lack of primary tendon healing.[21]

REFERENCES

The full complete reference list for this chapter appears in the digital version of the chapter, available at http://connect.springerpub.com/content/book/978-0-8261-5628-0/part/part04/chapter/ch36

CHAPTER 37

MUSCULOSKELETAL—LOWER LIMB

Theodora Lananh Swenson, James E. Gardner, and Aaron Yang

PELVIS AND HIP

Hip-Spine Syndrome

Differentiating between hip and lumbar spine pathologies can be challenging. The term *hip-spine syndrome* has been used to describe the overlapping symptoms between the two pathologies, which can often mimic one another.[1] Symptoms include low back/buttock, groin, and thigh pain. Classically, groin pain is associated with hip pathology, and low back/buttock pain is associated with lumbar spine pathology. Physical examination should include inspection for muscle atrophy and spinal alignment, palpation for areas of tenderness, and a thorough neurologic examination. Special tests can help clarify the etiology of symptoms as originating from the hip or the spine. Plain radiographs are the imaging modality of choice. For suspected hip pathology, anteroposterior (AP) and lateral views of the pelvis are standard, and frog-lateral radiographs of the hip are useful to assess the femoral head. For suspected spine pathology, AP and lateral radiographs of the spine are standard, and lateral flexionextension radiographs can be used to assess instability or spondylolisthesis. MRI and CT scan can be further obtained to evaluate soft tissue deformities. If the etiology of symptoms remains unclear, additional information may be obtained via electrophysiologic studies, vascular studies (anklebrachial index, duplex ultrasonography, magnetic resonance angiography), and intra-articular or epidural injections.

Sacroiliac Joint Pain

Sacroiliac joint (SIJ) pain is a common but underestimated cause of chronic low back pain that is due to irritation or inflammation of the SIJ. SIJ pain is usually localized to the buttocks but can also be referred to the upper or lower lumbar region, groin, abdomen, or even the foot.[2,3] No single physical examination or historical feature can reliably elucidate SIJ pain. Diagnosis often necessitates multiple provocative physical examination maneuvers, with varying sensitivities and specificities, or diagnostic nerve blocks.[4] Conservative management with physical therapy (PT), mobilization exercises, and nonsteroidal anti-inflammatory drugs (NSAIDs) may provide a viable option with fewer risks in the early course of treatment.[4] Referral for diagnostic or therapeutic interventions, including a corticosteroid injection into the SIJ, should be considered after conservative management has failed or for refractory pain.

Deep Gluteal Syndrome

Deep gluteal syndrome is a group of conditions producing posterior hip pain secondary to compression of the sciatic or pudendal nerve. This group of conditions includes piriformis syndrome, gemelli-obturator internus syndrome, ischiofemoral impingement syndrome, and proximal hamstring syndrome. Anatomically, the piriformis, superior gemellus, obturator internus, inferior gemellus, and quadratus femoris muscles are located in the deep gluteal space, and the superior and inferior gluteal, sciatic, posterior femoral cutaneous, and pudendal nerves traverse this region. It is thought that anomalous variations in the relationship between the piriformis muscle and the sciatic nerve pose a risk of development of deep gluteal syndrome and a total of 13 anatomic variations have been described.[5] After passing the piriformis, the sciatic nerve runs posterior to the obturator/gemellus complex and the quadratus muscle. It then passes between the ischial tuberosity and lesser trochanter, entering the posterior thigh at the lower margin of the quadratus femoris. Finally, proximal hamstring tendon pathologies can irritate the sciatic nerve due to their intimate relationship at the level of the ischial tuberosity. Symptoms include intermittent or persistent dysesthesias in the buttocks, posterior hip, and thigh without focal neurologic deficits. Pain is often caused by activities involving hip flexion (such as sitting or walking). MRI of the pelvis helps identify pathologic conditions entrapping the nerves. Treatment commonly includes conservative measures such as rest, PT, and avoidance of provoking factors. For patients with persistent or recurrent symptoms, surgical decompression may be recommended.

Greater Trochanteric Pain Syndrome

Greater trochanteric pain syndrome is classically due to inflammation of the trochanteric bursa. However, improved visualization of the hip via MRI and arthroscopy has shown that other etiologies exist, including gluteus medius or minimus tendinosis or tears and snapping hip syndrome. Symptoms include pain with walking, running, climbing stairs, sitting, and lying on the affected hip. Conservative treatment includes NSAIDs, an iliotibial band (ITB) stretching program, and hip abductor/extensor strengthening. If refractory to these measures, a steroid injection into the bursa can provide symptom relief. Various etiologies may be responsible for greater trochanteric region pain; therefore, musculoskeletal ultrasound (US) may become a valuable tool for both diagnostic and therapeutic reasons. For instance, true trochanteric bursitis can be blindly injected, but other bursas (such as the subgluteus medius bursa) will require US image guidance to reach the target.

Iliotibial Band Syndrome

ITB syndrome is often seen in conjunction with greater trochanteric bursitis, and potential causes include overtraining or running on uneven surfaces. Predisposing factors include genu varum, tibial varum, varus hindfoot, and foot pronation. Symptoms often include lateral knee pain, as the ITB slides over the lateral femoral condyle and inserts onto the Gerdy tubercle on the lateral tibia. The *Ober test* may be positive. Rehabilitation should be aimed at *stretching* the ITB, hip flexors, and gluteus maximus. Adductors may be strengthened to counteract the tight ITB, and hip abductor strengthening may also improve dynamic hip stability. Helpful *modalities* include ice, US, and phonophoresis. Foot pronation should be corrected; running only on even surfaces may help. A *steroid injection* into the area of the lateral femoral condyle may relieve pain. Symptoms can generally take 2 to 6 months to improve.

Femoral Acetabular Impingement

Femoral acetabular impingement (FAI) is due to abnormal contact between the femur and the acetabulum during range of motion (ROM). A cam lesion is the formation of extra bone on the head of the femur, causing pain when it impinges with the acetabulum. A pincer lesion occurs when the acetabulum extends too far over the femoral head, causing pain as it restrains normal hip ROM. Symptoms may be insidious and include groin pain with activity and after prolonged sitting with hips flexed to 90°. Patients may demonstrate location of their pain by grasping their hip with their palm, their thumb anterior, and their fingers over their buttocks to form a "C." FAI is a strong risk factor for hip osteoarthritis, and many cases of FAI have associated labral tears. Radiographs can visualize cam and/or pincer lesions, which are sufficient in aiding diagnosis. MRI helps visualize the soft tissue and magnetic resonance arthrogram can be used to demonstrate injury to the labrum. Treatment includes exercise-based rehabilitation. If conservative measures fail, orthopedic referral is indicated for surgical intervention.

KNEE

Pes Anserine Bursitis

The pes anserine bursa is located under the sartorius, gracilis, and semitendinosus tendons. Symptoms include pain and tenderness at the insertion of the medial hamstrings at the medial proximal tibia. Treatment should emphasize stretching the medial hamstrings and improving knee biomechanics. Athletes may wear protective knee padding. Steroid injections may be very effective, but US guidance should be considered since unguided injections rarely infiltrate the pes anserine bursa.[6]

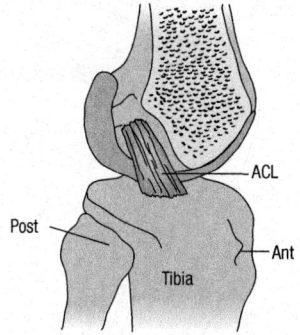

FIGURE 37.1 The anterior cruciate ligament.
ACL, anterior cruciate ligament; Ant, anterior; Post, posterior.

Anterior Cruciate Ligament

The anterior cruciate ligament (ACL) is composed of two major bundles, the posterolateral and the anteromedial bundle, and runs superiorly and posteriorly from its anterior medial tibial attachment to attach onto the medial aspect of the lateral femoral condyle (Figure 37.1). It prevents excessive anterior translation and abnormal external rotation of the tibia on the femur and prevents knee hyperextension. The ACL is most commonly injured due to extreme external rotation of the femur during excessive pivoting or cutting. Other mechanisms of injury include hyperextension, hyperflexion, or lateral trauma to the knee. A "pop" is often heard or felt at the time of injury. Immediate swelling due to hemarthrosis and a sense of instability usually follow. The medial collateral ligament (MCL) and the medial meniscus are commonly injured with the ACL, which is known as the terrible triad or the O'Donoghue triad.[7]

Nonoperative rehabilitation of ACL injury should concentrate on proprioceptive training and strengthening of the hamstrings to prevent anterior subluxation of the tibia. Bracing should limit terminal extension and rotation. Activity modification (e.g., avoiding cutting and pivoting sports) is extremely important to avoid injury to other intra-articular structures, such as the menisci.

The need for operative treatment depends on the amount of damage and degree of laxity, as well as patient-specific factors. A younger, more active patient is more likely to require surgical repair compared with an older, sedentary patient. Postoperative rehabilitation can last up to 6 to 9 months. Patients are typically weight-bearing as tolerated (WBAT) with an extension brace immediately after surgery. As with nonoperative rehabilitation, the emphasis is on strengthening the hamstrings and proprioceptive training. During the first 6 weeks, it is important to regain ROM (can be

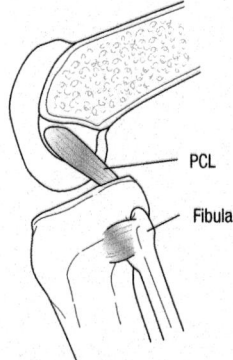

FIGURE 37.2 The posterior cruciate ligament (PCL).
Source: Adapted from Fu FH, Stone DA, eds. *Sports Injuries—Mechanisms, Prevention and Treatment.* 2nd ed. Williams & Wilkins; 2022. https://www.scribd.com/doc/36005808/Sports-Injuries-Mechanisms-Prevention-and-Treatment-2nd-Ed-F-Fu-D-Stone-Lippincott-1994-WW

assisted by continuous passive motion [CPM]) and enhance patellar mobility. The intensity and resistance should progressively increase between weeks 6 and 10. By week 10, there should be essentially no limitation in strengthening.

Prevention of these injuries is of utmost importance and has been a recent focus of sports medicine research. Young female athletes, especially those who play soccer and basketball, are at a much higher risk of ACL injury than their male peers. ACL injury prevention programs that incorporate proprioceptive and neuromuscular control training may reduce the risk of ACL injuries and therefore should be considered in high-risk athletes.[8]

Posterior Cruciate Ligament

The posterior cruciate ligament (PCL; Figure 37.2) is composed of two major bundles, the posteromedial and the anterolateral bundle, and runs anteriorly, superiorly, and medially from its posterior intercondylar tibial attachment to attach onto the medial femoral condyle. It prevents abnormal internal rotation (IR) and posterior translation of the tibia on the femur, which aids knee flexion. Injury of the PCL classically occurs secondary to a motor vehicle accident (MVA) when the tibia strikes the dashboard, forcing the tibia posteriorly. Injury also occurs with high valgus stress or falling on a flexed knee. Swelling is less common than in ACL injuries. MRI is the preferred imaging, although less sensitive for PCL pathology compared with ACL pathology; arthroscopy is more accurate in making the diagnosis. Treatment of a mild PCL sprain usually involves quadriceps strengthening without the need for bracing. Severe PCL injuries will often need to be repaired arthroscopically.

Meniscal Injury

The menisci are fibrocartilaginous structures of the intra-articular knee that increase the contact area between the femur and the tibia and can act as "shock absorbers" for the knee. Mechanisms of injury include excessive rotational stresses, typically the result of twisting a flexed knee. The medial meniscus is more often injured than the lateral meniscus. Knee locking, popping, and/or clicking are characteristic complaints. MRI may help confirm the clinical diagnosis and identify other injuries. Arthroscopy is the gold standard for diagnosis of a tear (Figure 37.3).

Treatment depends on the severity of injury. Nonsurgical treatment includes early management with RICE (rest, ice, compression, and elevation), NSAIDs, hamstring and ITB stretching, and a progressive resistive exercise program for quadriceps/hamstring/hip strengthening. A joint aspiration is sometimes useful to reduce effusion and relieve pain. Aquatic exercises can unload the affected meniscus. The intensity can be gradually increased with avoidance of activities involving compressive rotational loading. It may be reasonable to gradually resume sports activities once strength in the affected limb approaches 70% to 80% of that of the unaffected limb. Orthopedic referral for possible arthroscopic surgery is indicated if the patient is experiencing mechanical symptoms, including locking, buckling, or recurrent swelling with pain that has not responded to conservative treatment. Surgical treatment is evolving. Total meniscectomy is no longer considered an acceptable standard of care; efforts are now aimed at preserving as much cartilage as possible in order to prevent degenerative changes. The outer one-third of the menisci are vascular and may be repaired; the inner two-thirds are avascular and may need to be debrided. Following partial meniscectomy, full weight-bearing

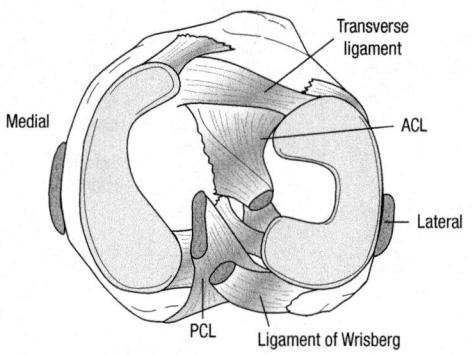

FIGURE 37.3 The menisci.
ACL, anterior cruciate ligament; PCL, posterior cruciate ligament.
Source: Adapted from Fu FH, Stone DA, eds. *Sports Injuries—Mechanisms, Prevention and Treatment.* 2nd ed. Williams & Wilkins; 2022. https://www.scribd.com/doc/36005808/Sports-Injuries-Mechanisms-Prevention-and-Treatment-2nd-Ed-F-Fu-D-Stone-Lippincott-1994-WW.

(WB) may occur once the patient is pain-free. Following meniscal repair, full WB may be delayed for up to 6 weeks. ROM exercises, stretching, and progressive strengthening of the lower limbs are the mainstays of postoperative therapy. Deep squatting is discouraged.

Patellofemoral Pain Syndrome

The etiology of patellofemoral pain syndrome (PFPS) is postulated to be a combination of overuse, muscular imbalance (e.g., hip abductor and external rotator weakness),[9] and/or biomechanical problems (e.g., pes planus or pes cavus, increased Q angle; Figure 37.4). Anterior knee pain may occur with activity and worsen with prolonged sitting or descending stairs. Acute management involves relative rest, ice, and NSAIDs. Prolonged sitting should be avoided. The mainstay of rehabilitation is to address the biomechanical deficits through a combination of quadriceps strengthening exercises with stretching of the quadriceps, hamstrings, ITB, and gastroc-soleus complex. Classically, short arc terminal knee extension (0°–30°) exercises were utilized with

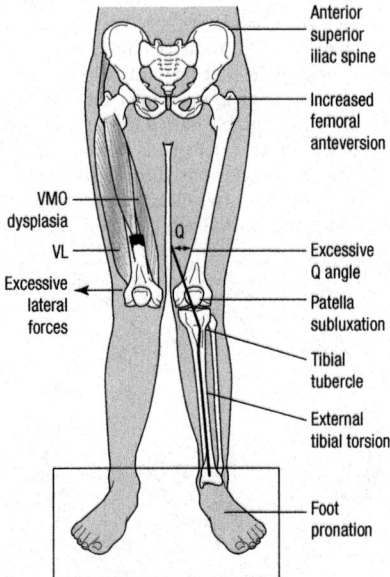

FIGURE 37.4 Sequelae of an increased Q angle. Normally, the male Q is 13°, while the female Q is 18°.

VL, vastus lateralis; VMO, vastus medialis obliquus.

Source: Adapted from Sports Injuries—Mechanisms, Prevention and Treatment. 2nd ed. Williams & Wilkins; 2022. https://www.scribd.com/doc/36005808/Sports-Injuries-Mechanisms-Prevention-and-Treatment-2nd-Ed-F-Fu-D-Stone-Lippincott-1994-WW.

the belief that they selectively strengthened the vastus medialis oblique (VMO). Currently, the idea of VMO selectivity is controversial. In general, short-arc (0°–45°), closed kinetic chain leg press exercises are recommended to strengthen all four heads of the quads, which are thought to be weakened in aggregate. Full-arc and open kinetic chain exercises should be avoided to reduce symptom aggravation.

Taping the patella so that it tracks properly (McConnell technique) may improve pain symptoms during exercise. Orthotics to correct pes planus or foot pronation and soft braces with patellar cutouts may provide modest symptomatic relief in appropriate cases. Surgery is rarely necessary and is reserved for recalcitrant instability or symptomatic malalignment.

Medial Tibial Stress Syndrome (Shin Splints) and Stress Fractures

Medial tibial stress syndrome is characterized by diffuse pain located along the medial tibia. Symptoms are exacerbated by exercise and believed to represent periostitis, usually of the posteromedial tibial border. Runners, gymnasts, and dancers are at risk, with causes including an increase in exercise intensity, inadequate footwear, hard surface training, or poor biomechanics. Local pain and tenderness are noted along the distal one-third of the tibia. Pain is often quickly relieved by rest. Radiographs are usually normal. Bone scan may be positive in severe cases and can help distinguish medial tibial stress syndrome from stress fracture. Treatment includes rest, NSAIDs, US, preactivity icing, and correction of aggravating factors.

Causes of tibial stress fractures (TSFs) are similar to those of tibial stress syndrome. Stress fractures are also common in the fibula and the metatarsals, especially the second metatarsal. Pain is initially only induced by exercise, but progresses to pain with WB or even at rest. There is often exquisite point tenderness along the distal or middle third of the tibia. The x-rays may be negative initially, but may show a clear fracture after several weeks (e.g., a positive "dreaded black line" on oblique radiograph, representing an anterior TSF). Bone scans are more sensitive, and MRI is often used to determine the severity of stress fracture. Medial TSFs can be treated with relative rest (e.g., crutches) for 4 to 6 weeks, NSAIDs, and transcutaneous electric nerve stimulation (TENS). Anterior TSFs may require several months of rest from sports activities and ongoing conservative treatment. Recalcitrant cases may eventually require a bone graft.

Chronic Compartment Syndrome

Chronic compartment syndrome of the leg includes pain that is felt after a specific period of exercise and can be associated with paresthesias, numbness, and weakness in the distribution of the nerve within the compartment. Electrodiagnostic studies are usually normal.

Resting and postexercise compartment pressures should be obtained. Resting pressures greater than 30 mmHg, 15-second postexercise pressures greater than 60 mmHg, or 2-minute postexercise pressures greater than 20 mmHg are all suggestive of chronic compartment syndrome. An initial conservative approach should include NSAIDs, proper footwear selection, and correction of training errors. If symptoms persist 1 to 2 months after a trial of conservative treatment, referral for surgical fasciotomy may be warranted.

Baker Cyst

A Baker cyst is a fluid collection within the posterior knee bursa located between the medial head of the gastrocnemius and the semimembranosus. Workup should include US to rule out deep vein thrombosis (DVT) or aneurysm prior to aspiration or excision.

FOOT AND ANKLE

Achilles Tendinitis

Overuse, overpronation, heel varus deformity, and poor flexibility of the Achilles tendon/gastroc-soleus/hamstrings may be contributing factors. The condition is often seen in basketball players, who may be particularly susceptible due to frequent jumping, and in runners who increase their mileage or hill training. Symptoms include pain and swelling in the tendon during and after activities. Examination may be significant for swelling, pain on palpation, a palpable nodule, and inability to stand on tiptoes. Chronic tendinosis may result in tendon weakness, potentially leading to rupture.

There is no consensus on the optimal mode of treatment, but most rehabilitation programs will likely begin with the PRICE (protection, rest, ice, compression, elevation) principle. Modalities, especially US, may be helpful. Plantar flexor strengthening is important. Downhill exercises should be emphasized; uphill running should be discouraged, especially early in the rehabilitation. Heel lifts may provide early relief but may lead to heel cord shortening with prolonged use. A properly fitted shoe, often with a stiff heel counter, is important. Steroid injections into the Achilles tendon are not recommended by many sources due to the risk of tendon rupture, as the Achilles tendon does not have a true synovial sheath. For severe or chronic cases, recovery to near-normal strength may take up to 24 months, even with good circulation. For this reason, novel treatments (e.g., platelet-rich plasma) are currently being studied, but the results are inconclusive.[10,11] Young, active persons with ruptured tendons usually undergo operative treatment; casting is an option for older, sedentary persons.

Ankle Sprains and Instability

Lateral ankle sprains are the most common type of ankle sprains and usually due to an inversion injury of a plantar-flexed foot. The anterior talofibular ligament (ATFL) is typically the first structure to be involved, followed by the calcaneofibular ligament (CFL) and the posterior talofibular ligament (PTFL). In the event of severe sprains, x-rays to check the tibiofibular syndesmosis may be necessary; these require surgical consultation.

Injuries of the medial (deltoid) ankle ligament due to an eversion injury are less common due to the strength of the deltoid ligament; an associated proximal fibula fracture (Maisonneuve fracture) should be ruled out.

Rehabilitation of ankle sprains involves three phases. Phase 1 normally lasts 1 to 3 days, until the patient is able to bear weight comfortably. This phase involves the RICE principle: rest (e.g., crutches), ice for 20 minutes three to five times a day, compression with ACE wrap, and elevation of the foot above the heart. Hot showers, alcohol, methyl salicylate counterirritants (e.g., Bengay), and other treatments that may increase swelling should be avoided during the initial 24 hours. Phase 2 usually lasts days to weeks. The goals during this phase are to restore ROM, strengthen the ankle stabilizers, and stretch/strengthen the Achilles tendon. Phase 3 is initiated when motion is near normal and pain and swelling are almost gone. Reestablishing motor coordination via proprioceptive exercises and endurance training is emphasized; these include balance board, running curves (figure of 8), and zigzag running.

Return to play guidelines vary. Some recommendations may be as follows: grade 1 (no laxity and minimal ligamentous tear): 0 to 5 days; grade 2 (mild to moderate laxity and functional loss): 7 to 14 days; grade 3 (complete ligamentous disruption and cannot bear weight): 21 to 35 days; and syndesmosis injury: 21 to 56 days. Recent literature has demonstrated that an early and accelerated rehabilitation program results in better short-term outcomes for grades 1 and 2 lateral ankle sprains.[12]

Plantar Fasciitis

Plantar fasciitis is commonly seen in athletes and in persons whose jobs require much standing or walking. In the acute phase, microtears of the plantar fascia can cause inflammation and heel or arch pain. In the chronic phase, the condition is more commonly termed plantar fasciopathy, as the fascia is less commonly inflamed, and instead degenerates. Biomechanical issues (e.g., an overpronated foot with increased tension on the fascia) are often the cause. Classic symptoms include medial heel pain and pain across the entire area of the plantar fascia, especially with the first few steps in the morning.

The key component of treatment is a home exercise program of routine, daily stretching of the plantar fascia (Figure 37.5) and Achilles tendon, which has proven to be superior to other treatment modalities.[13] Patients should be on relative rest from walking, running, and jumping, and consider switching to activities such as swimming or cycling to allow the fascia to heal. Proper footwear includes

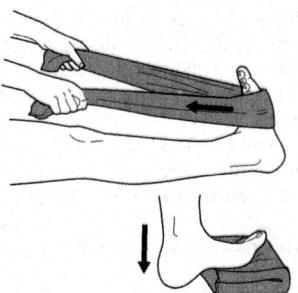

FIGURE 37.5 Stretching for plantar fasciitis.

well-cushioned soles, possible use of an extra-deep heel pad/cup insert, and avoiding high heels. Soft medial arch supports are generally preferable to rigid orthotics, which can exacerbate symptoms. NSAIDs and ice may help decrease inflammation. For patients not responding to other measures, splints may be useful to supply a gentle constant stretch across the sole of the foot and gastrocnemius at night while sleeping. Once the pain resolves, patients should gradually return to increased levels of activity while continuing their stretching program.

The majority of cases will improve with conservative measures within 6 to 12 weeks. In the rare, persistent case, a local corticosteroid injection may be considered. A potential complication of corticosteroid injection is necrosis of the fatty pad of the heel, which cannot be easily reversed or treated. Surgical intervention, which consists of a release of the involved fascia from its attachment to the calcaneus, can be considered if all other measures fail, but is rarely necessary.

Tarsal Tunnel Syndrome

Tarsal tunnel syndrome occurs due to entrapment of the posterior tibial nerve underneath the flexor retinaculum at the tarsal tunnel, which is the region behind the malleolus. Structures that pass underneath the tarsal tunnel include the tibialis posterior, flexor digitorum longus, tibial artery, tibial vein, tibial nerve, and the flexor hallucis longus. Symptoms include pain, numbness, and tingling at the medial foot. Workup includes radiographs to assess foot alignment, MRI to visualize space-occupying lesions, and electromyography/nerve conduction study. Treatment includes rest and NSAIDs. US-guided steroid injections may be considered if other measures fail, and surgical decompression may provide symptom relief in cases caused by space-occupying lesions.

REFERENCES

The full complete reference list for this chapter appears in the digital version of the chapter, available at http://connect.springerpub.com/content/book/978-0-8261-5628-0/part/part04/chapter/ch37

CHAPTER 38

MUSCULOSKELETAL—SPORTS AND PERFORMING ARTS MEDICINE

Daniel H. Blatz, G. Ross Malik, and Kevin Ozment

TEAM PHYSICIAN/COMPANY PHYSICIAN ROLES

Being a sports team or performing arts company physician requires a number of characteristics. Trustworthiness, good communication skills, organization, and medical knowledge are some of the main components.[1,2] The primary goal is to always ensure the athlete/artist is well cared for and you have that individual's best interests in mind. Furthermore, a physician in this role has to consider the team/company as a whole. Coaches, artistic directors, team/company managers, athletic trainers, and physical therapists are some of the essential parties who need to always be aware of the status of the athlete/artist. When dealing with under-age persons, the parents must also be aware of their status.

PREPARTICIPATION PHYSICAL EVALUATION

At the very beginning of each sporting and performance season, preparticipation physical evaluations (PPEs) are an often used means to evaluate overall health and readiness for sports/performing arts. Sports physicals or PPEs are presently required by all high schools in the United States, the National Collegiate Athletic Association (NCAA), and other organizations.[3] The main goals of a PPE include the following: (a) ensure safety and readiness for competition/participation; (b) identify medical and musculoskeletal conditions that could limit participation or lead to injury; (c) identify conditions that could lead to catastrophic injury or sudden death; (d) assess general health and fitness level; and (e) educate regarding healthy behaviors and answer health-related questions.[3]

The main components of the PPE include the following: (a) history review, including prior musculoskeletal issues, general medical history, and family history; (b) physical examination, including cardiac examination and assessment for signs of Marfan syndrome; and (c) determination of readiness for sports and performing arts.[3]

EMERGENCY ACTION PLAN

An emergency action plan (EAP) is a guide utilized to optimize a rapid and efficient response to medical, musculoskeletal, and/or environmental emergencies.[4,5] The EAP should have a number of characteristics and inclusions: (a) written out with well-defined roles and recommendations; (b) contact information of important personnel, as well as decision-making hierarchy; (c) list of necessary equipment that should be available and the location of the equipment; (d) general stepwise outline of what to do if an emergency arises; and (e) transportation and location of facilities to utilize if escalation of medical care arises, among other inclusions.[4,5]

The EAP is a document that needs to be reviewed and updated regularly in order to be accurate and to ensure that all personnel are aware of their roles.[4,5]

SPECIFIC EMERGENCY SITUATION AND READINESS

For many, if not all of the issues in Table 38.1, the EAP will help greatly in fine-tuning an efficient and effective response by the sports and performing arts physician. In the appropriate setting, additional useful equipment and medications to have available include an automated external defibrillator, EpiPen, bronchodilator/beta-agonist, stethoscope, rectal thermometer, ice baths, blood pressure cuff, pulse oximeter, oxygen, and oral and intravenous fluids.[4–9] With outdoor events, environmental conditions must always be taken into account.

CONCUSSION

Concussion (mild traumatic brain injury) is a clinical diagnosis involving a trauma to the head.[10,11] The most common symptoms are headache and dizziness; alterations in mood, behavior, vision, and memory may also be reported.[12] Athletes have elevated risk of concussions with previous concussions, history of headaches/migraines, learning disabilities, attention deficit disorder (ADD)/attention deficit hyperactivity disorder (ADHD), or depression/anxiety.[11,13]

Sideline examination can be challenging. The Sport Concussion Assessment Tool 5 (SCAT5) with Maddocks questions is commonly used to assess neurologic, cognitive, and balance status in athletes.[10,14,15] Tandem gait, finger-to-nose coordination, cranial nerve, vestibular, and oculomotor assessment can also be useful.[16] Diagnostic imaging such as CT is not indicated unless there is concern for intracranial hemorrhage.[11] Any athlete with suspected concussion should be removed from play, incorporating the "when in doubt, sit them out" mentality.[11] If any red flag symptoms are present, such as unequal pupil size, unconsciousness, neurologic deficit, seizing/posturing, and nausea/vomiting, the EAP should be initiated and the athlete should be transported to the emergency department immediately.[10,11,17,18] Consider cervical spine immobilization/cervical spine radiographs if indicated per the National Emergency X-Radiography Utilization Study (NEXUS) criteria.[19] Headaches >3 hours, retrograde amnesia, loss of consciousness, and immediate dizziness have been associated with more severe/prolonged injury.[20,21] Individuals with a

TABLE 38.1 Emergency Conditions[4-9]

Injury	Mechanism	Signs and Symptoms	Diagnosis and Treatment	Prognosis/Tools
Sudden cardiac arrest	HCM, coronary artery anomalies, myocarditis, arrhythmias/electrical abnormalities, atherosclerotic heart disease, commotio cordis	Sudden collapse, especially midactivity	Systolic murmur for HCM Follow ACLS guidelines Early defibrillation and CPR when indicated	Early defibrillation directly correlated with survival AED
PTX	Spontaneous or traumatic	Sudden dyspnea, unilateral chest pain, cough	Clinical assessment including auscultatory examination, chest x-ray to assess for tension PTX Needle decompression for tension PTX (second intercostal space in the midclavicular line)	Early detection = increased survival Stethoscope Large-bore needle Pulse oximeter
Exercise-induced anaphylaxis	Acute systemic hypersensitivity	Urticaria, angioedema, dyspnea, wheezing, gastrointestinal upset, dizziness, hypotension, rhinitis, headache	Attention to airway and breathing and circulation, EpiPen, IV fluids, beta-agonists	Early activation of emergency response system EpiPen
Exercise-induced asthma	Increase in airway resistance during or following exercise Associated with chronic asthma Also associated with allergic rhinitis or atopic dermatitis	Dyspnea, wheezing, cough, chest tightness/pain, difficulty speaking	Clinical history Auscultatory examination for wheezing Bronchodilator	Recognition and appropriate treatment lead to good outcomes Pulse oximeter

(continued)

TABLE 38.1 Emergency Conditions *(continued)*

Injury	Mechanism	Signs and Symptoms	Diagnosis and Treatment	Prognosis/Tools
Splenic/hepatic injury	Blunt abdominal trauma	Left (spleen) or right (liver) upper quadrant pain, pain with abdominal palpation, Kehr sign shoulder pain related to splenic injury, hypotension	Early ultrasound and/or CT imaging, close observation as appropriate	Recognition and appropriate assessment and monitoring lead to good outcomes Blood pressure cuff
Knee dislocation	High-velocity/traumatic injury Multiligamentous injury Possible neurovascular (popliteal artery, tibial nerve, peroneal nerve) injury	Swollen and painful knee, Often multidirectional instability May spontaneously reduce, so high index of suspicion in the appropriate scenario Assess neurovascular examination, but can be normal even with neurovascular injury	Early reduction Transport to appropriate setting for further testing, including anklebrachial index, CT Orthopedic and vascular consultation 24-hour observation in hospital to ensure limb is stable	Recognition and appropriate assessment and monitoring lead to good outcomes
Exertional heat stroke	Overexertion in warm, humid conditions Deconditioned athlete more at risk	Temperature ≥104°F/40°C Tachycardia, hypotension	Temperature ≥104°F/40°C Passive and active cooling Ice water immersion	Early recognition = good outcomes Cool first, transport later

ACLS, advanced cardiac life support; AED, automated external defibrillator; CPR, cardiopulmonary resuscitation; HCM, hypertrophic cardiomyopathy; IV, intravenous; PTX, pneumothorax.

Source: Data from Sideline preparedness for the team physician: Consensus statement. *Med Sci Sports Exerc.* 2012;44(12):2442–2445; Korey Stringer Institute. *Emergency action plans;* 2021. https://ksi.uconn.edu/prevention/emergency-action-plans; Andersen J, Courson RW, Kleiner DM, et al. National Athletic Trainers' Association position statement: Emergency planning in athletics. *J Athl Train.* 2002;37(1):99–104; Korey Stringer Institute. *Emergency conditions;* 2021. https://ksi.uconn.edu; May J, Crown L, Gaertner M. Field-side emergencies. In: O'Connor F, et al eds. *ACSM's Sports Medicine A Comprehensive Review.* Lippincott Williams & Wilkins; 2013:84–91; Boden B. Catastrophic sports injuries. In: O'Connor F, et al eds. *ACSM's Sports Medicine A Comprehensive Review.* Lippincott Williams & Wilkins; 2013:96–101.

TABLE 38.2 Graduated Return to Sport/School Following Concussion

Stage[a]	Graduated Return to Sport Activity	Graduated Return to School Activity
1[b]	Symptom-limited daily activities	Symptom-limited daily activities
2	Light exercise (walking/cycling)	School activities outside classroom
3	Sport-related exercise	Partial return to school (half day, breaks)
4	Training drills (noncontact)	Full return to school/academic activities
5	Full contact training activities	
6	Return to game play	

[a] Each stage should last a minimum of 24 hours.
[b] Stage 1 initiated after 1 to 2 days of cognitive/physical rest.

Source: Data from Herring S, Kibler W, Putukian M. Team Physician Consensus Statement 2013 update. *Med Sci Sport Exerc.* 2013;45(8):1618–22.

concussion are more susceptible to recurrent concussions for the first 7 to 10 days and/or the second impact syndrome, which can be lethal.[16,22]

An athlete with suspected concussion should be serially monitored for worsening symptoms.[10] The patient and the family should be educated on the importance of mental/physical rest, sleep hygiene, and avoidance of activities that worsen symptoms.[23] In the first 1 to 2 days, physical and cognitive rest is encouraged, with graduated return to play/school per Table 38.2.[10,13] Follow-up with a clinician should occur within 72 hours of injury.[10,24]

CERVICAL SPINE CLEARANCE

In preparation for possible catastrophic cervical spine injuries, one should secure the necessary medical equipment/personnel and rehearse the EAP.[25,26] This includes practicing manual stabilization of the cervical spine, repositioning/lifting the athlete, removal of athletic equipment, and spine immobilization.[26–28] Cervical spine stabilization should occur with any injury involving cervical spine point tenderness, altered consciousness, obvious visualized/palpated bony spinal deformity, or bilateral motor/sensory neurologic deficit.[27] Manual stabilization can be performed by positioning the fingertips below the mastoid process and grasping the occiput with both hands or by securing the head between one's forearms by grasping the trapezii.[27,29,30] The two most common techniques for spine stabilization are the "log-roll" and the "multi-person lift" methods.[31] If there are any physical barriers, such as helmet/face mask or pads, these should be removed with the proper tools if one can do so without compromising the stabilization/neutrality of the spine and without delaying appropriate medical care.[27,28,31–33]

TABLE 38.3 Unique Sport-Specific/Performing Arts-Specific Injuries[34-73]

Injury	Mechanism	Signs and Symptoms	Dx and Tx	Prognosis/RTP
American football				
Cervical sprain	Player vs. player collision, spearing technique	↓ neck ROM and pain, paravertebral spasms	Dx: cervical x-ray r/o fracture/instability Tx: NSAIDs, rest, PT	Full active ROM with little to no pain No neurologic findings or severe injuries
AC separation	Fall onto top/point of shoulder	AC joint TTP, resisted arm adduction pain, palpable step-off	Dx: shoulder x-ray Tx: grades I–II = PRICE, PT, anesthetic injection; grade III has evidence for either conservative or operative management grades IV–VI = fixation	After restoration of strength and ROM, RTP with AC joint padding
Soccer				
ACL tear	Noncontact twisting/cutting/jump landing Direct valgus blow	Hear/feel a pop Rapid effusion or hemarthrosis (+) Lachman, pivot shift, anterior drawer	Dx: x-ray (look for Segond fracture), MRI Tx: surgical repair: patellar > hamstring autograft	Average 9–12 months after surgery 65% return to preinjury level of participation
High ankle sprain (syndesmotic ankle injury)	Sudden ER of the ankle causing the talus to laterally rotate and separate the fibula from the tibia	Pain with WB Anterolateral or medial ankle pain Passive ER/DF pain Nonhealing "lateral" ankle sprain	Dx: standing stress/mortise x-ray, MRI if x-ray inconclusive Tx: non-WB boot for 2–3 weeks, PT; surgery if instability, fracture, or refractory Tx	Tolerates jog and single-leg hop Position-specific drills with no symptoms Nonoperative: highly variable, 2–4 weeks Operative: 3–4 months, non-WB 6–12 weeks postoperatively

Basketball

Achilles tendon rupture	Push-off during running or hard lateral movement; typically third-/fourth-decade males Prevalence 4× higher than the next sport	Audible "pop" Feels as if was kicked Loss of PF Heel pain and ecchymosis Palpable gap	Dx: MRI or US Tx: nonoperative: PF immobilization, progress to DF and early PT Surgical: tendon suture repair	80% will RTP Average time to RTP = 6 months
FDP avulsion (jersey finger)	DIP forced extension during active DIP flexion → FDP tendon rupture; ring finger most common	Finger extended with hand at rest No active DIP flexion	Dx: MRI or US; x-rays to r/o bony avulsion Tx: immediate hand surgeon referral	Soft tissue: 12 weeks protected before gripping Bony avulsions: 4-6 weeks protected activity

Wrestling

Shoulder dislocation (anterior glenohumeral instability)	Direct posterior shoulder trauma Fall with arm abducted, extended, ER	Acute pain, weakness, instability Arm held in fixed slight ER and abduction	Dx: postreduction x-rays, MRI-Bankart lesion Tx: swift reduction; sling for 3-6 weeks if first occurrence, PT RTC/shoulder girdle strengthening	Full RTC strength, no apprehension Redislocation rate 90% for <20 years old RTP after surgical stabilization = 4-6 months
Herpes gladiatorum skin infection (herpes simplex virus 1)	Skin-to-skin contact Repetitive skin trauma with prolonged exposure	Primary: systemic symptoms 1-2 days, multidermatomal vesicles Secondary: burning and itching 2-3 days, then dermatomal vesicles	Dx: viral cultures within 1-2 days and PCR test Tx: oral valacyclovir 500 mg BID × 7 days	First-degree outbreak: NFHS: 10-14 days NCAA: no new blisters × 72 hours and complete antivirals Recurrent outbreak: Antivirals completed; lesions scabbed over

(continued)

TABLE 38.3 Unique Sport-Specific/Performing Arts-Specific Injuries (*continued*)

Injury	Mechanism	Signs and Symptoms	Dx and Tx	Prognosis/RTP
Ice hockey				
Core muscle injury (sports hernia, athletic pubalgia)	Poorly understood Overuse abdominal muscle injury resulting in fascia failure, posterior inguinal wall deficiency, muscle or aponeurosis injury Male > female	Exercise-related unilateral low abdomen and groin pain Worse with sudden acceleration, resisted hip adduction and abdominal curl	Dx: history and examination most important, MRI or dynamic US Tx: in-season = 4 weeks of rest with closed-chain lower body exercises, NSAIDs, ± steroid injections; surgery after nonoperative Tx failure	Nonoperative: 6–12 weeks, can be self-limiting and variable, RTP after completing functional sport assessment Open repair: 97% RTP 10–12 weeks Laparoscopic: RTP 2–3 weeks
FAI	Abnormal femoral head and acetabular contact with labral impingement due to cam/pincer/mixed deformities Goalie "butterfly" style	Limited HF and IR ROM with groin and hip pain Pain with repeated HF while skating	Dx: x-ray, MRI to evaluate the labrum and cartilage Tx: restrict HF, PT, NSAIDs; surgery: correct bone deformity and labral repair	Nonoperative: 3 months, variable prognosis Operative: RTP >90% at 6 months, most return to preoperative level
Baseball				
UCL injury	Repetitive valgus stress with pitching or throwing causing tensile strain on UCL	Insidious medial elbow pain during cocking and early acceleration Acute rupture: pop while throwing	Dx: x-ray-bony avulsions, spurs, calcifications; MRI/MR arthrogram Tx: throwing cessation and PT, gradual throwing program; complete tear: UCL reconstruction ("Tommy John" procedure)	Nonoperative: variable outcomes Operative: season ending, RTP 9–12 months postoperatively, 80% return to preinjury level

Hook of hamate fracture	Heel of bat impact while batting, or grip of golf club, or racket	Palmar pain with grip or impact while batting	Dx: x-ray-carpal tunnel view, CT if x-ray negative Tx: nondisplaced = cast; surgical excision if fails conservative Tx	RTP once tenderness resolved Operative: RTP at 6 weeks
Tennis				
TFCC tear	Fall on outstretched hand Degeneration due to repetitive racket swing	Painful clicking of ulnar wrist Pain with ulnar fovea and with ulnar deviation	Dx: x-ray and MRI; gold standard = arthroscopy Tx: bracing, wrist strengthening, reduce wrist twisting; arthroscopic debridement/repair if refractory	Nonoperative: variable, weeks to months Operative: immobilize 4 weeks, then 2–4 weeks PT
Medial head of gastrocnemius tear (tennis leg)	Forceful gastrocnemius contraction with knee extended and foot DF	Typically 35–50 years old Acute midcalf pain, swelling, WB pain Snapping sensation	Dx: US (MRI if unclear) Tx: almost always conservative; surgery if compartment syndrome	RTP: weeks to 3–4 months depending on grade/extent of injury
Alpine skiing				
Skier's thumb/UCL injury	Fall on abducted thumb while gripping ski pole Majority tear distally on proximal phalanx	Pain, swelling, ecchymosis at the ulnar aspect of the thumb MCP joint Valgus laxity	Dx: anteroposterior (AP)/lateral x-ray to r/o avulsion fracture, MRI or US (look for Stener lesion) Tx: partial tear = nonoperative with MCP immobilization × 4 weeks, PT; complete tear = surgical repair	7% of all ski-related injuries Operative: RTP in 3 months, 90% with good outcomes Nonoperative: RTP 1–2 months

(continued)

TABLE 38.3 Unique Sport-Specific/Performing Arts-Specific Injuries (*continued*)

Injury	Mechanism	Signs and Symptoms	Dx and Tx	Prognosis/RTP
Tibial shaft fracture	Most common lower extremity fracture in skiers (63%) Valgus/ER impact, ER forces on the ski Use of "carving" technique	Pain, deformity, swelling, unable to WB Open fractures common Neurovascular compromise possible	Dx: examination, x-ray, CT Tx: nondisplaced = long leg cast; displaced = reduce, immobilize, and surgical referral; open = surgical referral; monitor for compartment syndrome	2%–10% risk of nonunion Closed fracture: union by 10–13 weeks 92% RTP after surgery, 67% RTP for nonsurgical
Gymnastics				
Pars interarticularis stress fracture (spondylolysis)	Repetitive lumbar hyperextension and shear forces L5 common	Low back pain worse with extension, running, rotation, side bends ± radicular pain	Dx: x-ray, MRI if x-ray (−) Tx: rest (no extension for 6 weeks), short-duration lumbar orthosis, PT core strengthening	Acute: 75%–100% heal Early bilateral lesion: 50% heal Chronic: little to no healing
Distal radius epiphysitis (Gymnast's wrist)	Distal radial physeal stress injury due to repetitive wrist WB Loads 2–16 × the body weight on the wrist can be seen	TTP over distal radial physis Pain with wrist hyperextension and axial loading	Dx: x-ray (bilaterally to compare), ± MRI Tx: stop wrist WB until pain gone (at least 6 weeks), wrist brace, gradual return to activity; operative if severe growth arrest	Generally good if no physis growth arrest Up to 12 weeks for pain to resolve Serial x-rays for up to 1 year are important

Dancers

Fifth metatarsal fracture (Dancer's fracture)	Inversion injury while dancing "en pointe" Spiral fracture of the fifth metatarsal shaft	Pain/swelling lateral forefoot Difficulty walking	Dx: x-ray Tx: short walking boot, shoe cast, WB as tolerated	Great prognosis with nonoperative Tx, even for displaced fractures Average RTP = 19 weeks
Flexor hallucis tendonitis (dancer's tendonitis)	Ballet dancers Excessive stress with repetitive toe-off	Activity/dance-related pain at the medial or posterior ankle Pain with resisted great toe flexion	Dx: x-ray (look for os trigonum), MRI Tx: stretch, rest, night splints, NSAIDs; surgical release of tendon if refractory	Responds well to conservative Tx Good prognosis to RTP
Anterior ankle impingement	Aggravated by pliés positioning Often an osteophyte at the margin of the anterior tibia and dorsal talus	Pain with repeated stressful DF Anterior ankle swelling/pain, TTP anterior joint line DF may be limited	Dx: examination, lateral foot x-ray in DF, ± MRI Tx: avoid demi-plié, shoe mod, kinetic chain PT, steroid injection; arthroscopy is effective	Good prognosis with conservative Tx Best surgical outcomes in those without arthritis or chondral lesions

(continued)

TABLE 38.3 Unique Sport-Specific/Performing Arts-Specific Injuries (*continued*)

Musicians

Injury	Mechanism	Signs and Symptoms	Dx and Tx	Prognosis/RTP
Thoracic outlet syndrome	Compression of neurovascular structures, brachial plexus (lower trunk common), subclavian artery or vein	Typically bowed string players. Pain/paresthesias from neck down the arm. Arm/hand feels cold. Worse with holding instrument or overhead activity	Dx: difficult to definitively diagnose, often diagnosis of exclusion of other conditions. Tx: postural correction, PT; surgery only if failed conservative Tx >3–4 months	50%–90% recovery with conservative Tx. Limited evidence for surgical outcomes; first rib resection most dependable
Focal motor dystonia	Unclear mechanism (altered basal ganglia circuitry, lack of sensory-motor inhibitions, stress/anxiety, etc.)	Involuntary spasm of affected body part. Fingers often involved. Task-specific movement disorder	Dx: history and examination, exclude other conditions with MRI, EMG. Tx: botox injections, behavioral training, constraint-induced movement therapy	Overall poor prognosis

AC, acromioclavicular; ACL, anterior cruciate ligament; DF, dorsiflexion; DIP, distal interphalangeal joint; Dx, diagnosis; EMG, electromyography; ER, external rotation; FAI, femoroacetabular impingement; FDP, flexor digitorum profundus; HF, hip flexion; IR, internal rotation; MCP, metacarpophalangeal joint; MR, magnetic resonance; NCAA, National Collegiate Athletic Association; NFHS, National Federation of High Schools; NSAIDs, nonsteroidal anti-inflammatory drugs; PCR, polymerase chain reaction; PF, plantarflexion; PRICE, protect, rest, ice, compression, elevation; PT, physical therapy; r/o, reverse oblique; ROM, range of motion; RTC, rotator cuff; RTP, return to play; TFCC, triangular fibrocartilage complex; TTP, tenderness to palpation; Tx, treatment; UCL, ulnar collateral ligament; US, ultrasonography; WB, weight-bearing.

SPORT-SPECIFIC/PERFORMING ARTS-SPECIFIC INJURIES

Athletes and artists, at all levels of competition, are at risk of developing a wide variety of sport-specific injuries. Injuries more commonly occur during competition than practice.[34] The list of possible injuries is extensive and can differ depending on a multitude of factors, including the sport, the position played, gender, and age.[35] Various injuries have a higher prevalence in certain sports/performing arts based on their mechanism of injuries. These are highlighted in Table 38.3 with their presentation, workup, and treatment in order to return the athlete to play safely.

RETURN TO PLAY CONSIDERATIONS

Following injury, illness, and time away from sport and performance, certain criteria should be met to ensure the athlete/artist is ready for the physical stress of their sport/performing art. Certainly there will be variability in return to play guidelines depending on the specific injury and the requirements of their sport. General criteria include the following: (a) minimal to pain-free range of motion (ROM); (b) 85% to 100% strength of prior strength or contralateral strength; and (c) 85% to 100% baseline ROM or contralateral ROM.[74] This ideally should be evaluated outside of a competitive/performance setting. Additionally, regardless of injury duration, the individual needs to demonstrate they can do all the required movements of their position at the required speed and intensity. Once these criteria are met, release to sport/performing arts can be granted.

REFERENCES

The full complete reference list for this chapter appears in the digital version of the chapter, available at http://connect.springerpub.com/content/book/978-0-8261-5628-0/part/part04/chapter/ch38

CHAPTER 39

PERIPHERAL NERVE CONDITIONS

Kevin Huang, Benjamin Washburn, and Marco Masci

MONONEUROPATHIES OF THE UPPER EXTREMITY

Median Neuropathy at the Wrist (Carpal Tunnel Syndrome)

Median nerve entrapment at the wrist is the most common entrapment neuropathy (For less common upper extremity mononeuropathies, see Table 39.1.). It occurs as the median nerve and flexor tendons pass between the transverse carpal ligament and the carpal bones. It is more common in females, often occurring bilaterally, with the dominant hand more severely affected.

Signs/symptoms: It presents with paresthesias in the median nerve distribution (medial thumb, index, middle, and radial aspect of the ring finger). Symptoms may be localized to the wrist and hand, although can also radiate to the forearm, arm, and rarely shoulder. Symptoms are provoked with wrist flexed or extended. Aggravating activities often include holding a phone, a book, or grasping the steering wheel while driving. Nocturnal symptoms are commonly associated with prolonged wrist flexion or extension, which improves by shaking the hands out. Patients may describe difficulty opening jars, turning doorknobs/keys, or buttoning shirts.[1,2]

Examination: Examination shows hypoesthesia in a median distribution. Comparison of the radial aspect of the fourth finger (median-innervated) with the ulnar aspect of the fourth finger (ulnar-innervated) can be helpful. Sensation over the thenar eminence is *spared* as the palmar cutaneous sensory branch arises proximally to the carpal tunnel. Motor examination may reveal thumb abduction and opposition weakness. In more severe cases, atrophy of the thenar eminence may be noted. Special tests suggestive of carpal tunnel syndrome (CTS) include Tinel sign (tapping over the median nerve at the wrist), Phalen maneuver (the wrists held passively flexed, with symptoms typically provoked in 30 seconds to 2 minutes), and reverse Phalen maneuver (the wrists held passively extended, with symptoms typically provoked in 30 seconds to 2 minutes).[1]

Electrodiagnostic findings: Nerve conduction studies (NCS) show median sensory and/or motor nerve slowing across the wrist. When routine studies are normal, the combined sensory index (CSI) can increase the sensitivity of diagnosing a mild demyelinating CTS.

Management: Conservative management includes neutral nocturnal wrist splint, occupational therapy, glucocorticoid injection, and oral

TABLE 39.1 Other Upper Extremity Peripheral Mononeuropathies

Nerve	Symptoms	Causes
Axillary (C5, C6)	Weakness of shoulder abduction and external rotation (deltoid, teres minor) Numbness over lateral shoulder (axillary sensory nerve)	Trauma (e.g., shoulder dislocation, fracture of proximal humerus) Entrapment of the quadrilateral space (compression of axillary nerve and posterior humeral circumflex artery)[5]
Musculocutaneous (C5, C6)	Weakness of elbow flexion and supination (biceps brachii, brachialis, coracobrachialis) Numbness of anterolateral forearm (lateral antebrachial cutaneous) Absent biceps reflex	Strenuous physical activity (e.g., weightlifting, rowing) Surgery Pressure during sleep
Ulnar (wrist: "Guyon Canal")	Weakness of hand intrinsics, hypothenar muscles Numbness of digit 5 and ulnar aspect of digit 4 + *spares the dorsal ulnar cutaneous*	Ganglion cyst, repetitive pressure (e.g., biker's palsy), repetitive activities (e.g., laborers using hand tools)
Proximal median	Weakness of thumb abduction/opposition + *thenar sensory involvement, wrist flexion weakness, thumb flexion weakness* Numbness in the first three digits and radial side of the fourth digit	Multiple possible compression sites in the region of antecubital fossa: ligament of Struthers, lacertus fibrosus, between two heads of pronator teres, flexor digitorum superficialis arch (sublimis bridge) External compression: trauma, casting, venipuncture
Anterior interosseous (pure motor branch from the median nerve in the forearm)	Weakness of thumb flexion (flexor pollicis longus), pronation (pronator quadratus), flexion of distal interphalangeal joints of digits 2 and 3 Inability to do "OK" sign Numbness: none	Crush injury, trauma, neuralgic amyotrophy

(continued)

TABLE 39.1 Other Upper Extremity Peripheral Mononeuropathies (continued)

Nerve	Symptoms	Causes
Posterior interosseous (pure motor branch from the radial nerve)	Weakness of wrist extension, finger extension Numbness: none	Nerve entrapment most commonly at the arcade of Frohse
Suprascapular (C5, C6)	**Suprascapular notch (more common):** weakness in shoulder abduction (supraspinatus) and external rotation (infraspinatus), atrophy of the supraspinous and infraspinous fossae **Spinoglenoid notch:** weakness in shoulder external rotation (infraspinatus), atrophy of infraspinous fossa Numbness: none	Compression by mass effect (e.g., ganglion cysts, cancerous lesions), neuralgic amyotrophy, activities with repetitive shoulder abduction/protraction (e.g., weightlifting, volleyball, baseball pitchers, dancers) thought to increase risk[1,5]
Long thoracic (C5, C6, C7)	Medial scapular winging (isolated serratus anterior involvement) which is most evident with active shoulder flexion Numbness: none[1,6]	External compression or stretch Neuralgic amyotrophy Iatrogenic (surgery)[1,6]
Spinal accessory (cranial nerve XI)	Lateral scapular winging (isolated trapezius involvement) which is most evident with active shoulder abduction Numbness: none	Trauma/stretch to posterior cervical triangle Cervical lymph node biopsy

glucocorticoids. Approximately two-thirds of patients have successful outcomes with conservative management. Surgical management includes surgical decompression. Referral for decompression rather than conservative management should be considered in those with significant axonal degeneration on NCS or active and chronic denervation on needle electromyography (EMG).

Ulnar Neuropathy at the Elbow

Ulnar neuropathy at the elbow (UNE) is the second most common entrapment neuropathy of the upper extremity. It is more common in men and more commonly involves the nondominant side. UNE is thought to occur from compression or mechanical stretch around the elbow, most commonly at the cubital tunnel and retrocondylar groove.

Signs/symptoms: Symptoms include paresthesias in the fourth/fifth digits, nocturnal symptoms, and medial elbow pain, which may radiate to the medial forearm into the hypothenar region. In severe cases, it can present with weakness in the intrinsic hand muscles (decreased pinch and grip strength), sometimes without significant sensory symptoms. Aggravating factors include sustained elbow flexion (e.g., talking on the phone), leaning on the elbow, sustained grip, or repetitive pronation/supination. Symptoms often improve with straightening of the elbow.

Examination: Examination shows hypoesthesia in the volar and dorsal fifth digit, medial fourth digit, and medial aspect of the hand (note: the medial forearm is spared as involvement would imply a more proximal plexus injury). Hypoesthesia over the dorsal medial hand implies dorsal ulnar cutaneous nerve involvement. In severe cases, atrophy of the hypothenar and thenar eminences (adductor pollicis and deep head of the flexor pollicis brevis are ulnar-innervated) can occur. Motor examination may reveal weakness in the hand intrinsics and finger flexors, with the first dorsal interosseous most affected. Symptoms may be provoked by applying pressure to the retrocondylar groove, with elbow flexion, and Tinel at the cubital tunnel/retrocondylar groove. Additional physical examination signs may include the Benediction posture (the ring and pinky finger metacarpophalangeal joints hyperextended and the proximal/distal interphalangeal joints flexed), Wartenberg sign (passively abducted pinky), and Froment sign (when trying to pinch a piece of paper, the long flexors of the thumb and index finger create a flexed thumb/index finger posture to compensate for intrinsic hand muscle weakness).[1]

Electrodiagnostic findings: A pure demyelinating process tends to be localizable, with focal slowing of ulnar motor nerve conduction velocities across the elbow. Inching studies, although technically demanding, may better localize the sites of compression. If pathology is primarily axonal, then localization may not be possible.

Management: Conservative management includes activity modification (avoid leaning on elbows and avoid sustained elbow flexion), soft foam elbow pad to prevent direct compression, and splints limiting elbow flexion to 45° to 90° at night (given poor compliance, wrapping the elbow with a towel may be better tolerated). Surgical management includes transposition or surgical decompression if the site of pathology is localizable (decompression is generally preferred over transposition).[3]

Radial Neuropathy

Radial nerve entrapment can occur at multiple locations along the path of the nerve, most often at the spiral groove followed by the axilla, which are the sites vulnerable to compression.

Signs/symptoms: At the spiral groove, it characteristically occurs when a person has the arm draped over a chair during deep sleep ("Saturday Night Palsy") or in the setting of humerus fracture, and presents with paresthesias in the dorsum of the radial side of the hand and proximal phalanges with wrist/finger drop. At the axilla, it can occur with inappropriate crutch use due to direct pressure. It has similar findings as the spiral groove, with the addition of paresthesias of the posterior arm and weakness of elbow extension.

Examination: Examination at the spiral groove shows decreased sensation in superficial radial sensory nerve distribution (lateral dorsum of the hand and dorsal proximal phalanges of the thumb, index, middle, and ring fingers), decreased brachioradialis reflex, marked finger and wrist drop, mild weakness of supination (supinator) and elbow flexion (brachioradialis), and full elbow extension strength as SPARES the triceps. Examination findings at the axilla are the same as spiral groove compression, plus elbow extension weakness and decreased sensation more proximally into the posterior forearm and arm, and will additionally show decreased triceps reflex.

Electrodiagnostic findings: Both lesions at the spiral groove and axilla typically have abnormal radial sensory nerve action potentials (SNAP) and compound muscle action potential (CMAP), but can be localized to the axilla if the triceps or anconeus are abnormal on needle EMG.[1]

Management: Conservative management includes physical therapy and wrist/finger splinting in extension. Surgical management is usually reserved for severe/acute injuries such as nerve laceration.[4]

Brachial Plexopathy

Causes of brachial plexopathy include traumatic brachial plexopathy (stretch, crush, penetrating injuries, etc.), neuralgic amyotrophy, iatrogenic, malignancy/mass lesions, and radiation injury (Table 39.2).[1]

TABLE 39.2 Brachial Plexopathy

Plexus Location	Signs
Panplexus	Complete sensory loss, weakness, and reflex loss in the entire arm (serratus anterior and rhomboids spared as these come directly off of the root level)
Upper trunk (C5–C6) "Erb palsy"	Weakness of deltoid, biceps, brachioradialis, rotator cuff muscles Partial weakness in those with partial C6 innervation Decreased sensation in the lateral arm, forearm, and first three and a half digits Decreased biceps and brachioradialis reflexes
Middle trunk (C7)	Weakness primarily in triceps, flexor carpi radialis, and pronator teres Decreased sensation in the posterior arm, forearm, and primarily third digit Decreased triceps reflex
Lower trunk (C8–T1) "Klumpke palsy"	Weakness of hand intrinsics, ulnar wrist deviation/flexion (all ulnar innervation) Decreased sensation in the medial arm, forearm, and medial aspect of the fourth digit and the whole fifth digit No reflex abnormalities
Lateral cord	Weakness in musculocutaneous/median nerve distributions: weakness in elbow flexion, wrist pronation, and wrist flexion Decreased sensation in the lateral forearm, hand, and first three fingers Decreased biceps reflex
Posterior cord	Weakness in radial/axillary/thoracodorsal distributions: weakness in shoulder abduction *and* adduction, elbow extension, wrist extension, and finger extension Decreased sensation in the lateral and posterior arm, posterior forearm, and dorsal hand Decreased brachioradialis and triceps reflexes
Medial cord	Weakness in all ulnar-innervated and C8–T1 median-innervated muscles which *spares* C8 radial distribution Weakness in hand intrinsics and flexors with sparing of finger extensors Sensory decreased in the medial arm, forearm, hand, and fourth/fifth digits Normal reflexes
Thoracic outlet syndrome (neurogenic)	Most cases of neurogenic thoracic outlet syndrome thought to be caused by compression from a fibrous band from anomalous cervical rib to first thoracic rib Affects C8–T1 but often preferentially affects T1 fibers with thenar > hypothenar wasting Leads to weakness in the hand intrinsics, finger flexors, and finger extension Decreased sensation in the medial arm, forearm, hand, and fourth/fifth digits Normal reflexes

MONONEUROPATHIES OF THE LOWER EXTREMITY

Peroneal/Fibular Neuropathy

Peroneal/fibular neuropathy is the most common entrapment neuropathy of the lower extremity. Compression of the common peroneal/fibular nerve most often occurs at the fibular neck.

Signs/symptoms: It presents with foot/toe drop and ankle eversion weakness, and sensory disturbances of the lateral leg, dorsum of the foot, and the first web space. Patients report toe dragging and foot slapping, which increase the risk of tripping and inversion ankle sprains. Risk of nerve entrapment increased with habitual crossed-leg posture, squatting, kneeling, trauma (e.g., knee dislocations, fibular fractures), and total knee replacements.

Examination: Examination shows decreased sensation of the lateral leg, dorsum of the foot, and the first web space; decreased strength in ankle dorsiflexion, great toe extension, and ankle eversion; steppage gait compensating for foot slap/toe drag; difficulty standing on heel on the affected side; and may have positive Tinel at the fibular neck provoking paresthesias.[1]

Electrodiagnostic findings: In demyelinating neuropathy, studies will show conduction block/slowing of peroneal/fibular motor studies across the fibular neck, normal superficial peroneal/fibular SNAP, and normal peroneal/fibular CMAP. In axonal neuropathy, studies will show decreased superficial peroneal/fibular SNAP and peroneal/fibular motor CMAP.[1]

Management: Conservative management includes bracing (e.g., ankle foot orthosis [AFO]), physical therapy, activity modification, padding of the fibular head, and ultrasound-guided hydrodissection.[6] Surgical management includes surgical decompression or repair.[7]

Femoral Neuropathy

Isolated lesions of the femoral nerve are uncommon and may need to be differentiated from more proximal L2 to L4 nerve root lesions. Known causes include positioning or compression during surgery, intra-abdominal/pelvic surgery, complication after total hip arthroplasty (anterior approach), compression at the inguinal ligament, and inguinal hematomas after femoral catheterization. Isolated femoral neuropathies should be further localized as being proximal or distal to the inguinal ligament.[1]

Signs/symptoms: If distal to the inguinal ligament, it presents with knee buckling from quadriceps weakness, with decreased sensation in the anteromedial thigh and medial leg. If proximal to the inguinal ligament, same as distal to the inguinal ligament, plus dragging of the leg from iliopsoas weakness.

Examination: If distal to the inguinal ligament, there is weakness of knee extension, decreased sensation in the anteromedial thigh and medial leg, and decreased patellar reflex. If proximal to the inguinal ligament, same as distal to the inguinal ligament, plus hip flexor weakness.[8]

Electrodiagnostic findings: Findings will show decreased femoral motor CMAP and saphenous SNAP. EMG for lesions proximal to the inguinal ligament should reveal abnormalities in the iliopsoas in addition to quadriceps muscles.[1]

Management: Conservative management includes physical therapy, drainage, or correction of coagulopathy for compressive hematomas.

Sciatic Neuropathy

Sciatic neuropathy, although uncommon, is the second most common nerve entrapment syndrome of the lower extremity. It presents similarly to the more common peroneal/fibular neuropathy and L5 radiculopathy, which often present with foot drop. Etiologies include posterior hip dislocation, hip replacement surgery, mass lesions, vasculitis, and trauma (compression or penetrating injury).[8]

Signs/symptoms: Complete sciatic neuropathy presents with weakness of the knee flexors and all movements of the ankle and toes and sensory disturbances involving the leg/foot distal to the knee, although initially may present with foot drop and associated toe dragging and foot slapping with gait.

Examination: Examination shows decreased sensation in the lateral knee (lateral cutaneous nerve of the knee), lateral thigh and leg, as well as the dorsum of the foot and the first web space (superficial/deep peroneal nerve), the posterior calf, lateral foot, and plantar aspect of the foot (tibial nerve). There is weakness of knee flexion, ankle dorsiflexion/plantarflexion and inversion/eversion, and toe flexors/extensors. Hip abduction strength should be normal (would be abnormal in L5 radiculopathy) and there is decreased Achilles reflex.[1]

Electrodiagnostic findings: Findings will show decreased superficial peroneal/fibular SNAP, sural SNAP, peroneal/fibular CMAP, and tibial CMAP if axonal injury, as well as prolonged H-reflex. EMG should be abnormal in the short head of the biceps femoris (normal in peroneal/fibular neuropathy) and normal for the gluteus maximus, medius, minimus, and tensor fascia lata (abnormal in L5–S1 lumbosacral radiculopathy).[1]

Management: Management includes physical therapy, bracing (e.g., ankle AFO), and treatment directed at the underlying cause (e.g., steroids and immunotherapy for vasculitis).

LUMBOSACRAL PLEXOPATHY

The lumbosacral plexus is anatomically divided into the upper lumbar plexus and the lower lumbosacral plexus. Each plexus is divided into anterior and posterior divisions (Table 39.3). Symptoms of lumbosacral plexopathies include weakness, pain, and sensory abnormalities in the lower extremity. Common causes include retroperitoneal hemorrhage, tumors and other mass lesions, neuralgic amyotrophy, radiation injury, and postpartum obstetric injuries. Treatment will depend on the underlying etiology and may include physical therapy, nonsteroidal anti-inflammatory drugs (NSAIDs) and neuropathic agents to manage pain, and surgery to relieve mechanical compression due to structural lesions.[1]

TABLE 39.3 Lumbosacral Plexopathy

Plexus Location	Signs
Upper lumbar plexus (ventral rami of L1–L4 roots)	Weakness of the iliopsoas, quadriceps, and adductor muscles
Anterior division: L2–L4 roots, obturator nerve (hip adductors)	Reduced or absent patellar tendon reflex
Posterior division: L2–L4 roots, femoral nerve (hip flexors and knee extensors) and the LCNT	Pain that radiates from the pelvis to the anterior thigh
Terminal branches: iliohypogastric nerve, ilioinguinal nerve, genitofemoral nerve	Sensory loss and paresthesias over the lateral, anterior, and medial thigh, as well as the medial lower leg (saphenous nerve)
	Isolated lesions of the LCNT (meralgia paresthetica) present with purely sensory signs of pain and numbness in well-circumscribed distribution of the anterolateral thigh
Lower lumbosacral plexus (ventral rami of L4–S1 nerve roots)	Weakness of the hip extensors, abductors, and internal rotators; hamstrings and muscles innervated by tibial and peroneal nerves (may be preferential involvement of peroneal nerve fibers leading to isolated foot drop)
Anterior division: L5–S2 roots, tibial division of the sciatic nerve (knee flexors) and tibial nerve (plantarflexors and inverters)	
Posterior division: L5–S2 roots, peroneal division of the sciatic nerve (short head biceps femoris) and peroneal nerve (dorsiflexors and evertors)	Absent ankle reflex
	Pain radiating from the pelvis to the posterior thigh and posterolateral lower leg
Terminal branches: superior and inferior gluteal nerves	Sensory loss and paresthesias over the posterior thigh and posterolateral leg to the foot

LCNT, lateral femoral cutaneous nerve of the thigh.

RADICULOPATHY

Radiculopathy can involve any of the spinal nerve roots, most commonly in the cervical and lumbosacral regions (Tables 39.4 and 39.5). Symptoms include pain in a radicular pattern, dermatomal sensory abnormalities, and myotomal weakness. It is commonly caused by mechanical compression from nearby tissues, such as intervertebral disc or bony abnormalities due to spondylosis or acute injury. Less common causes include a local mass or infection.

Management: Nonsurgical treatments include activity modification, physical therapy, medications such as NSAIDs, muscle relaxants, neuropathic agents, and corticosteroid injections. Surgery is typically reserved for symptoms refractory to conservative management or cases of progressive or disabling motor and/or sensory deficits. Symptoms of saddle anesthesia, progressive balance difficulties, and bowel/bladder incontinence would be suggestive of a compressive cord lesion or cauda equina syndrome, which would warrant emergent surgical evaluation.

Electrodiagnostic findings: Findings will show normal SNAP due to the distal location of the dorsal root ganglia, and decreased CMAP amplitude may be present in more severe/chronic cases. EMG may reveal active denervation and/or chronic neuropathic findings in the affected myotomes. Paraspinals are the earliest muscles affected, although may reinnervate and therefore appear normal in cases of chronic radiculopathy.

PERIPHERAL NEUROPATHY

Peripheral neuropathies comprise numerous disease processes that affect the myelin and/or axons of all or many of the peripheral nerves. Their etiologies are diverse and can be categorized into inherited or acquired. Inherited peripheral neuropathies are rare and include Charcot-Marie-Tooth disease (a hereditary motor and sensory neuropathy). Acquired peripheral neuropathies may be secondary to toxic, medication-induced, inflammatory, endocrine, vitamin deficiency, infectious, paraneoplastic, critical illness and idiopathic etiologies, with the most common cause being diabetes mellitus. Their presentation may be acute, subacute, or slowly progressive depending on their underlying etiologies (Table 39.6).[1]

Electrodiagnostic findings: Electrodiagnostic studies are useful in identifying the presence and severity of a peripheral neuropathy. They are used to identify patterns of demyelination versus axonal loss in the sensory and/or motor peripheral nerves, which can help guide further workup to identify the underlying etiology and determine treatment options and prognosis.

Management: Management involves identifying and treating the underlying cause of the peripheral neuropathy, as well as rehabilitative management to treat associated impairments. This may include physical therapy, orthotics for foot drop, and treatments for neuropathic pain (medications, alternative therapies such as acupuncture, transcutaneous electrical nerve stimulation [TENS], and other modalities).

TABLE 39.4 Cervical Radiculopathy

Nerve Root	Pain Distribution	Sensory Deficit	Motor Deficit	Key Muscles	Reflex Deficit
C4	Lower neck, trapezius	"Cape-like" distribution	N/A	N/A	N/A
C5	Neck, shoulder, lateral arm, scapula	Lateral shoulder and lateral arm	Shoulder abduction and external rotation, elbow flexion	Deltoid, supraspinatus, infraspinatus, rhomboids, biceps, brachioradialis	Biceps, brachioradialis
C6	Neck, shoulder, dorsal/lateral arm and forearm, thumb	Lateral forearm, thumb, index finger	Wrist extension, shoulder abduction, elbow flexion, forearm pronation	Deltoid, supraspinatus, infraspinatus, biceps, brachioradialis, triceps pronator teres, FCR, ECR	Biceps, brachioradialis
C7	Neck, dorsal/lateral forearm, middle finger	Dorsal forearm, middle finger, index finger	Elbow extension, wrist flexion, forearm pronation	Triceps, pronator teres, latissimus dorsi, FCR, ECR	Triceps
C8	Neck, medial forearm, hand, ring and small fingers	Medial forearm, ring and small fingers, hypothenar eminence	Finger abduction, hand grip	Hand intrinsics, finger flexors and extensors	N/A
T1	Neck, axilla, medial arm and forearm, chest	Medial forearm, medial arm, axilla	Thumb abduction	FDS and FDP to index and middle fingers, APB, FPL	N/A

APB, abductor pollicis brevis; ECR, extensor carpi radialis; FCR, flexor carpi radialis; FDP, flexor digitorum profundus; FDS, flexor digitorum superficialis; FPL, flexor pollicis longus; N/A, not applicable.

TABLE 39.5 Lumbosacral Radiculopathy

Nerve Root	Pain Distribution	Sensory Deficit	Motor Deficit	Key Muscles	Reflex Deficit
L1	Inguinal region	Inguinal region	N/A	N/A	Cremasteric
L2	Groin, anterior thigh	Anterolateral thigh	Hip flexion, hip adduction	Iliopsoas	Cremasteric
L3	Anterior thigh to knee, groin	Medial thigh and knee	Knee extension, hip flexion, hip adduction	Quadriceps, iliopsoas, hip adductors	Patellar (variable)
L4	Anterior thigh, medial lower leg	Medial lower leg	Knee extension, hip flexion, hip adduction	Quadriceps, tibialis anterior, hip adductors	Patellar
L5	Lateral thigh, anterolateral lower leg, dorsal foot	Dorsal/lateral lower leg, dorsal foot, great toe	Ankle dorsiflexion, inversion, and eversion, great toe extension, hip abduction	Tibialis anterior, tibialis posterior, peroneus longus and brevis, EHL, gluteus medius, TFL	Medial hamstring
S1	Posterior thigh, calf, heel	Lateral foot, toes, and ankle, sole of foot	Ankle plantarflexion, knee flexion, hip extension	Gastrocnemius, soleus, hamstrings, gluteus maximus	Achilles
S2-S4	Posterior thigh (S2), medial buttocks	Medial buttocks, perineal and perianal region	Ankle plantarflexion, knee flexion, and hip extension (S2), anal contraction (S2-4)	Gastrocnemius, soleus, medial hamstrings, gluteus maximus, external anal sphincter	Bulbocavernosus, anal wink

EHL, extensor hallucis longus; N/A, not applicable; TFL, tensor fasciae lata.

TABLE 39.6 Peripheral Neuropathy

Type of Peripheral Neuropathy	Signs and Symptoms
Axonal loss (most peripheral neuropathies including diabetes, B_{12} deficiency, thyroid disorders, alcohol and other toxins, critical illness, connective tissue)	Symmetric and length-dependent onset of symptoms involving sensory changes in a stocking/glove distribution Distal weakness and reduced or absent distal reflexes
Mononeuropathy multiplex (vasculitis, diabetes, inflammatory demyelinating polyneuropathy, Lyme disease, leprosy, HIV, sarcoid, lymphoma/leukemia)	Asymmetric presentation with stepwise progression of motor and sensory symptoms
Charcot Marie Tooth (most common inherited peripheral neuropathy)	Presents at an early age with slowly progressive muscle weakness, muscle atrophy, and development of pes cavus and hammertoes Other hereditary polyneuropathies present primarily with autonomic and sensory loss or primarily motor symptoms
Acute demyelinating ("Guillain-Barré syndrome" or acute inflammatory demyelinating polyneuropathy)	Symmetric, ascending paralysis Motor symptoms more prominent than sensory Occurs over days to weeks Usually preceded by upper respiratory infection or gastroenteritis
CIPD	Slowly progressive, symmetric motor predominant with both proximal and distal weakness, impairments in vibration and proprioception, hyporeflexia Can follow stepwise progression or relapsing and remitting course Usually presents in fifth to sixth decade

CIPD, chronic inflammatory demyelinating polyneuropathy.

REFERENCES

The full complete reference list for this chapter appears in the digital version of the chapter, available at http://connect.springerpub.com/content/book/978-0-8261-5628-0/part/part04/chapter/ch39

CHAPTER 40

PELVIC HEALTH REHABILITATION

Sarah Hwang

INTRODUCTION

The pelvic floor is a group of muscles, fascia, and ligaments that support the pelvic organs, aid in stabilization, help provide bowel and bladder control, and are important in sexual function. The pelvic floor muscles function as part of the core.

Pelvic floor disorders include a wide range of conditions that can significantly affect a person's quality of life. Pelvic floor disorders can result in myofascial pelvic pain, bowel and bladder dysfunction, dyspareunia, and pelvic organ prolapse (POP). Any person can develop pelvic floor disorders, although females are at an increased risk due to their pelvic anatomy and biomechanics. A 2014 study demonstrated a prevalence of approximately 25% of symptomatic pelvic floor disorders in women in the United States.[1] Urinary incontinence is also seen in men, most notably post prostatectomy.

Chronic pelvic pain (CPP) can affect both men and women and can result from a variety of causes, including musculoskeletal, gynecologic, urologic, gastrointestinal, neurologic, and psychosocial conditions. Oftentimes, CPP can be multifactorial; thus, a multidisciplinary approach to treatment is favored. Physiatrists have knowledge in pain, neurogenic and musculoskeletal disorders, and bowel and bladder management and thus are well-suited to direct care for patients with pelvic floor disorders and CPP.[2]

PELVIC FLOOR DYSFUNCTION

When the pelvic floor muscles are functioning correctly, the muscles can voluntarily and involuntarily contract and relax.[3] Pelvic floor dysfunction is the inability to properly contract and relax the pelvic floor muscles. In general, underactive or noncontracting pelvic floor cannot voluntarily contract when desired,[3] resulting in conditions such as stress urinary incontinence, fecal incontinence, and POP. High-tone or overactive pelvic floor muscles do not relax properly[3] and typically result in pain, dyspareunia, constipation, and urinary frequency/urgency. Noncontracting, nonrelaxing pelvic floor occurs when the muscles are hypertonic but also weak.

Urinary Incontinence

Urinary incontinence is defined as the involuntary leakage of urine. It is further subdivided into three types:

- *Stress urinary incontinence (SUI):* occurs with an increase in intra-abdominal pressure in the setting of deficiencies in the pelvic floor muscles, urethra, bladder, and/or sphincter, resulting in difficulty maintaining urethral closure pressures
- *Urge urinary incontinence (UUI):* occurs with a sudden urge to void that cannot be overcome, resulting in urinary leakage, and can occur from both iatrogenic and neurologic causes
- *Mixed urinary incontinence:* occurs when a person experiences both SUI and UUI

Fecal Incontinence

Fecal incontinence (FI) is the involuntary loss of stool. The incidence of FI increases with age. FI can result from many different causes, including neurologic disease, gastrointestinal disorders, weakness of or injury to the pelvic floor, pelvic surgery, or pelvic radiation.[4]

Pelvic Organ Prolapse

POP occurs when the structural support of the pelvis is compromised, resulting in descent of the internal organs into the vagina. There are three major types of POP:

- *Cystocele:* the most common type of POP which occurs when the bladder descends into the vagina
- *Rectocele:* occurs when the rectum descends into the vagina
- *Uterine prolapse:* occurs when the uterus descends into the vagina

Pelvic Myofascial Pain

Pelvic floor myofascial pain is defined as a regional condition of myofascial pain and tightness caused by chronic muscle contraction. It is characterized by tender points, taut bands, and trigger points within the pelvic floor muscles.[5]

Dyssynergic Defecation

Dyssynergic defecation occurs as a result of pelvic floor dysfunction, where there is inability to coordinate the relaxation needed in order to defecate.

Treatment of Pelvic Floor Dysfunction

Pelvic floor physical examination includes evaluation of the pelvic muscles, nerves, and bony structures. Individualized pelvic floor physical therapy should be incorporated into the treatment of pelvic floor dysfunction. Therapy should not only be prescribed to address the pelvic floor, but should also include treatment for other contributing conditions, including lumbar spine pathology and pelvic girdle pathology. Bowel and bladder retraining and education should be a focus in patients experiencing these issues. Appropriate referrals to urogynecology, urology, and gastroenterology to rule out other causes of symptoms should be included as well.

CHRONIC PELVIC PAIN

CPP is defined as noncyclic pain of greater than 6 months in duration that localizes to the pelvis, anterior abdominal wall at or below the umbilicus, or the buttocks and is sufficient in severity to cause functional disability or require medical care.[6] CPP can be multifactorial in nature and can arise from multiple organ systems, including the musculoskeletal and neurologic systems. Myofascial pelvic pain is one cause of CPP. This condition is often seen alongside other diagnoses of CPP. Other common causes of CPP include endometriosis, vulvodynia, irritable bowel syndrome, interstitial cystitis, chronic prostatitis, central sensitization, anxiety, depression, and a history of trauma or sexual abuse.

Pelvic nerve injuries should also be considered when evaluating patients with CPP. The border nerves (ilioinguinal, iliohypogastric, genitofemoral nerves) and the pudendal nerves most commonly contribute to pelvic pain symptoms. Injuries to the border nerves can occur after pelvic surgeries, including gynecologic surgeries and inguinal hernia repairs. Injuries to the pudendal nerves can occur after vaginal delivery, pelvic surgeries, and cycling, with chronic straining during defecation or during anal intercourse.[7]

Treatment of Chronic Pelvic Pain

A multidisciplinary approach to treatment of CPP may include multiple medical specialties (physical medicine and rehabilitation, gynecology, urogynecology, urology, gastroenterology, colorectal surgery, neurology, primary care, and psychiatry). In addition, treatment may include pelvic floor physical therapy, sex therapy, and pain psychology. Medications can be utilized to reduce pain, treat anxiety, and restore restful sleep. Injections can be utilized to treat pelvic floor myofascial pain, including trigger point injections and botulinum toxin injections.

REFERENCES

The full complete reference list for this chapter appears in the digital version of the chapter, available at http://connect.springerpub.com/content/book/978-0-8261-5628-0/part/part04//chapter/ch40

INDEX

AAC. *See* augmentative alternative communication
ABI. *See* acquired brain injury
achilles tendinitis, 320
ACL. *See* anterior cruciate ligament
acquired brain injury (ABI), 231
activities of daily living (ADLs), 50
acupuncture, 62–63
acute inflammatory demyelinating polyneuropathy (AIDP), 225
acute inpatient rehabilitation, 4
AD. *See* autonomic dysreflexia
adaptive equipment (AE), 55–57
adhesive capsulitis, 308
ADLs. *See* activities of daily living, 50
AE. *See* adaptive equipment
ALS. *See* amyotrophic lateral sclerosis
The Americans With Disabilities Act
    accessible office and policies, 32, 33
    communication, 32
    physical examination, 32
    requirements, 29–30
amputations
    acquired, 69–70
    congenital limb deficiencies, 70
    lower extremity, 73–74
    prosthesis. *see* Prosthesis
    upper extremity, 70–73
amyotrophic lateral sclerosis (ALS)
    electromyography (EMG), 223
    nerve conduction studies (NCS), 223
    physical examination findings, 223, 224
anemia, 106–107
ankle sprains and instability, 320–321
antalgic gait, 36
anterior cord syndrome, 181
anterior cruciate ligament (ACL), 315–316
AOS. *See* apraxia of speech
aphasia
    causes, 251
    communication-based therapy, 252
    impairment-based therapy, 251–252
    types of, 251, 253–254
apraxia, 8–9
apraxia of speech (AOS), 255
ataxia, 222
athetosis, 222
atrial fibrillation, 88
augmentative alternative communication (AAC), 252
autonomic dysreflexia (AD), 184–186
axial pain
    discogenic pain, 301–302
    facet (zygapophyseal) joint pain, 299–300
    sacroiliac joint dysfunction, 301
axonotmesis, 277

Baker cyst, 320
Borg's Rating of Perceived Exertion (RPE) Scale, 87
braces, 50
brachial plexopathy, 340–341
Brown-Séquard syndrome, 180
burn rehabilitation
    community reintegration, 103

contractures, 100
epidemiology, 97
heterotopic ossification (HO), 102
hypermetabolic response, 101
pruritus, 101–102
psychiatric complications, 102
scarring, 100–101

cachexia, 104–105
calcium pyrophosphate deposition disease (CPPD), 134
cancer rehabilitation
bone metastases, 106
CIPN, 107–108
CRF, 105–106
epidemiology, 104
hematologic changes, 106–107
hormonal/endocrine therapy, 108–109
immunotherapy and cellular therapies, 109–110
lymphedema, 112
radiation therapy (RT), 111
surgery, 111–112
cancer-related fatigue (CRF), 105–106
cardiac rehabilitation (CR)
atrial fibrillation with rapid ventricular response, 88
cardiac precautions, 89
contraindications, 83, 85
epidemiology, 83
exercise physiology and prescription, 84–87
heart failure exacerbation, 87–88
phases, 83, 84
sternal precautions, 89
ventricular assist devices, 88–89
carpal tunnel syndrome, 336–339
cauda equina syndrome (CES), 181
central cord syndrome, 180
cerebral palsy (CP)
associated disorders, 161
classification, 160–161
definition, 160
diagnosis, 160
etiology, 160
HINE score, 162
treatment, 161
cervical spine
radiculopathy, 345–346
spurling maneuver, 18
CES. *See* cauda equina syndrome
Charcot Marie Tooth (CMT), 165–166
chemotherapy-induced peripheral neuropathy (CIPN), 107–108
Chiari malformations, 163
chorea, 222
chronic compartment syndrome, 319–320
chronic inflammatory demyelinating polyneuropathy (CIPD), 225–226
chronic pelvic pain, 351
chronic obstructive pulmonary disease (COPD), 91–92
CILT. *See* constraint-induced language therapy
CIPD. *See* chronic inflammatory demyelinating polyneuropathy
CIPN. *See* chemotherapy-induced peripheral neuropathy
CIS. *See* clinically isolated syndrome
clinically isolated syndrome (CIS), 211
CMT. *See* Charcot Marie Tooth
cognitive impairment
definition, 230
differential diagnosis, 231–232
domains and processes, 230–231
imaging, 234
laboratory testing, 233–234

neuropsychological test, 234
screening tools, 233
treatment, 234–235
color perception, 12
coma, 193
complex regional pain syndrome (CRPS), 288–290
concussion
    assessment tools and questionnaires, 200
    CT imaging, 202
    definition, 198
    epidemiology, 198
    history, 198–200
    management, 202–203
    molecular basis, 198, 199
    physical examination, 200–201
    symptoms, 201
    vestibular changes, 201–202
constraint-induced language therapy (CILT), 251
contractures, 100
conus medullaris syndrome, 181
COPD. *See* chronic obstructive pulmonary disease
corticospinal tract (CST), 177
COVID-19 rehabilitation
    autonomic dysfunction, 144
    cardiovascular complications, 144
    cognitive impairment, 143
    dysphagia, 145
    exercise prescription and therapy intervention, 146–147
    fatigue, 143–144
    headache, 142
    hypercoagulability, 144–145
    neuropathy and myopathy, 142
    peripheral compression neuropathies, 142
    pressure ulcers, 145
    psychiatric disorders/sleep, 145–146
COPD. *See* chronic obstructive pulmonary disease

Cozen test, 20
CP. *See* cerebral palsy
CPPD. *See* calcium pyrophosphate deposition disease
CR. *See* cardiac rehabilitation
cranial nerves
    abducens, 10
    facial, 10–11
    glossopharyngeal, 11
    hypoglossal, 12
    oculomotor, 10
    olfactory, 9–10
    optic, 10
    spinal accessory, 11–12
    trigeminal, 10
    trochlear, 10
    vagus, 11
    vestibulocochlear, 11
CRF. *See* cancer-related fatigue
CRPS. *See* complex regional pain syndrome
cryotherapy, 60
CST. *See* corticospinal tract

Daily Adjusted Progressive Resistance Exercise (DAPRE) method, 65
day rehabilitation, 4
debility and immobility
    cardiopulmonary, 120
    definition, 119
    endocrine, 121
    gastrointestinal and genitourinary, 121
    integumentary, 121
    musculoskeletal, 120–121
deep gluteal syndrome, 313
deep venous thrombosis
    chemoprophylaxis based on ASIA grading, 125
    DOACs, 124
    low-molecular-weight heparin (LMWH), 124
    risk factors, 123
    total hip or knee arthroplasty (THA/TKA), 124–125

unfractionated heparin (UFH), 123–124
warfarin (vitamin K antagonist), 124
delirium, 232
DeLorme axiom method, 65
dementia, 231
de Quervain Tenosynovitis, 310
dermatomyositis (DM), 227–228
detrusor sphincter dyssynergia (DSD), 245–246
digital Stenosing tenosynovitis (Trigger Finger), 311
direct oral anticoagulants (DOACs), 124
disability
  acceptable *vs.* unacceptable language, 26–27
  biomedical model, 27
  definition, 26
  International Classification of Functioning (ICF), 28–29
  person-centered care, 30–31
  shared decision-making, 31
  social model, 27–28
  social security administration, 29
  supported decision-making, 31
  worker's compensation, 29
discogenic pain, 301–302
DM. *See* dermatomyositis
DOACs. *See* direct oral anticoagulants
dorsal root ganglion (DRG) stimulation, 292
DSD. *See* detrusor sphincter dyssynergia
dual antiplatelet therapy (DAPT), 208
dynamic elastic response (DER) foot, 81
dysarthria, 255, 257
dysarthria-clumsy hand syndrome, 205
dysphagia, 145
  aspiration, 256
  cranial nerve functions, 258
  esophageal phase, 256
  etiology, 256, 258
  instrumental assessment, 259
  management and treatment, 259–261
  medications side effect, 258
  oral phase, 256
  penetration, 256
  pharyngeal phase, 256
dyspnea, 141–142
dyssynergic defecation, 350
dystonia, 220–222

EDx. *See* electrodiagnostic testing
elbow
  lateral epicondylitis, 20, 309–310
  medial epicondylitis, 20, 309–310
  ulnar neuropathy, 339–340
electrodiagnostic testing (EDx)
  definition, 265
  electromyography, 272–278
  history and physical examination, 266
  nerve conduction study, 266–272
  pathology patterns, 278–279
  patient considerations, 265–266
  relative contraindications/ precautions, 265
  report, 279
electromyography
  concentric, 272–273
  monopolar, 272
  motor unit action potential features, 273–275
  Seddon classification, 277–278
  waveforms, 275–277
exercise prescription
  aerobic and anaerobic, 66
  components, 63–64
  effectiveness, 64
  recommendations, 63

strength training exercises.
see Strength training exercises
extraocular movements, 12–13

facet (zygapophyseal) joint pain, 299–300
FAI. *See* femoral acetabular impingement
falls, 129–130
femoral acetabular impingement (FAI), 314
femoral neck fracture, 153–154
femoral neuropathy, 342–343
fibromyalgia, 135–136
finger-to-chin test, 16–17
foot, ankle, and lower leg
  achilles tendinitis, 320
  anterior drawer test, 25
  gout, 133–134
  peroneal/fibular neuropathy, 342
  plantar fasciitis, 321–322
  rheumatoid arthritis, 132–133
  sciatic neuropathy, 343
  sprains and instability, 320–321
  tarsal tunnel syndrome, 322
frailty, 119

gait
  analysis, 17
  ankle dorsiflexors, 34
  ankle plantar flexors, 34
  cane basics, 40
  components of, 34, 35
  crutch basics, 40–42
  gastrocnemius, 36
  gluteus maximus (extensor lurch), 37
  gluteus medius–minimus (Trendelenburg), 36–37
  hip abductors, 34
  hip extensors/hamstrings, 35
  hip flexors, 34
  knee extensors, 35
  muscle-deficit, 36–38

  neuromuscular impairments, 39
  standing, 35–36
  quadriceps (back knee) gait, 37–38
  walker basics, 42–43
GBS. *See* Guillain–Barré syndrome
gout
  clinical manifestations, 133–134
  laboratory and imaging findings, 134
  treatment, 134
Graded Symptom Checklist (GSC), 200
greater trochanteric pain syndrome, 313
GSC. *See* Graded Symptom Checklist
Guillain–Barré syndrome (GBS), 94

heart failure exacerbation (HFE), 87–88
heat (thermotherapy), 58–60
heel-to-shin test, 17
hemiballismus, 222
hemiparesis-hemiataxia syndrome, 206
hemiplegic gait, 39
hemispatial neglect, 13
hereditary motor and sensory neuropathy (HMSN), 165
heterotopic ossification (HO), 102, 187, 196
  symptoms, 122
  treatment, 122–123
HHR. *See* humeral head replacement
hip
  deep gluteal syndrome, 313
  FABER / Patrick test, 23
  FADIR, 23
  femoral acetabular impingement, 314
  femoral neck fracture, 153
  femoral neuropathy, 342–343

greater trochanteric pain syndrome, 313
iliotibial band syndrome, 314
intertrochanteric fractures, 153–154
osteoarthritis (OA), 131–132
sacroiliac joint pain, 312–313
stinch field resisted hip flexion, 23
total hip arthroplasty, 151–152
hip-spine syndrome, 312
home health, 5
humeral head replacement (HHR), 150–151
HMSN. *See* hereditary motor and sensory neuropathy
HO. *See* heterotopic ossification
hypercoagulability, 144–145
hypermetabolic response, 101

IBM. *See* inclusion body myositis
ILD. *See* interstitial lung disease
iliotibial band syndrome, 314
inclusion body myositis (IBM), 228
insomnia
  medications, 128–129
  sleep barriers, 128
intensive care unit (ICU) rehabilitation
  ABCDEF bundle, 157–158
  delirium, 157
  PADIS guidelines, 156
  physical therapists role, 158
  speech therapy, 158
International Standards for Neurological Classification of Spinal Cord Injury (ISNCSCI), 178–180
interstitial lung disease, 93–94
intertrochanteric fractures, 153–154
iontophoresis, 61–62
ISNCSCI. *See* International Standards for Neurological Classification of Spinal Cord Injury

jersey finger (flexor digitorum profundus rupture), 311
JIA. *See* juvenile idiopathic arthritis
joint replacement rehabilitation
  hip, 151–152
  knee, 148–149
  shoulder, 149–151
juvenile idiopathic arthritis (JIA), 172–173

Karvonen formula, 86
Kennedy disease. *See* X-linked spinobulbar muscular atrophy
knee
  anterior cruciate ligament (ACL), 315–316
  anterior drawer test, 24
  Baker cyst, 320
  chronic compartment syndrome, 319–320
  Lachman test, 24
  McMurray test, 24
  medial tibial stress syndrome, 319
  meniscal injury, 317–318
  osteoarthritis (OA), 131–132
  patellofemoral pain syndrome (PFPS), 318–319
  pes anserine bursa, 314
  pseudogout, 134
  single-leg squat, 25
  stress fractures, 319
  total knee arthroplasty, 148–149
  Valgus stress test, 23

Lambert-Eaton myasthenic syndrome (LEMS), 227
Lateral medullary (Wallenberg) syndrome, 205
LEMS. *See* LambertEaton myasthenic syndrome

long-term acute care hospital (LTACH), 4
LTACH. *See* long-term acute care hospital
lumbar spinal fusion, 154–155
left ventricular assist device [LVAD] implantation, 88–89
lumbosacral spine and pelvis
 Fortin finger, 22
 Kemp test, 22
 lumbosacral plexopathy, 344
 radiculopathy, 345, 347
 seated slump, 22
 straight leg raise, 22
lymphedema, 112

mallet finger (distal extensor tendon rupture), 311
manager/social worker (MSW), 5
massage, 61
MCS. *See* minimally conscious state
medial and lateral epicondylitis, 309–310
medial tibial stress syndrome, 319
melodic intonation therapy (MIT), 252
meniscal injury, 317–318
MG. *See* myasthenia gravis
minimally conscious state (MCS), 193
MIT. *See* melodic intonation therapy
mobility
 gait. *see* gait
 wheelchairs. *see* wheelchairs
motor neuron diseases
 amyotrophic lateral sclerosis. *see* amyotrophic lateral sclerosis (ALS)
 demyelinating polyneuropathies, 225–226
 Kennedy disease, 224
 myopathy, 227–229
 neuromuscular junction disorders, 226–227
 spinal muscular atrophy, 224–225
motor speech disorders
 apraxia of speech, 255
 dysarthria, 255, 257
 neurogenic stuttering (NS), 255–256
movement disorders
 hyperkinetic, 220–222
 Parkinson disease. *see* Parkinson disease
MS. *See* multiple sclerosis
MSW. *See* manager/social worker
multiple sclerosis (MS)
 chronic fatigue, 215
 cognitive impairment, 215
 diagnosis and clinical features, 211–212
 disease-modifying therapy (DMT), 214–215
 epidemiology, 211
 gait impairment, 215
 IV corticosteroids, 213–214
 prognosis, 216
 RRMS, 212–213
muscle stretch reflexes
 Babinski, 16
 grading, 14, 15
 pathologic conditions, 15, 16
 primitive reflexes, 16
muscular dystrophy
 childhood inflammatory myopathies, 169
 Duchenne muscular dystrophy *vs.* Becker muscular dystrophy, 167–168
 Emery Dreifuss muscular dystrophy (EDMD), 168
 facioscapulohumeral muscular dystrophy (FSHD), 168
 myotonic muscular dystrophy, 169
musculoskeletal examination

cervical spine, 18
elbow, 19–20
foot, ankle, and lower leg, 25
hip and thigh, 22–23
knee, 23–25
lumbosacral spine and pelvis, 21–22
shoulder, 18–19
wrist and hand, 20–21
myasthenia gravis (MG), 226–227
myoclonus, 222
myopathy, 227–229

nerve conduction study
anomalous innervations, 271
setup, 268–271
terminology, 266–268
troubleshooting, 271–272
Neurobehavioral Symptom Inventory (NSI), 200
neurogenic bladder
bladder distention, 243
bladder innervation, 243, 244
functional classification, 244–245
neuroanatomy, 243
sacral or infrasacral lesions, 247
suprapontine lesions, 246
suprasacral lesions, 246–247
neurogenic bowel
classification of, 248, 249
management, 249–250
neuroanatomy, 247
parasympathetic innervation, 247, 248
somatic innervation, 248
sympathetic innervation, 248
neurogenic stuttering (NS), 255–256
neuromuscular respiratory failure, 94–95
neurologic examination
balance and coordination, 16–17
cognition, 8–9
cranial nerves. *see* cranial nerves
funduscopic, 12–13
MSRs. *see* muscle stretch reflexes
muscle strength grading, 14
muscle tone, 13–14
sensation, 16
speech and language, 9
neuropraxia, 277
neuropsychologist/rehabilitation psychologist, 5
neurotmesis, 277–278
neutropenia, 107
noninvasive ventilation (NIV), 95
NS. *See* neurogenic stuttering
NSI. *See* Neurobehavioral Symptom Inventory

OA. *See* osteoarthritis
occupational therapy (OT), 50, 133, 290
OP. *See* osteoporosis
oral reading for language in aphasia (ORLA), 251
ORLA. *See* oral reading for language in aphasia
orthoses
adaptive equipment (AE), 55–57
lower extremity, 50, 53–54
upper extremity, 50–52
orthotist, 6
osseointegration, 76–77
osteoarthritis (OA), 306
clinical manifestations, 131
laboratory and imaging findings, 131
risk factors, 131
treatment, 131–132
osteoporosis (OP), 187
laboratory and imaging findings, 136–137
risk factors, 136
screening, 137
treatment, 138–139
OT. *See* occupational therapy
outpatient rehabilitation, 4–5

pain medicine
  cannabinoids, 296
  complex regional pain syndrome (CRPS), 288–290
  equianalgesic opioid conversion, 297–298
  implanted drug delivery systems/pumps, 292–294
  lidocaine/ketamine infusions, 296
  muscle relaxants, 295–296
  neuromodulation techniques, 290–292
  neuropathic pain, 294–295
  nonopioid analgesics, 295
  pathophysiology, 288
Parkinson disease (PD)
  causes of disability, 217, 218
  incidence and prevalence, 217
  motor and nonmotor symptoms, 217, 218
  pathophysiology, 217
  severity of disease, 217, 218
  treatment, 218–220
Parkinsonian gait, 39
paroxysmal sympathetic hyperactivity (PSH), 196
patellofemoral pain syndrome (PFPS), 318–319
patient care technician (PCT), 6
PCL. *See* posterior cruciate ligament
PD. *See* Parkinson disease
peak exercise capacity, 86–87
pediatric rehabilitation
  botulism, 166
  cancer, 172
  cerebral palsy (CP), 160–162
  congenital brachial plexus palsy, 171
  juvenile idiopathic arthritis (JIA), 172–173
  muscular dystrophy. *see* Muscular dystrophy
  myasthenia gravis, 166
  postinfectious and metabolic polyneuropathies, 166
  SCIs, 169–170
  scoliosis, 170–171
  therapy services, 174
  traumatic brain injuries (TBIs), 171
pelvic floor dysfunction
  dyssynergic defecation, 350
  fecal incontinence (FI), 350
  pelvic myofascial pain, 350
  treatment of, 350–351
pelvic health rehabilitation
  CPP, 351
  pelvic floor dysfunction, 349–351
peripheral nerve stimulation (PNS), 291–292
peripheral neuropathy, 345, 348
peroneal/fibular neuropathy, 342
pes anserine bursitis, 314
PFPS. *See* patellofemoral pain syndrome
phonophoresis, 61
physiatrist, 5
physiatry
  interdisciplinary team, 5–6
  levels of care, 3–5
  patient-centered approach, 3
  training and board certification, 7
physical therapist (PT), 5
physical therapy (PT), 50
plantar fasciitis, 321–322
PNS. *See* peripheral nerve stimulation
polymyositis (PM), 227–228
post acute sequelae of COVID-19 (PASC). *See* COVID-19 rehabilitation
Post-Concussion Symptom Scale (PCSS), 200
posterior cruciate ligament (PCL), 316
posttraumatic agitation, 195
posttraumatic amnesia (PTA), 191
posttraumatic headache, 202–203
posttraumatic hydrocephalus (PTH), 196
posttraumatic seizures, 195–196

posttraumatic syringomyelia (PTS), 188
PR. *See* pulmonary rehabilitation
pressure injury
   blanchable and nonblanchable erythema, 125
   deep tissue, 127
   definitions, 125
   full-thickness skin loss, 126
   medical device-related, 127
   mucosal membrane, 127
   partial-thickness loss, skin, 126
   prevention and treatment, 127–128
   tissue loss, 126
   unstageable, 126
promoting aphasics' communication effectiveness (PACE), 252
pronator drift, 17
prosthesis
   benefits, 77
   bilateral TF amputations, 76
   complications, 81
   DER, 80–81
   exclusion criteria, 77
   fluid-controlled knee, 79–80
   gait, 81–82
   HD socket designs, 75–76
   MPC knee, 79–80
   multiaxial foot, 80
   osseointegration, 76–77
   partial foot socket designs, 76
   polycentric knee, 79
   SACH, 80
   single-axis foot, 80
   TT suspension, 75, 77
   weight-activated stance-control (WASC) knee, 79
prosthetist, 6
pruritus, 101–102
PSH. *See* paroxysmal sympathetic hyperactivity
pseudodementia, 231
pseudogout, 134
PTA. *See* posttraumatic amnesia
PTH. *See* posttraumatic hydrocephalus
PTS. *See* posttraumatic syringomyelia
pulmonary rehabilitation (PR)
   goal, 91
   neuromuscular respiratory failure, 94–95
   obstructive disorders, 91–93
   restrictive disorders, 93–94
   spinal cord injury (SCI), 90–91
   tracheostomy management, 95–96
pupillary light response, 12

quadriceps (back knee) gait, 37–38

radial neuropathy, 340
radiation therapy (RT), 111
radicular pain
   radiculopathy, 302–303
   spinal stenosis, 303–304
radiculopathy, 302–303, 345–347
rapid ventricular response (RVR), 88
rehabilitation nurse (RN), 5
relapsing remitting multiple sclerosis (RRMS), 212–213
respiratory therapist (RT), 6
reverse total shoulder arthroplasty (RTSA), 151
RHD. *See* right hemisphere disorder
rheumatoid arthritis
   clinical manifestations, 132
   laboratory and imaging findings, 132–133
   treatment, 133
right hemisphere disorder (RHD), 252
Romberg test, 17
RRMS. *See* relapsing remitting multiple sclerosis
RT. *See* respiratory therapist
RTSA. *See* reverse total shoulder arthroplasty
RVR. *See* rapid ventricular response

sacroiliac joint (SIJ)
  dysfunction, 301
  pain, 312–313
sarcopenia, 105
scaphoid fractures, 310–311
scapular dyskinesis, 309
sciatic neuropathy, 343
SCI. *See* spinal cord injury
scoliosis, 170–171
semantic feature analysis (SFA), 252
seronegative spondyloarthropathies, 134–135
shoulder
  acromioclavicular joint separation, 306, 307
  adhesive capsulitis, 308
  anterior dislocation, 19
  anterior shoulder instability and labral injuries, 307–308
  (long-head) bicipital tendinitis, 308–309
  cross-arm adduction, 19
  empty can test, 19
  Hawkins Kennedy impingement, 19
  humeral head replacement (HHR), 150–151
  Neer impingement, 19
  reverse total shoulder arthroplasty, 150
  rotatory cuff pathology, 306–307
  speed test (biceps), 19
  scapular dyskinesis, 309
  total shoulder arthroplasty, 149–150
SIADH. *See* Syndrome of inappropriate antidiuretic hormone
SIJ. *See* sacroiliac joint
skilled nursing facility (SNF), 4
sleep wake disturbances (SWD), 194–195
SLP. *See* speech language pathologist

SMA. *See* spinal muscular atrophy
solid ankle cushioned heel (SACH) foot, 80
spasticity, 14
  assessment scales, 236, 237
  botulinum toxin dose, 239, 240
  chemodenervation and neurolysis, 238
  definition, 236
  early and frequent mobilization, 237
  heat modalities, 238
  intrathecal baclofen (ITB) therapy, 240
  medications, 238, 239
  noxious stimuli addressing, 236
  onabotulinumtoxin A dosing, 239, 241
  positioning, 236–237
  pumps and surgical replacement, 242
spastic paraplegia or diplegia/ crouched gait, 39
speech language pathologist (SLP), 5–6
spina bifida
  Chiari malformations, 163
  incidence of, 162
  limb deformities, 163
  rehabilitation issues, 163–164
spinal cord injury (SCI)
  autonomic dysreflexia, 184–186
  bone metabolism, 187
  cardiovascular disease (CVD), 187–188
  classification, 178–180
  clinical syndromes, 180–181
  epidemiology, 177
  expected functional outcomes, 183–184
  nerve transfer surgery, 189
  pediatric rehabilitation, 169–170
  posttraumatic syringomyelia (PTS), 188

prognosis and recovery, 182–183
sexual function and fertility, 188–189
tendon transfer surgery, 189
tracts, 177–178
treatment, 181–182
urinary tract surveillance, 188
venous thromboembolism (VTE), 184
spinal cord stimulation, 290–291
spinal muscular atrophy (SMA), 165, 224–225
spinal stenosis, 303–304
spine
axial pain, 299–302
epidural injections, 304–305
lumbar spinal fusion, 154–155
radicular pain, 302–304
radiofrequency nerve ablation (RFA), 305
seronegative spondyloarthropathies, 134–135
treatment, 304
vertebroplasty/kyphoplasty, 305
splints, 50
sports and performing arts medicine
cervical spine clearance, 327
concussion, 324, 327
emergency action plan, 323–324
emergency conditions, 324–326
preparticipation physical evaluations (PPEs), 323
return to play considerations, 335
team and company physician role, 323
unique injuries, 328–335
sternal precautions, 89
steroid myopathy, 229
strength training exercises
concentric contractions *vs.* eccentric contractions, 65
DAPRE method, 65
isokinetic, 65
isometric, 64
isotonic, 64–65
plyometric movement, 65
progressive resistive exercise:, 65
stroke
Aspirin administration, 206
dual antiplatelet therapy (DAPT), 207
endovascular interventions, 206
epidemiology and risk factors, 204
functional outcomes, 209–210
ischemic stroke syndromes, 204-205
motor recovery, 208
NASCET, 207
patent foramen ovale (PFO), 207
post acute medical complications, 207
therapy approaches, 208–209
tissue plasminogen activator (tPA), 205–206
SWD. *See* sleep wake disturbances
Syndrome of inappropriate antidiuretic hormone (SIADH), 197

tardive dyskinesia, 222
targeted muscle reinnervation (TMR), 73
tarsal tunnel syndrome, 322
TBI. *See* traumatic brain Injury
TCU. *See* transitional care unit
TENS. *See* transcutaneous electrical nerve stimulation
tetraplegia, 189
therapy prescription
modalities, 58–63
patient's diagnosis, 58
thrombocytopenia, 107
tibialis anterior gait, 38

tibial stress fractures (TSFs), 319
tracheostomy, 95–96
total body surface area (TBSA) burns
  pediatric patients, 97, 99
  rule of nines, 97
total hip arthroplasty (THA), 151–152
total knee arthroplasty, 148–149
total shoulder arthroplasty (TSA), 149–150
Tourette syndrome, 220
traction, 60–61
transcutaneous electrical nerve stimulation (TENS), 61
transfemoral (TF) amputation, 70
transhumeral (TH) amputation, 69
transitional care unit (TCU), 4
transplant rehabilitation
  cardiac transplantation, 117–118
  common indications, 113, 114
  deconditioning and frailty, 117
  end-organ dysfunction, 113
  immunosuppression therapy, 115–117
  medical complications, 115, 117
  pretransplant considerations, 113–115
transradial (TR) amputation, 69
transtibial (TT) amputation
traumatic brain Injury (TBI)
  acute care management, 193
  cerebral contusion, 190
  classification, 191–192
  diffuse axonal injury (DAI), 190
  disorders of consciousness, 191–193
  epidemiology, 190
  recovery and outcomes, 197
  rehabilitation history, 194
  subdural hemorrhages (SDHs), 190–191
  symptoms and medical complications, 194–197
  vasogenic and cytogenic edema, 191
tremor, 220

ulnar neuropathy at the elbow (UNE), 339–340
ultrasound (US)
  image optimization/knobology, 281
  interventional applications, 285–286
  normal and pathologic structures, 283–285
  physics, 280
  sonographic artifacts, 282
  standard orientation, 281
  transducer movement, 281–282
  transducer selection, 280–281
UNE. *See* ulnar neuropathy at the elbow
upper extremity amputations
  below-elbow prosthesis, 71, 72
  bilateral, 71
  congenital limb differences, 71
  externally powered myoelectric prostheses, 72
  partial hand amputations, 71
  TH amputation, 72–73
  unilateral, 70, 71
upper motor neuron (UMN) injury, 12–13
urinary incontinence, 349–350

vegetative state/unresponsive wakefulness syndrome (VS/UWS), 192–193
venous thromboembolism (VTE), 184
visual acuity, 12
visual field deficits, 12, 13
vocational rehabilitation specialist (VR), 6

voice disorder, 256
VR. *See* vocational rehabilitation specialist
VS/UWS. *See* Vegetative state/unresponsive wakefulness syndrome
VTE. *See* venous thromboembolism

wheelchairs
  axle, 45–46
  camber, 46
  casters, 46
  components of, 44, 45
  cushions, 46–47
  frame and weight, 44–45
  handrims, 46
  mag *vs.* wire-spoked wheels, 46
  pneumatic *vs.* rubber tires, 46
  power, 48–49
  recline/tilt-in-space, 47
  scooters, 48
  special and modified, 47–48
wrist and hand
  de Quervain Tenosynovitis, 310
  digital stenosing tenosynovitis (Trigger finger), 311
  Finkelstein (Eichhoff) test, 21
  jersey finger, 311
  mallet finger, 311
  median neuropathy, 336–339
  osteoarthritis (OA), 131–132
  rheumatoid arthritis, 132–133
  scaphoid fractures, 310–311
  stenosing tenosynovitis, 21
  tinel sign, 21

X-linked spinobulbar muscular atrophy, 224